Skin Diseases in the Immunocompromised

John C. Hall

Editor

Skin Diseases in the Immunocompromised

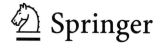 Springer

Editor
John C. Hall
St. Luke's Hospital
Kansas City
Missouri
USA

ISBN 978-1-4471-6478-4   ISBN 978-1-4471-6479-1   (eBook)
DOI 10.1007/978-1-4471-6479-1
Springer London Heidelberg New York Dordrecht

Library of Congress Control Number: 2014947336

For my father, William E. Hall PhD, who inspired me to write books.
A special thanks to editor Cheryl Winters-Tetreau and all the authors who made this book a reality.

Preface

Skin Diseases in the Immunocompromised

(What all clinicians need to know.)

As the number of surviving immune-suppressed patients continues its rapid increase, the skin manifestations have become increasingly important. AIDS patients survive longer and in increasing numbers. Renal, heart, liver, bone marrow, and lung transplant patients are surviving longer and the numbers are climbing rapidly. Diabetes is exploding in this country and offers its own unique brand of immune-suppressed skin diseases.

Immunosuppressive drugs are being used more frequently. Newer biologics and tyrosine kinase drugs have added new categories of immune-suppressed patients. Newborn premature patients are surviving more frequently and are immune suppressed.

The skin may be the earliest sign of these conditions and be the organ showing the most profound, earliest, and treatment-limiting side effects. We hope to clearly elucidate the signs of immune-suppressed skin diseases to afford early diagnosis and management of this ever-increasing diverse group of illnesses.

Kansas City, MO, USA   John C. Hall

Abbreviations

AA	Alopecia areata
AD	Atopic dermatitis
AFP	Alpha-fetoprotein
AGEP	Acute generalized exanthematous pustulosis
AIN	Anal intraepithelial neoplasia
AKs	Actinic keratoses
ALA	Aminolevulinic acid
AML	Acute myeloid leukemia
ART	Antiretroviral therapy
AT	Ataxia-telangiectasia
ATM	Ataxia telangiectasia mutated
ATP	Adenosine triphosphate
bbUVB	Broadband ultraviolet B
BCC	Basal cell carcinoma
BTK	Bruton's tyrosine kinase
c-AMP	Cyclic adenosine monophosphate
CEA	Carcinoembryonic antigen
CGD	Chronic granulomatous disease
CHS	Chediak-Higashi syndrome
CIA	Chemotherapy-induced alopecia
CMC	Chronic mucocutaneous candidiasis
CMV	Cytomegalovirus
CRP	C-reactive protein
CT	Computed tomographic
CTCAE	Common terminology criteria for adverse events
CTCL	Cutaneous T-cell lymphoma
CVID	Common variable immunodeficiency
DFA	Direct fluorescent antibody
EBV	Epstein-Barr virus
EGFR	Epidermal growth factor receptor
EM	Erythema multiforme
EORTC	European Organization for Research and Treatment for Cancer
EPF	Eosinophilic pustular folliculitis
ESR	Erythrocyte sedimentation rate
FCAS	Familial cold autoinflammatory syndrome
5FU	5-Fluorouracial

FDA	Food and Drug Administration
GA	Granuloma annulare
GPCR	G-protein coupled receptor
GVHD	Graft-versus-host disease
HAART	Highly active antiretroviral therapy
HBV	Hepatitis B virus
HCT	Hematopoietic cell transplantation
HCV	Hepatitis C virus
HER 2	Human epidermal growth factor receptor 2
Hh	Hedgehog [signaling pathway]
HHV-8	Human herpesvirus 8
HIES	Hyper immunoglobulin E syndrome
HIV	Human immunodeficiency virus
HLA	Human leukocyte antigens
HPV	Human papilloma virus
HSC	Hematopoietic stem cells
HSCT	Hematopoietic stem cell transplantation
HSV	Herpes simplex virus
HZ	Herpes zoster
IGD	Interstitial granulomatous dermatitis
IGRT	Image-guided radiation therapy
IL	Interleukin
IMIDs	Immune-mediated inflammatory diseases
IMRT	Intensity-modulated radiation therapy
IRIS	Immune reconstitution inflammatory syndrome
KA	Keratoacanthoma
KS	Kaposi's sarcoma
LAD	Leukocyte adhesion deficiency
LCV	Leukocytoclastic vasculitis
LP	Lichen planus
MAL	Methyl aminolevulinate
mALA	Methyl-esterified ALA
MAPK	Mitogen activated signaling pathway
MCC	Merkel cell carcinoma
MCV	Molluscum contagiosum virus
MDT	Multidrug therapy
5-MOP	5-methoxypsoralen
8-MOP	8-methoxypsoralen
MPD	Minimal phototoxic dose
MRI	Magnetic resonance imaging
MRSA	Methicillin-resistant *Staph. aureus*
MSSA	Methicillin-sensitive *Staph. aureus*
mTOR	Mammalian target of rapamycin
MWS	Muckle-Wells syndrome
nbUVB	Narrowband ultraviolet B
NCI	National Cancer Institute
NEH	Neutrophilic eccrine hidradenitis
NF	Necrotising fasciitis

NMSC	Non-melanoma skin cancer
NSCLC	Non-small cell lung cancer
OTR	Organ transplant recipients
PAMPs	Pathogen-associated molecular patterns
PASI	Psoriasis Area and Severity Index
PCR	Polymerase chain reaction
PDGFR	Platelet derived growth factor receptor
PDT	Photodynamic therapy
PIDs	Primary immunodeficiencies
PNI	Perineural invasion
PRRs	Pattern recognition receptors
PTC	Papillary thyroid carcinomas
PTCH1	Patch 1
PUVA	Psoralen plus ultraviolet A
RA	Rheumatoid arthritis
RCT	Randomized clinical trial
RET	Rearranged during transfection
ROS	Reactive oxygen species
RSV	Respiratory syncytial virus
RTOG	Radiation Therapy Oncology Group
SCC	Squamous cell carcinoma
SCCIS	Squamous cell carcinoma in situ
SCID	Severe combined immunodeficiency
SD	Seborrheic dermatitis
SG	Sebaceous glands
SLE	Systemic lupus erythematosus
SLNB	Sentinel lymph node biopsy
SM	Smoothened
SPF	Sun protection factor
SSSI	Serious skin and soft tissue infection
SSSSS	Superficial staphylococcal scalded skin syndrome
TB	Tuberculosis
TGF	Transforming growth factor
TKI	Tyrosine kinase inhibitors
TLRs	Toll-like receptors
TNF	Tumor necrosis factor
TSS	Toxic shock syndrome
UDA	Urticaria-deafness-amyloidosis [syndrome]
UV	Ultraviolet
UVA	Ultraviolet A
UVB	Ultraviolet B
VEGFR	Vascular endothelial growth factor receptor
VZV	Varicella zoster virus
WAS	Wiskott–Aldrich syndrome

Contents

Part I Disease Specific

1 Skin Disorders in Immunocompromised
   Diabetes Patients   3
   Nasirah Atiq and Hok Bing Thio

2 Skin Disorders of AIDS Patients   13
   Eduardo Castro-Echeverry

3 Skin Disorders in Patients with Primary Immunodeficiencies   31
   Natasha Klimas and Travis W. Vandergriff

4 Cancer Patients and Skin Disease   45
   John C. Hall

Part II Transplant Patients

5 Skin Disease in Solid Organ Transplant Patients   55
   John C. Hall

6 Graft vs Host Disease and Skin Manifestations   61
   Min Kin Derek Ho and Noah Scheinfeld

Part III Drug Related

7 Cutaneous Reactions to the Biologics   71
   David J. Chandler and Anthony P. Bewley

8 Cutaneous Reactions to Chemotherapy   87
   Jessica A. Savas and Reshma L. Mahtani

9 Cutaneous Reactions to Corticosteroids   99
   Peniel Zelalem

10 Cutaneous Reactions to Tyrosine Kinase Inhibitors   107
   Barbara Melosky

Part IV   Age Related

11 Cutaneous Manifestations of Aging
    and Immunodeficiency................................ 123
    Robert A. Norman and Zachary Henry

Part V   Radiation

12 UVA and UVB Therapy: Practical Applications
    and Implications for the Immunosuppressed Patient
    and Skin Disease 141
    James R. Coster and Joseph A. Blackmon

13 Skin Cancer in the Immunocompromised 155
    Ting Wang, Daniel J. Aires, and Deede Liu

14 Radiation Therapy for Non-melanoma Skin Cancer
    in Immunosuppressed Patients and Cutaneous Toxicity
    from This Therapy 171
    Adam D. Currey, Edit B. Olasz, J. Frank Wilson,
    and Zelmira Lazarova

Index 183

Contributors

Daniel J. Aires, MD, JD Division of Dermatology, Department of Internal Medicine, University of Kansas School of Medicine, Kansas City, KS, USA

Nasirah Atiq, MD Internal Medicine, Medisch Centrum Leeuwarden, Leeuwarden, Friesland, The Netherlands

Anthony P. Bewley, MB, ChB, FRCP Department of Dermatology, Barts Health NHS Trust, London, UK

Joseph A. Blackmon, MD Department of Dermatology, University of Kansas, Kansas City, KS, USA

Eduardo Castro-Echeverry, MD, MPH Pathology Resident, PGY-3, Anatomic and Clinical Pathology, Scott & White Memorial Hospital – Texas A&M Health Sciences Center, Temple, TX, USA

David J. Chandler, MB, ChB, DTM&H, MSc Department of Dermatology, Human Immunology Unit, Weatherall Institute of Molecular Medicine, University of Oxford, Oxford, UK

James R. Coster, MD Department of Radiation Oncology, University of Kansas, School of Medicine, Kansas City, KS, USA

Adam D. Currey, MD Department of Radiation Oncology, Medical College of Wisconsin, Milwaukee, WI, USA

John C. Hall, MD St. Luke's Hospital, University of Missouri Medical School, Kansas City Care Clinic (Free Health Clinic), Kansas City, MO, USA
Truman Medical Center, Kansas City, MO, USA

Zachary Henry Lake Erie College of Osteopathic Medicine, OMS IV, Bradenton, FL, USA

Min Kin Derek Ho, BS Department of Dermatology, SUNY Downstate College of Medicine, Brooklyn, NY, USA

Natasha Klimas, BS Department of Dermatology, University of Texas Southwestern Medical Center, Dallas, TX, USA

Zelmira Lazarova, MD Department of Dermatology, Medical College of Wisconsin, Milwaukee, WI, USA

Deede Liu, MD Division of Dermatology, Department of Internal Medicine, University of Kansas Medical Center, Kansas City, KS, USA

Reshma L. Mahtani, DO Division of Hematology/Oncology, University of Miami, Deerfield Beach, FL, USA

Barbara Melosky, MD, FRCPC Division of Medical Oncology, British Columbia Cancer Agency Vancouver, Vancouver, BC, Canada

Robert A. Norman, DO, MPH Professor of Dermatology, Nova Southeastern Medical School, Tampa, FL, USA

Private Practice, Tampa, FL, USA

Edit B. Olasz, MD, PhD Department of Dermatology, Medical College of Wisconsin, Milwaukee, WI, USA

Jessica A. Savas Division of Hematology/Oncology, University of Miami, Deerfield Beach, FL, USA

Noah Scheinfeld, MD, JD Department of Dermatology, Weil Cornell Medical College, New York, NY, USA

Hok Bing Thio, MD, PhD Department of Dermatology, Erasmus University Medical Centre, Rotterdam, Zuid-Holland, The Netherlands

Travis W. Vandergriff, MD Department of Dermatology, UT Southwestern Medical Center, Dallas, TX, USA

Ting Wang, MD, PhD Division of Dermatology, Department of Internal Medicine, University of Kansas Medical Center, Kansas City, KS, USA

J. Frank Wilson, MD Department of Radiation Oncology, Medical College of Wisconsin, Milwaukee, WI, USA

Peniel Zelalem, MD Internal Medicine, University of Kansas Medical Center, Kansas City, KS, USA

Part I

Disease Specific

Skin Disorders in Immunocompromised Diabetes Patients

Nasirah Atiq and Hok Bing Thio

Abstract

Immunity and diabetes is a complicated subject and many skin-related problems may be involved. From the clinician's standpoint, there are five dermatologic conditions related to immunity and diabetes that need special note: the diabetic foot, mucormycosis, necrotizing fasciitis, candidiasis, and recurrent cellulitis of the lower extremities. These illnesses seem uniquely associated with diabetic immune dysregulation.

Keywords

Diabetic foot • Necrotizing fasciitis • Mucormycosis • Candidiasis • Cellulitis • Candida sepsis

Introduction

Immunity and diabetes is a complicated subject and many skin-related problems may be involved. There are five dermatologic conditions related to immunity and diabetes that need special note. The five conditions are the diabetic foot, mucormycosis, necrotizing fasciitis, candidiasis, and recurrent cellulitis of the lower extremities. These illnesses seem uniquely associated with diabetic immune dysregulation.

N. Atiq, MD
Internal Medicine, Medisch Centrum Leeuwarden,
Leeuwarden, Friesland, The Netherlands

H.B. Thio, MD, PhD (✉)
Department of Dermatology, Erasmus University
Medical Centre, Burgemeester's Jacobplein 51,
Rotterdam, Zuid-Holland 3015CA, The Netherlands
e-mail: h.thio@erasmusmc.nl

Diabetes mellitus is a metabolic disease characterized by chronically elevated blood glucose levels, known as hyperglycemia. The hyperglycemic state in diabetes is due to defects in secretion or action of insulin, or more commonly, both. Diabetes affects millions of people worldwide. In the U.S. an estimated 26 million people are affected. The International Diabetes Federation Atlas reports that the prevalence of diabetes in the year 2012 was 8.3 % for all ages. That means that in 2012, 371 million people were living with diabetes worldwide. In 2030 it will be about 552 million. In many poor countries in Africa and in South East Asia, diabetes is undiagnosed in about half of the population.

Although there are many forms of diabetes mellitus, the majority of cases can be assigned to type I or type II diabetes. Approximately 80–90 % of patients have type II diabetes and about 10 % have type I diabetes.

J.C. Hall (ed.), *Skin Diseases in the Immunocompromised*,
DOI 10.1007/978-1-4471-6479-1_1, © Springer-Verlag London 2014

Type I diabetes is characterized in patients by an absolute lack of insulin since the pancreatic beta cells have been destroyed by mainly T lymphocytes. Normally these pancreatic beta cells, in the islet of Langerhans, secrete insulin but in type I diabetes the islet are under attack by mainly T lymphocytes. As type I diabetes is an autoimmune disease, it is also related to other autoimmune diseases such as thyroid disease, Addison's disease, and celiac disease. Type I diabetes usually develops in childhood and is progressive with the age.

Type II diabetes is caused by insulin resistance or dysfunction of the pancreatic beta cells which results in reduction of insulin secretion (relative insulin deficiency). Normal glucose uptake, metabolism, and storage are affected. These progressive and irreversible changes in the glucose homeostasis are due to insulin resistance. The dysfunction of pancreatic beta cells is their failure to adapt to increased insulin demands caused by long-term insulin resistance and hypersecretion of insulin. The four key risk factors for type II diabetes are obesity, increasing age, ethnicity, and family history.

Diabetes mellitus does not leave any organ of the body unaffected. It is a major cause of mortality and morbidity from long-term complications including cardiovascular diseases, renal failure, stroke, blindness, and amputations. Since this metabolic dysregulation is associated with secondary damages to all our essential organ systems, it is not surprising that diabetes type I and type II also affect the skin. The incidence and severity of many skin disorders are increased in patients with diabetes mellitus.

There are many studies which suggest that not only diabetes type I, but also type II, is a disease of the immune system. The immune system defends the body against various microbial, chemical, and physical injuries such as microorganisms and foreign substances to which we are constantly exposed. It comes in action when the natural barriers of the body fail. The skin and mucosa are examples of the mechanical barrier. The immune system has evolved into a complex and sophisticated system, consisting of a nonspecific (congenital) body's first-line defense innate immune system and a specific (acquired) adaptive immune system.

The innate immunity is the early and rapid pro-inflammatory immune response which was initially thought to be non-specific. But now it is known that the innate immune system has specificity that is directed against components of microorganisms, called pathogen-associated molecular patterns (PAMPs). The pattern recognition receptors (PRRs), for example toll-like receptors (TLRs), are host cellular receptors which recognize PAMPs. Endothelial cells, adipocytes, and macrophages identify threats via the PRRs and release pro-inflammatory cytokines like interleukin (IL)-6 and tumor necrosis factor (TNF)-α. These cytokines, also known as inflammatory markers, stimulate production of acute phase proteins like C-reactive protein (CRP). Several inflammatory markers are increased in diabetes type II as well. As the diabetes continues, there is also an increase in acute phase proteins. Another evidence of the role of innate immune system in diabetes type II is that the characteristic diabetes dyslipidemia is an acute phase response to injury and illness. There are more than 20 studies which illustrate that increase of circulating concentrations of inflammatory markers, like CRP and IL-6, predicting the chance of developing diabetes type II.

Hundal et al. showed that a 2-week treatment of diabetes type II patients with aspirin will decrease the fasting blood-glucose level by about 25 % and CRP by 17 %. The insulin sensitivity was increased by 30 %. So there is a link between inflammatory and metabolic pathways in which anti-inflammatory drugs reduce high levels of blood-glucose and lower the inflammatory markers. For that reason there is possibly activation of the innate immune system in diabetes type II in which there is a chronic, cytokine mediated inflammation.

Now there is evidence that not only diabetes type I, but also in type II and metabolic syndrome, there is activation of the innate immune system. There is increasing evidence indicating that about 90 % of patients with diabetes type II, without having any evident immune mediated inflammatory disease, have innate immune system dysfunction. The associations between diabetes type II, insulin resistance, and innate immune system might be the result of the body's response to chronic tissue injury that occurs in diabetes mellitus type II.

The etiological factors which lead to skin disorders in diabetes patients can be categorized into metabolic, infectious, vascular, neuropathic, or diabetes-associated disorders including necrobiosis lipoidica diabeticorum, diabetic bullae, and diabetic foot. Some of the skin disorders in diabetes patients can also be caused by the treatment of diabetes. Opportunistic infections caused by bacteria, fungi, viruses and protozoa are the most common skin disorders in immunocompromised patients.

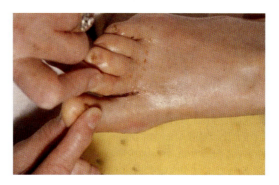

Fig. 1.1 The diabetic foot is related to a synergistic combination of vasculopathy, neuropathy, and immune compromise. Note the lack of hair over toes, blanched skin, and yellow crusting indicating impetiginization. Tinea pedis can be the initial skin infection leading to ulceration, as seen between the first and second toes. The patient had to have a below-knee amputation. Treating the tinea prophylactically and the bacteria as soon as signs develop could have resulted in saving the leg

Skin Manifestations of Diabetes Mellitus Associated with Immunosuppression

Dry skin is a common skin problem in about 50 % of diabetes patients. It is more frequent in type II diabetes than in type I. It is caused by abnormal structures of keratinocytes and thickening of stratum corneum. Moisturization of the top of stratum corneum layer is impaired. The skin barrier function is interrupted.

Furthermore, dry skin can be the result of autonomic neuropathy which causes decreased perspiration. Diabetic xerosis appears to be associated with micro-angiopathy. Diabetic xerosis is involved in the pathogenesis of foot ulcers as well. To improve skin surface, hydration treatment with emollients and moisturizers is necessary.

Among the various complications of diabetes, including retinopathy, nephropathy, and neuropathy, is the diabetic foot. It is associated both with neuropathy and microangiopathy. These lead to compromise of the epidermal barrier function and immunosuppression. This leaves the diabetic foot (Fig. 1.1) more susceptible to infections with several organisms. Staphylococcus and streptococcus are almost always the organisms implicated. The neuropathy leads to more trauma and burns due to lack of sensation. Interdigital tinea pedis leads to openings in the skin that allow bacteria

to enter and cause cellulitis. Other skin disorders associated with diabetes are listed below.

Skin disorders associated with diabetes:
- Acanthosis nigricans
- Acquired perforating dermatosis
- Acrochordons (skin tags)
- Bullosis diabeticorum
- Calciphylaxis
- Cellulitis
- Diabetic foot
- Diabetic rubeosis
- Diabetic thick skin
- Eruptive xanthoma
- Erysipelas
- Granuloma annulare
- Infectious skin diseases
- Lichen ruber planus
- Necrobiosis lipoidica diabeticorum
- Periungual telangiectasia
- Pretibial pigmentation
- Pigmented purpura
- Scleroedema adultorum of Buschke
- Vitiligo
- Yellow nails

Infectious diseases causing skin disorders in diabetes patients, such as diabetic foot, will be more severe in immunocompromised patients. There are no reliable statistics about the incidence of skin cancer in diabetic patients.

Skin Diseases in Immunocompromised Diabetic Patients

At the moment there is an increased use of immunosuppressive drugs and biologicals which suppress the immune system. Immunosuppression is generally used after an organ transplantation to prevent rejection. Besides this, immunosuppressive drugs are also prescribed for auto-immune diseases likes rheumatoid arthritis or for skin disorders such as psoriasis. Immunosuppression results in a rising prevalence of (opportunistic) infections worldwide. These infections can manifest in the skin. Because the immune system of diabetes patients is not optimal, these immunosuppressed patients are at an additional risk for infections.

Bacteria

Staphylococcus

Immunocompromised and diabetic patients are predisposed to infection with methicillin-sensitive staphylococcus aureus (MSSA) and methicillin-resistant staphylococcus aureus (MRSA). Staphylococcus epidermidis is a normal colonizer of the skin and is not considered a pathogen in the skin. However staphylococci are generally colonized on the normal skin. MSSA and MRSA are more common and often more severe in diabetics. MRSA often quickly forms an abscess and surgical intervention needs to be done immediately. Cutaneous manifestations of infection by staphylococci include cellulitis, furunculosis, blistering distal dactylitis (Fig. 1.2), abscesses, ecthyma, bullous impetigo, and superficial staphylococcal scalded skin syndrome (SSSSS). Early recognition and treatment with antibiotics is required for all of these conditions.

Group B Streptococcus

Although group B streptococcus infection is most frequent in pregnant women and neonates, it also occurs regularly in immunocompromised and elderly diabetic patients. This usually causes a cellulitis of the lower extremity (Fig. 1.3).

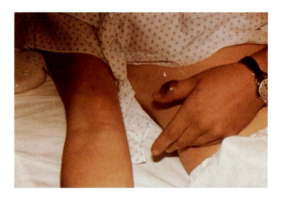

Fig. 1.2 Blistering dactylitis of the thumb due to methicillin-sensitive staphylococcus aureus. Every streptococcal and staphylococcal skin infection is more common and recurrent in diabetics

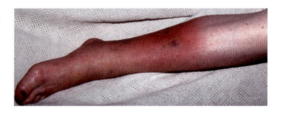

Fig. 1.3 Erythema, increased warmth, pain, and tenderness seen on the lower leg. This is usually due to staphylococcus aureus (methicillin-sensitive or -resistant) but can be due to group A beta hemolytic streptococci alone or in combination with staphylococcus. In diabetics this tends to be recurrent, and prophylactic antibiotics should be considered

Co-infection with Staphylococcus aureus is very frequent. The main signs of this infection are cellulitis, erysipelas, infected ulcers, necrotizing fasciitis, and toxic shock syndrome (TSS). TSS is a potentially fatal disease that requires quick recognition and treatment.

Clostridium perfringens

Clostridium perfringins is a anaerobic, Gram-positive bacteria. Clostridial myonecrosis (gas gangrene) is related to immunosuppression. It presents with suddenly rigorous pain that progresses rapidly in the involved location. The skin is blanched and edematous, where later hemorrhagic bullae will be developing. Diabetic patients with clostridium bacteria can present with a cellulitis-like skin abnormalities. It is important to recognize this infection, as it spreads quickly and can be fatal in 24–48 h. The treatment of choice is a high-dose intravenous penicillin with surgical debridement.

Klebsiella

Klebsiella pneumonia is a Gram-negative bacterium which is present in the mouth and intestines, and on the skin. It is an opportunistic bacterium that causes infection in immunosuppressed individuals. In these individuals Klebsiella presents with acral hemorrhagic bullae. Cellulitis caused by Klebsiella has also been reported in several cases. Diabetes patients may develop cellulitis and bullae in the lower extremities, which may progress to necrotizing fasciitis. Lesions resembling impetigo have been reported in immunosuppressed diabetic patients.

Mycobacterium Tuberculosis

Mycobacterium tuberculosis is the bacterium that causes tuberculosis. Cutaneous tuberculosis is a rare skin condition. Cutaneous tuberculosis may present as cutaneous tuberculous gummas and cutaneous tuberculous scrofuloderma. Cutaneous tuberculous gummas, also known as metastatic tuberculous abscesses and are the result of hematogenous spreading of bacilli. It is associated with diabetes mellitus and immunosuppressive medications.

Escherichia Coli

This is an aerobic Gram-negative bacterium in the gastrointestinal tract, however, infection with E. coli is more common in the urinary tract. It may form infectious abscesses anywhere in the body, including the skin. In diabetic patients, cutaneous infections caused by E. coli are found at the locations where insulin injections occurred. Also, E. coli infection of ulcers or wounds in the extremities are reported.

Another cutaneous sign of E. coli infection in diabetic or immunosuppressed patients is cellulitis, which resembles cellulitis due to streptococcal infection. Development of bullae at the place of infection may be seen.

Morganella

Morganella morganii is a Gram-negative bacterium that is part of the normal flora. It is a rare cause of opportunistic infections in immunocompromised individuals. But there are some case reports in which the authors mention cellulitis and hemorrhagic bullae due to M. morganii in diabetic patients. An untreated cellulitis caused by M. morganii may lead to septic shock.

Other bacteria, such as Salmonella and Enterobacteriaceae, rarely cause cellulitis in diabetic or immunocompromised patients.

Mycosis

Candidiasis

Candidiasis is a very common fungal infection that occurs in immunosuppressed and diabetes patients. It is also the most common cause of fungal infection in all organ-transplanted patients. Other diseases which are predisposing to candidiasis are hematologic malignancy, neutropenia, chemotherapy, use of immunosuppressive drugs such as cyclosporine, heroin use, and prolonged use of antibiotics. Localized infection is by far the most common manifestation. This can be localized around the nail on the proximal and lateral nail folds (paronychia) and, when severe, can cause nail destruction (Fig. 1.4). Localized candida is most common in the intertriginous areas but in the right clinical setting, especially in hospitals, it can occur at any site (Fig. 1.5).

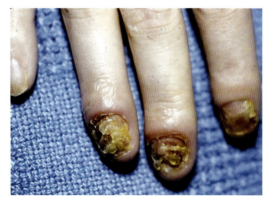

Fig. 1.4 Candida of the nails usually present with redness, tenderness, and swelling to the proximal and lateral nail folds as shown here. In more immunecompromised patients it can lead to nail destruction with yellowish hyperkeratotic debris as also is shown here. Paronychia should always be considered a possible sign of underlying diabetes

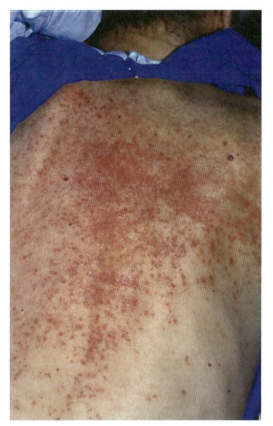

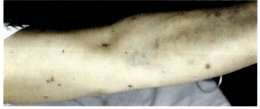

Fig. 1.6 Erythematous macronoudles over the arm of an immune-compromised patient indicating candida sepsis. Candida was seen on skin biopsy and also cultured from the blood

Fig. 1.5 Candida is most commonly seen as an intertrigo in genital, under abdominal panniculus, and axiallae. This figure shows the typical satellite papuls and pustules of candida on the back (an atypical location) of an immune-suppressed hospitalized patient who has been lying on his back, creating a warm, moist environment for Candida growth. Candida is not contagious but an opportunistic normal inhabitant of the mucous membranes and inter-triginous areas

Candida sepsis is a potentially fatal form of candida and is associated with diabetes. Candida albicans is responsible for about 50 % of all systemic candida infections. The other 50 % of all systemic candidiasis infections is caused by C. glabrata, C. tropicalis, C. krusei, and C. parapsi-losis. In systemic candidiasis with skin lesions, C. tropicalis is the most common cause of the infection.

In about 10 % of patients with candida sepsis the skin is affected. An early recognition of the skin lesions in these patients may lead to earlier diagnosis and treatment of the candidiasis. The skin lesions usually appear when the patient is ill,

febrile, and does not respond to several antibiotics. These skin lesions can be diffused or localized, and multiple or single. Usually they are on the (proximal) extremities and the trunk. The skin lesions that occur in patients with candidiasis infection are typically erythematous papules or papulonodules (Fig. 1.6). Usually they are not pruritic. Further skin manifestation of candidiasis includes necrotic pustules and papules, ulcerative lesions, cellulitis-like purpuric lesions, nummular hyperpigmented lesion, nodular abscesses, and nodular folliculitis.

Apart from the skin, systemic candidiasis also affects the eyes and the musculoskeletal and visceral organs. The triad of muscle abscesses caused by candida infection is papular skin lesion, fever, and diffuse muscle sensitivity. Although mortality is decreased since antifungal prophylaxis and antifungal therapy for patients at risk, the mortality rate of C. tropicalis fungemia is still about 70 %. The mortality rate of C. albicans and C. krusei are respectively 49 and 38 %.

The first-choice treatment for candidiasis is fluconazole. The other antifungal drugs that are used for treatment of candidiasis are amphotericin B, cariconazole, and echinocandin. The spectrum of the echinocandins includes also candida species, against which azoles and amphotericins are not effective. Echinocandins seem to be effective and the side effects are limited.

Zygomycosis

Zygomycosis, also known as mucormycosis, is caused by a group of opportunistic fungi of the Zygomycetes class, of the order of Mucorales. The respiratory tract is the main route of entry of zygomycetes. These organisms are found in fruit and bread and can be present in throat, nasal, or stool cultures. After candidiasis and aspergillosis, the zygomycosis are the most frequent opportunistic mycosis, with about 500 new cases each year.

Zygomycosis occurs generally in uncontrolled diabetic patients, in patients with leukemia, after an organ transplantation, and in other states of immunosuppression. Patients may present with pulmonary, cutaneous, rhinocerebral, gastrointestinal, or disseminated disease. Cutaneous zygomycosis presentation varies from slowly progressive infection to an infection with gangrene and hematogenous distribution. This infection is usually present in the nose and can spread to the central nervous system very fast.

There are two types of cutaneous zygomycosis: primary and secondary. The primary cutaneous zygomycosis is a rare cutaneous disease that usually occurs in severe immunocompromised patients. Most cases are reported in acute or chronic leukemia. The skin signs of the infection can be observed on the face, arms, legs, and the trunk. The lesions may be indurated and reddish purple, which then become necrotic with an erythematous halo. Brown or black discoloration of the lesions is common as the fungus produces cutaneous infarction. These lesions have a tendency to ulcerate and drain an exudate. If the infection progresses, it may affect the bones, muscles, tendons, and fascia.

The secondary cutaneous zygomycosis is more common than the primary type. Disseminated and rhinocerebral zygomycosis may result in secondary cutaneous zygomycosis. This type of cutaneous zygomycosis is more frequent in uncontrolled diabetes patients and in metabolic acidosis. The lesions associated with secondary cutaneous zygomycosis are large, painful, reticular purpuric maculae. Lesions may progress and lead to necrotizing fasciitis or bull's-eye cutaneous infarct, which is characterised by purpuric rim and central yellow crusting.

Other cutaneous manifestations of zygomycosis include edema and induration with central black blisters, annular necrotic ulcers, and an erythematous plaque with necrosis and pustules.

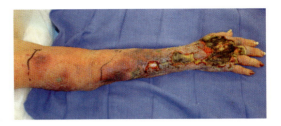

Fig. 1.7 Gangrenous changes exposing tendons over the hand, which resulted in amputation of the arm. This illustrates two conditions associated with diabetes and a decreased immune system function: necrotizing fasciitis and the underlying cause in this case of mucormycosis

Rarely it is associated with necrotizing fasciitis (Fig. 1.7). Necrotizing fasciitis is usually polymicrobic or due to streptococci and is increased in diabetic patients.

Rhinocerebral mucormycosis is the most frequent sign of systemic infection. In general, the brain, maxillary sinus and cavernous sinus are affected. Orbital cellulitis is a common presentation of rhinocerebral mucormycosis. Individuals with poorly controlled diabetes or ketoacidosis are at risk for orbital cellulitis.

Cutaneous mucormycosis needs a combination of surgical debridement, correction of the metabolic disorders, and antifungal drugs such as amphotericin B or posaconazole. Voriconazole does not cover the mucormycosis organisms.

Cryptococcosis

Infection with Cryptococcus neoformans type D is associated with cutaneous lesions. Serotypes A, B, and C are not often linked to skin diseases. Cryptococcus usually affects the central nervous system. The second most commonly affected organ is the skin. In immunocompromised individuals, distribution of Cryptococcus may also occur in the bones, skin, meninges, and kidneys.

Diabetes mellitus, immunosuppression, hematologic malignancy, AIDS, and chemotherapy are predisposing factors to cryptococcal infection. Cryptococcosis is more frequent in non-HIV immunosuppressed individuals.

In non-HIV immunocompromised individuals, cellulitis and ulcers are the most common cutaneous manifestations of cryptococcal infection. Also TNFα inhibitors are linked to cryptococcosis. In

HIV patients, the skin manifestations of crypto-coccosis includes herpes simplex-like lesions, ulcerations, and molluscum contagiosum-like papules.

Cryptococcal cellulitis has the same symptoms as bacterial cellulitis, such as tenderness, warmth, and erythema. Cellulitis in immunocompromised patients may also present with bullae, vesicles, and cutaneous abscesses. Cryptococcal infection may lead to necrotizing fasciitis in patient with diabetes and individuals who are immunesuppressed.

Some skin lesions of cryptococcal infection are similar to other dermatologic disorders such as herpes simplex, Kaposi sarcoma, eczema, pyoderma gangrenosum or keloid. Untreated infection with Cryptococcus will be fatal. The best antifungal drug for cryptococcosis is amphotericin B. Continued antifungal therapy is recommended as cryptococcosis is a latent infection and may reactivate when the immune system is suppressed.

Coccidioidomycosis

Coccidioidomycosis, also known as Valley fever, is caused by Coccidioides immitis. The infection presents typically with subacute respiratory symptoms and usually it is self-limiting. Diabetes patients, immunocompromised patients such as HIV-patients, and pregnant women are at risk for this infection. Also, patients using biologic agents like etanercept or infliximab are at risk for coccidioidomycosis.

Secondary coccidioidomycosis may present with skin abnormalities. Skin signs of coccidioidomycosis is separated into two groups: reactive and reactive interstitial granulomatous dermatitis. Reactive skin disorders include acute generalized exanthema, erythema multiforme-like eruptions, erythema nodosum, and Sweet syndrome. These skin disorders are rare in immunocompromised individuals, because a disseminated coccidioidomycosis is rapidly fatal before the skin signs are present. Toxic erythema and erythema nodosum, which are hypersensitivity reaction of the skin to the coccidioidal infection, are rare in immunocompromised individuals as well.

The most common coccidioidomycosis-related skin lesions in immunocompromised individuals includes papulopustles, erythematous plaques, erythema and edema of distal fingers, (necrotizing) cellulitis, multiple nodules, and verrucous nodules. Immunocompromised individuals with coccidioidomycosis can be treated with fluconazole, itraconazole, or amphotericin B. In HIV-positive patients and immunosuppressed individuals such as organ transplant patients, continued antifungal therapy is recommended.

Sporotrichosis

Sporotrichosis is caused by Sporothix schenkii, which is found on wood, soil, and plants. Infection with Sporothix schenkii occurs through inhalation of spores or direct inoculation. Gardeners, florists, farmers, forestry workers, and veterinarians are at risk for this infection.

Sporothix schenkii can cause disease in immunocompromised and immunocompetent individuals. This fungal presents in the skin through direct innoculation as a painless papule or pustule that becomes a nodule. It causes ulcerates and purulent fluid. It can stay in this chancre form but usually progresses with nodules proximally up the lympatics especially on the upper extremity. Disseminated infection with Sporothix schenkii is rare but more common in immunocompromised patients or patients with diseases like diabetes, sarcoidosis, or HIV infection. In HIV-positive patients, sporotrichosis can be fatal. In this group of patients prolonged treatment with itraconazole is recommended.

Localized cutaneous signs of sporotrichosis can be treated with itraconazole or potassium iodide. The best antifungal drug for disseminated sporotrichosis is amphotericin B.

Viral

Herpes Simplex

Infections caused by herpes simplex virus are very frequent in immunocompromised individuals, particularly individuals with HIV. It is not clear whether prevalence of herpes simplex infection is higher in diabetic patients than in the general population.

Herpes Zoster

Herpes zoster is due to reactivation of infection with the varicella-zoster virus. The primary varicella zoster infection manifests as chicken pox. The virus remains latent in the dorsal root ganglions or in the cranial nerve ganglions. Reactivation occurs when the immune system is suppressed. It presents with cutaneous painful dermatomal erythematous patches with vesicles. Generally less than three dermatomes are affected.

In immunosuppressed patients the incidence of herpes zoster is increased in the both disseminated and dermatomal herpes zoster. A recent study in Spain suggests that incidence of herpes zoster in diabetic patients is increased with relative risk of 2.1–3.7.

Algae

Protothecosis

Protothecosis is an opportunistic infection caused by Prototheca algae. It is a rare pathogen, but may cause chronic infection in immunosuppressed and diabetic patients. Prototheca colonize the respiratory and gastrointestinal tract, the skin and the nails. In the immunocompetent individual Prototheca infection presents as a painless papule or nodular lesion that grows and becomes edematous. It may progress to dermatitis or bursitis.

Cutaneous manifestation of protothecosis in immunocompromised patients is different compared to the immunocompetent individuals and it may present with painful ulcers, papules, nodules, and cellulitis. Cellulitis is a common manifestation of this infection in diabetic and immunosuppressed individuals. The clinical presentation of protothecosis may be very variable and difficult to recognize. The diagnosis is made by seeing the algae on histologic examination of biopsy tissue.

Cutaneous protothecosis can be treated with intravenous amphotericin B in combination with surgical debridement and intravenous itraconazole.

Parasites

Myiasis may occur in diabetes patients, especially in their ulcers and wounds. Patients with lack of mobility, necrotic tissue, and poor hygiene are at risk for myiasis.

Conclusion

Diabetes causes an overall increased risk of infections. This risk is magnified by the circulatory and neurogenic pathology of the lower extremities that is a major part of diabetes morbidity an mortality. Appropriate foot care, especially of tinea pedis and onychomycosis, can be limb saving and even life saving since it is a major risk factor for more serious bacterial infections. Certain infections are particularly high risks in diabetics, most notably necrotizing fasciitis, mucromycosis, and cellutiis of the foot and lower extremities. Early recognition and therapy can be as important and controlling insulin requirements.

Suggested Reading

Alavi A, Sibbald RG, Mayer D, Goodman L, Botros M, Armstrong DG, et al. Diabetic foot ulcers Part I. Pathophysiology and prevention. J Am Acad Dermatol. 2014a;70(1):e1–18.

Alavi A, Sibbald RG, Mayer D, Goodman L, Botros M, Armstrong DG, et al. Diabetic foot ulcers Part II. Management. J Am Acad Dermatol. 2014b;70(1):e21–4.

Al-Mutairi N, Sharma AK, Al-Sheltawi M. Cutaneous manifestations of diabetes mellitus. Study from Farwaniya hospital, Kuwait. Med Princ Pract. 2006;15(6):427–30.

Bristow I. Non-ulcerative skin pathologies of the diabetic foot. Diabetes Metab Res Rev. 2008;24 suppl 1:S84–9.

Hall JC, Hall BJ. Hall's manual of skin as a marker of underlying disease. Shelton, CT, USA; 2011. p. 245–60.

Pavlović MD, Milenković T, Dinić M, Misović M, Daković D, Todorović S, et al. The prevalence of cutaneous manifestations in young patients with type I diabetes. Diabetes Care. 2007;30(8):1964–7.

Skin Disorders of AIDS Patients

2

Eduardo Castro-Echeverry

Abstract

Cutaneous manifestations of HIV and AIDS have been described in several cohorts over the past 30 years. This chapter describes clinical presentation, diagnosis, and treatment of cutaneous disorders that are unique or more common in AIDS patients. They can be divided into infectious, inflammatory, and neoplastic diseases. Infectious diseases consist of viral infections, bacterial infections, fungal infections, and parasitic infections. Viral infections include HSV, HPV, VZV, molluscum contagiosum, EBV, and CMV. Bacterial infections include staphylococcal infections, syphilis, bacillary angiomatosis, and mycobacterial infections. Fungal infections include deep cutaneous fungal infections. Parasitic infections include scabies, both common and crusted. Neoplastic disorders include Kaposi Sarcoma, HPV-related anal squamous cell carcinoma, and cutaneous lymphoproliferative disorders, including plasmablastic lymphoma. Inflammatory disorders include eosinophilic pustular folliculitis, also known as Ofuji's disease, and various drug reactions due to highly active antiretroviral therapy. Without exception, these disorders show more severe clinical presentations, last longer, and show greater resistance to therapy in this patient population than in immunocompetent individuals. In most instances, treating the underlying immunosuppression leads to an improved outcome.

Keywords

AIDS • HSV • HPV • Zoster • Molluscum contagiosum • Syphilis • Lymphoma • AIN • Anal carcinoma • HAART

E. Castro-Echeverry, MD, MPH
Pathology Resident, PGY-3, Anatomic
and Clinical Pathology, Scott & White Memorial
Hospital – Texas A&M Health Sciences Center,
2401 S. 31st St., Temple, TX 76504, USA
e-mail: ecastro82@gmail.com

Introduction and Historical Perspective

More than 30 years ago, the CDC published a report of 50 previously healthy, young homosexual men with Kaposi's sarcoma involving lymph nodes, viscera, mucosa and skin. With the benefit of hindsight, it seems only natural that the first known reports of AIDS coincide with the first reported cutaneous manifestations of AIDS, as the skin represents one of our principal and most visible immunologic barriers. Since that time, a host of different infectious, neoplastic and inflammatory cutaneous disorders have been reported and linked with both HIV and AIDS. This is thanks in large part to a handful of landmark cohort studies from around the United States and the world (Boston, Baltimore, San Francisco, Brazil, Cote D'Ivoire, Spain, Thailand) conducted from the mid-1980s through the late 1990s. In the early stages of its spread, the disease preferentially affected homosexual and bisexual men, so the study populations described were heavily weighted toward this subgroup.

Since the advent of Highly Active Antiretroviral Therapy (HAART), the natural history of HIV in developed countries has changed considerably, and consequently the incidence of AIDS-related cutaneous disorders in the United States has decreased. While this is certainly welcome news, AIDS remains a significant concern in the developing world. Data from the Joint United Nations Programme on HIV/AIDS (UNAIDS) states that approximately 68 % of the 22.5 million HIV-infected individuals reside in Sub-Saharan Africa. With some of the most impoverished healthcare systems in the world, availability of HAART in this region is fairly limited. Thus, the population at risk for developing AIDS has effectively shifted from homosexual and bisexual men to heterosexual couples and their families, including an estimated 2.5 million children. With this in mind, the original cohorts describing cutaneous manifestations of AIDS have limited applicability to this population. To this end, several studies from Tanzania, Zimbabwe, Ethiopia, and South Africa have been published more recently and further describe and delineate the cutaneous manifestations of AIDS in these previously underrepresented populations.

In this chapter we will discuss the wide variety of cutaneous conditions that preferentially affect AIDS patients, as well as cutaneous conditions that are considered AIDS-defining illnesses.

While a comprehensive list of cutaneous disorders associated with AIDS can seem daunting, there are several guiding principles that allow us to simplify and understand the range of cutaneous diseases with an increased prevalence in this patient population. In terms of etiology, we can divide these conditions, with some natural overlap, into infectious, inflammatory, and neoplastic. We can further subdivide infectious etiologies into bacterial, viral, fungal, and parasitic/protozoal; inflammatory disorders into drug-induced and acquired; and neoplastic disorders into epithelial, lymphoproliferative, and mesenchymal/vascular. The majority of diseases described here are not exclusive to AIDS. Without exception, however, AIDS patients present with more frequent and severe manifestations of these diseases, requiring longer, more aggressive, and, in some cases entirely different, treatments, as well as prophylaxis following successful therapy. Also common to all of the entities described below is the fact that treating the underlying condition by way of HAART therapy will usually lead to the best possible outcome. Wherever possible, the emphasis of this chapter is on particular clinical features that are unique or more common in the context of AIDS.

AIDS-Defining Illnesses

HIV survives and replicates by impairing its host's ability to effectively identify and eliminate infectious microorganisms. It preferentially infects, replicates, and destroys CD4 helper T cells, and their progressive decrease in number correlates with the host's immunocompetence. Once the CD4 count drops below 200 cells/mm^2, or constitutes less than 15 % of the T cell population, the host's immunosuppression is such that the individual is considered susceptible to a wide variety of microorganisms, including less virulent organisms—termed opportunistic infections—that would otherwise be colonizers. It is at this point that an HIV-positive individual is said to suffer from AIDS.

While CD4 count is an invaluable parameter in assessing the immunocompetence of an

HIV-positive person, it is ultimately the host's ability to ward off disease that is a direct measure of immune status, and for this reason there are a number of conditions that are considered "AIDS-defining" illnesses, such that the presence of one of these diseases indicates a level of immunosuppression worthy of the term AIDS. According to the CDC, the following mucocutaneous lesions are considered AIDS-defining illnesses in individuals whose HIV status is unknown and who have no other cause for immunodeficiency:

- Candidiasis of the esophagus, trachea, bronchi, or lungs
- Cryptococcosis with hematogenous dissemination to the skin
- Herpes simplex virus mucocutaneous ulcer persisting for longer than 1 month
- Kaposi's sarcoma in a patient younger than 60 years of age

In an individual who is HIV-seropositive, the following additional lesions are considered AIDS defining:

- Coccidioidomycosis or histoplasmosis with hematogenous dissemination to the skin
- Kaposi's sarcoma at any age

Infectious Etiologies

Infections are defined as an imbalance in the interaction between a host and a microbe that favors parasitic growth of the latter to the detriment of the host's well-being. Whether or not an infection develops depends on the immunocompetence of the host, the number of microorganisms present, and the virulence of the organism. Not surprisingly, the catalogue of AIDS-related infections is composed mostly of microorganisms that normally constitute the flora of an individual. Alternatively, they may represent previous infections that have persisted dormant in the host.

Viral Infections

Herpes Simplex Virus (HSV)

It is estimated that a substantial proportion of sexually active adults are seropositive for HSV1

or HSV2, such that the majority of patients who progress to AIDS already have been exposed and harbor the virus in a latent stage of replication. Not surprisingly, HSV flare-ups are one of the most common dermatologic complaints in this population.

Clinical Features

In AIDS patients, herpes lesions are common, persistent and particularly resistant to treatment. Any painful ulceration in an AIDS patient should be considered and treated as HSV until proven otherwise. In fact, with severe immunosuppression (CD4 < 50 cells/mm^2), 58 % of all ulcerations, and 2/3 of all perianal ulcerations contain HSV. Conversely, the presence of HSV in the company of risk factors is a marker for unsuspected, undiagnosed HIV. Where a herpetic lesion persists for more than 1 month, advanced HIV should be suspected, as evidenced in Fig. 2.1. Diagnosis is difficult in these cases as there may be a chronic ulcer with no vesicles and no herpetiform (grouped lesions) configuration. Culture with a swab or tissue examination may be falsely negative and tissue culture may be necessary to make the final diagnosis. Clinically, patients tend to present with tender, painful, ulcerative lesions of the penis, perianal area and lip. Multiple scattered lesions may be seen. Periungual lesions and follicular facial lesions may be misdiagnosed as bacterial infections. Although cutaneous HSV lesions are common in AIDS patients, disseminated HSV is relatively rare.

Diagnosis

Definitive diagnosis can be achieved by a Tzanck smear, a viral swab culture, or direct fluorescent antibody (DFA) staining of skin scrapings. Specimens should be obtained from the base of an intact lesion or from the advancing border of the lesion. Should results prove negative, a skin biopsy from the ulcer margin will demonstrate the characteristic histopathologic features. If a biopsy is obtained, it should be submitted for viral culture. Occasionally, in the context of histologically atypical, culture-negative lesions, immunohistochemistry or PCR for HSV may assist in diagnosis. Additional stains for AFB

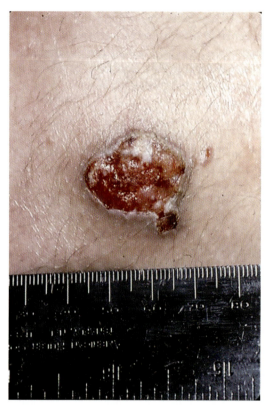

Fig. 2.1 Three-cm ulcer with one satellite lesion present for 18 months on the anterior thigh (which is an atypical location) of an AIDS patient. Diagnosis was made only after tissue culture. It was exquisitely painful and did not respond to any medical treatment regimens. Wide excision was curative

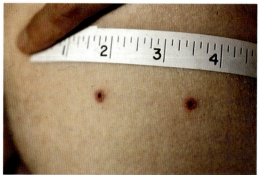

Fig. 2.2 Ecthymatous papules with central hemmorhagic crust and surrounding erythema that was diagnosed as chronic (months) varicella in an AIDS patient

and Fungi should be performed to rule out other synchronous cutaneous infections.

Resistance to acyclovir is naturally occurring in the herpesvirus, and thus the likelihood of selecting a resistant strain increases with the size of the lesion. As AIDS patients can present with extensive areas of cutaneous involvement, they have a greater tendency to suffer from acyclovir-resistant HSV. Failure to heal after appropriate diagnosis and treatment should prompt susceptibility testing.

Treatment

Oral acyclovir, 200–800 mg five times daily or intravenous acyclovir at 5 mg/kg three times daily is the preferred treatment regimen. Dosing may vary depending on the severity and response of the lesion. Should the lesion prove resistant to acyclovir, intravenous trisodium phosphonoformate

(Foscarnet) should be administered until the ulcers heal. In rare instances, the lesion may prove resistant to Foscarnet therapy, in which case a combination of ACV and foscarnet or a 6-week-long continuous infusion of parenteral acyclovir along with topical treatment with (S)-1-1(3-hydroxy-2-phosphonylmethoxypropyl) cytosine or trifluorothymidine may be indicated.

Once lesions heal, indefinite prophylactic treatment with acyclovir is indicated.

Varicella Zoster Virus (VZV) and Herpes Zoster (HZ)
Clinical Features

Herpes zoster is more common in HIV-infected individuals with CD4 counts around 315 cells/mm^2. In AIDS patients, there may be a primary varicella eruption arising concurrently with dermatomal zoster. Crucially, disseminated VZV may precede or follow a typical zosteriform vesicular eruption. Thus, in the context of AIDS, dermatomal HZ should prompt evaluation for systemic, disseminated VZV. Clinically, lesions follow the typical pattern of successive crops of vesicular lesions with surrounding erythema ("dewdrops on a rose petal"). Unusual patterns reported in this population include ecthymatous, shown in Fig. 2.2; crusted, punched-out ulcerations; and verrucous lesions. Importantly, these unusual patterns tend to be associated with acyclovir resistance. Should cutaneous HZ occur in the distribution of the nasociliary branch of the ophthalmic nerve—extending from the forehead

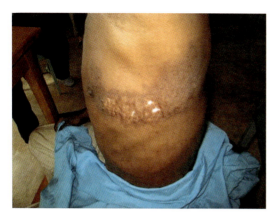

Fig. 2.3 Severe trunkal scar formation seen in an AIDS patient in Kenya. The patient still has severe postherpetic neuralgia at the scar sight months after the blisters from herpes zoster have faded (Thanks to Scott Stanley for photographs)

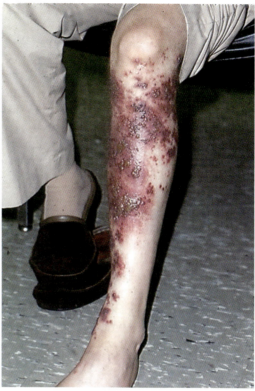

Fig. 2.4 Severe, hemorrhagic, exquisitely painful, dermatomal, linear bullae on a red base, indicating herpes zoster. This was the presenting sign in this AIDS patient (Thanks to Scott Stanley for photographs)

to the side or tip of the nose, with or without conjunctivitis—an ophthalmologic consultation to exclude uveitis and/or keratitis is indicated.

Post-herpetic neralgia can be severe in these patients even if younger that 60 years of age, which is the commonest age of post-herpetic neralgia in the general population. Dramatic scar formation may occur, as seen in Fig. 2.3 More extensive dermatomal disease, seen in Fig. 2.4, and disseminated varicella should prompt a search for AIDS in any patient, especially those with other risk factors.

Diagnosis

Classic clinical morphology and distribution is sufficient to initiate treatment. The diagnosis can be confirmed by a Tzanck smear, a viral swab, or DFA staining. Where rapid diagnostic tests prove equivocal, a biopsy may be indicated. A biopsy is useful for histologic examination, to exclude another pathogen, and for susceptibility testing.

Treatment

Whether it represents primary infection or reactivation, careful evaluation for systemic involvement is warranted. Where pulmonary, hepatic, or other systemic disease is present, aggressive treatment should be pursued. Suggested treatment regimens include IV acyclovir at 10 mg/kg every 8 h, adjusted for renal function; and oral acyclovir, 800 m g every 4 h with careful monitoring. If

there is ocular involvement, intravenous acyclovir is always indicated along with steroids. In the absence of systemic or ocular involvement, treatment is determined by the overall immune status of the individual and the location of the lesion. Where acyclovir resistance is suspected, foscarnet is effective. In general, cutaneous lesions due to VZV take longer to heal than HSV.

Vaccination with the live attenuated virus should be reserved for immunocompetent patients, and has been shown to be safe in pediatric patients with HIV and CD4 counts greater than 14 % and/or greater than 200 cells/mm^2. Conversely, disseminated VZV as a result of vaccination has been reported and suggested as an AIDS-defining illness.

Cytomegalovirus (CMV)

Primary CMV infection is usually asymptomatic, although some cases may present with a mononucleosis-like syndrome. This phase is followed by latent infection, in which viral shedding occurs in saliva, semen, and/or urine. Seroprevalence for CMV approaches 100 % in homosexual and bisexual males. Disseminated CMV is especially common with CD4 counts of less than 100 cells/mm^2. A persistent question regarding CMV has been its specific role in the pathogenesis of these symptoms—whether it actually causes these symptoms or is simply an incidental finding.

Clinical Features

In patients with disseminated CMV, there may be pulmonary, ocular, gastrointestinal, and neurologic involvement. Generalized wasting syndrome, pneumonitis, and encephalitis may follow. Reported mucocutaneous presentations of CMV include perianal and oral ulcers, macular purpura of the extremities associated with leukocytoclastic vasculitis, and small, keratotic, verrucous lesions, 1–3 cm in diameter, scattered on the trunk, limbs, and face.

Diagnosis

A biopsy demonstrating specific cytopathic changes suggestive of CMV, possibly supported by immunohistochemical studies, is useful in arriving at this diagnosis.

Treatment

Treatment includes ganciclovir and foscarnet. Resolution of lesions following therapy supports CMV as the causative agent.

Epstein-Barr Virus (EBV)

While the majority of adults harbor EBV, oral hairy leukoplakia caused by EBV is exclusive to HIV patients. EBV infects epithelial cells, leading to hyperkeratotic thickening. It is estimated that as many as 25 % of HIV-infected individuals may be affected, and prevalence appears to correlate with immunosuppression.

Clinical Features

Oral hairy leukoplakia presents as white verrucous confluent plaques most commonly located on the lateral aspects of the tongue that do not scrape off with a tongue depressor. Usually,

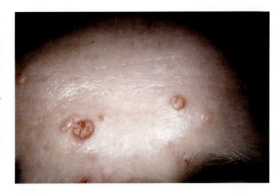

Fig. 2.5 Discrete umbilicated papules on the forehead of an AIDS patient with some crusting. It would be uncommon to see an adult male with molluscum in this location

lesions are asymptomatic but may cause dysphagia with advanced disease. Histologically, vacuolated cells or koilocytes may be seen in the stratum spinosum of the squamous epithelium.

Diagnosis

Clinical findings in the appropriate context are sufficient for definitive diagnosis, although a biopsy may be required to rule out malignancy in an atypical lesion. (Chatis et al. 1989; Johnson et al. 1985; Kaplan et al. 1987).

Treatment

Oral hairy leukoplakia does not require therapy. Topical therapy with podophyllin, surgical resection, or systemic antivirals is effective initially, although recurrence is seen in 75–100 % of patients.

Molluscum Contagiosum

Molluscum contagiosum is a large 200-by-300 nm double-stranded DNA poxvirus of the Poxviridae family that selectively infects epidermal cells. It occurs most commonly in the head, as seen in Fig. 2.5, and neck area of patients with CD4 lymphocyte counts of less than 200 cells per mm^2. Numerous lesions or lesions involving multiple sites imply CD4 counts of less than 50 cells per mm^2. These trends make molluscum a useful cutaneous marker of advanced HIV infection. Molluscum lesions produce significant morbidity in AIDS patients due to physical disfigurement,

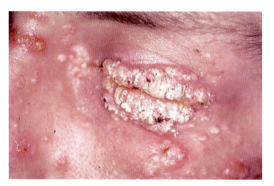

Fig. 2.6 Disfiguring molluscum on the eyelid of an AIDS patient. Umbilicated papules around the eyelids form a fungating, crusted mass over the eyelid itself

as seen in Fig. 2.6, and their potential to induce pruritus and eczematous reactions. Not surprisingly, they are the most common cutaneous manifestation prompting outpatient dermatologic care in this population.

Clinical Features
Molluscum lesions begin as discrete, pearly to flesh-colored, dome-shaped papules 3–10 mm in diameter with central umbilication. They are usually grouped together but may disseminate widely. In AIDS patients, giant lesions as seen in Fig. 2.7 with cutaneous horns have been reported.

Diagnosis
Several clinical features suggest this diagnosis. In addition to their distinct clinical morphology, expression of a white, curdlike core from beneath the surface of an umbilicated lesion is consistent with this diagnosis. Staining with toluidine blue or Giemsa will show characteristic viral inclusions known as molluscum bodies. Biopsies will show a downgrowth of epidermal cells with large eosinophilic molluscum bodies.

Treatment
With a limited number of lesions, cryotherapy or electrodessication and curettage may be effective. With hundreds of lesions, destructive therapy is generally ineffective. In these cases, the only reported effective therapy is to treat the underlying condition with HAART.

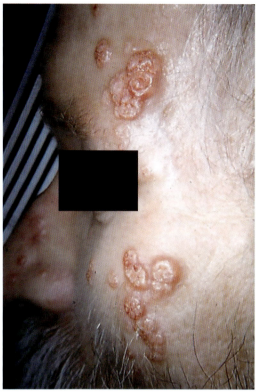

Fig. 2.7 Giant molluscum in an AIDS patient, forming plaques of umbilicated nodules. This can mimic crytococcus neoformans in AIDS patients

Human Papillomavirus (HPV) and Anal Cancer
Patients with AIDS/HIV have a higher prevalence of HPV infection resulting in both nongenital and genital warts. With advanced immunosuppression, warts become more numerous and refractory to treatment. Particularly in homosexual and bisexual men, high-risk HPV infection is associated with an increased incidence of anal intraepithelial neoplasia (AIN) and anal cancer.

Clinical Features
Typically, the lesions are regular or flat warts. Occasionally, extensive verruca plana, as seen in Fig. 2.8, and tinea versicolor-like warts may be seen. Condyloma acuminata occurring at anal/perianal sites in male individuals is associated with homosexual anogenital intercourse, and

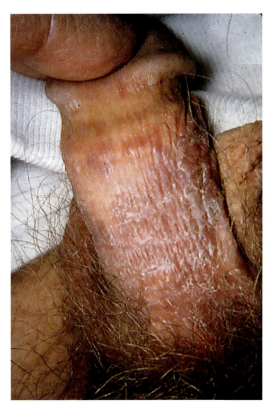

Fig. 2.8 Flat-topped shiny papules forming a sheath-like plaque over the shaft of the penis. This mimics seborrhea or psoriasis, but the biopsy showed squamous cell carcinoma-in-situ in an AIDS patient that has most likely been induced by the human papilloma virus of the 16,18, 31, or 32 subtype

Anal carcinoma may consist of anal squamous cell carcinoma or primary adenocarcinoma of the anus. Malignancies may be found in the anal canal or in the anal margin. Currently, it appears that HPV 16 is associated with anal canal carcinoma, while other high-risk HPV types are associated with anal margin carcinomas. High-grade anal dysplasia can progress to anal carcinoma in less than a year.

Diagnosis

In diagnosing anogenital warts in immunocompetent individuals, classic clinical presentation is sufficient for diagnosis. In the context of AIDS, a biopsy is recommended, as verrucous lesions are not necessarily synonymous with HPV infection. Histologically, demonstration of koilocytic changes on biopsy is sufficient. Additionally, a biopsy permits evaluation for intraepithelial neoplasia and PCR analysis for high-risk HPV.

Treatment

With advanced immunodeficiency, complete eradication of the lesions is unlikely. Aggressive treatment with carbon dioxide laser surgery may be counterproductive as there is a high failure rate and significant morbidity. Isotretinoin and interferons may prove helpful. HAART tends to improve the common verrucous lesions, although it has little to no effect on AIN or anal cancer. In the presence of intraepithelial neoplasia, electrocautery followed by 85 % trichloroacetic acid or imiquimod is effective.

Carcinomas of the anal margin can be treated with surgical excision and adjuvant radiation. Small case series have shown a good prognosis with no recurrence following treatment. Carcinomas of the anal canal, on the other hand, are treated with chemoradiation therapy as well as surgical excision, and have a tendency to recur.

Owing to the similarity between HPV-related anal carcinoma in homosexual and bisexual men and HPV-related cervical carcinoma in sexually active women, there is a proposal to emulate the well-established cervical cancer screening algorithms currently in place, with periodic high-resolution anoscopy, cytology, and subsequent biopsies of suspicious lesions, as well as HPV

leads to increased risk of HIV infection as well as development of anal neoplasia and cancer. There is an association between decreased CD4 counts and increased intraepithelial neoplasia of the vulva, penis, and anus.

AIN and anal carcinoma have received particular attention in recent years owing to the fact that HIV-positive homosexual and bisexual men have a markedly increased incidence of anal cancer. In fact, recent data shows the highest incidence of non-AIDS defining malignancies is anal carcinoma. All forms of AIN and anal carcinoma are associated with high-risk HPV, which consists of subtypes 16, 18, 26, 31, 33, 35, 39, 45, 51–53, 56, 58, 59, 66, 68, 73, and 82. High-grade anal dysplasia and anal carcinoma, in particular, are almost exclusively associated with high-risk HPV.

subtype analysis. Such efforts, however, are currently in their embryonic stage, and may or may not prove effective in preventing anal carcinoma.

Fungal Infections

Oral Candidiasis

Mucosal candidiasis likely occurs in all HIV-infected individuals at some point during the course of their illness. Oropharyngeal candidiasis is the most common site of involvement. Extension into the esophagus and tracheobronchial tree is considered an AIDS-defining illness.

Clinical Features

Oropharyngeal candidiasis is usually asymptomatic. Patients may complain of soreness or burning sensation of the mouth, sensitivity to spicy foods, and reduced or altered sense of taste. Four different patterns have been identified: pseudomembranous, atrophic, hyperplastic, and angular cheilitis. With the exception of atrophic oral candidiasis, these patterns are easily recognizable. Atrophic oral candidiasis presents as patches of erythema on the vault of the mouth and/or soft palate.

Diagnosis

Because demonstration of pseudohyphae is usually interpreted as an incidental finding in specimens of the oral mucosa, clinical presentation is sufficient for diagnosis.

Treatment

Treatment is directed at control of symptoms rather than a definitive cure. Topical treatments requiring administration four to five times daily are preferred to systemically absorbed agents.

Onychomycosis

This is not particularly increased in AIDS patients, but it has a characteristic clinical presentation.

Clinical Features

The fungal nail infection in AIDS patients can affect a fingernail and not affect the toenails, which is very uncommon in the general popula-

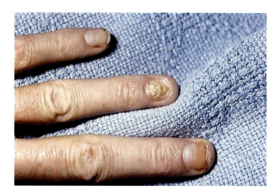

Fig. 2.9 Single nail dystrophy in an AIDS patient that began from a proximal subungual location. The nail is replaced by keratotic white/yellow debris. The adjacent nails may be showing early involvement with slight yellowish discoloration

tion. It also often affects only one fingernail, as seen in Fig. 2.9, and begins in a proximal subungual location. The nail becomes dystrophic and become completely replaced with keratotic yellow/white debris.

Diagnosis

False-negative cultures are common. The best way to diagnosis is to send a nail plate to the laboratory for a PAS stain, which will show septated branching hyphae. If a culture is positive it usually grows trichophytun rubrum.

Treatment

Treatment is the same as for non-AIDS patients, with topical ciclopirox or oral terbenifine.

Cutaneous Manifestations of Systemic Infections

Identification of invasive fungal infections in cutaneous lesions is highly suggestive of concurrent systemic infections. The three most common fungal organisms involved are discussed below, although a wide array of fungal organisms have been reported and may be ultimately responsible. While histopathologic examination of the organism may suggest an etiology, fungal culture is necessary for definitive identification of the organism.

Cryptococcosis

Cryptococcosis may arise in asymptomatic patients and typically resembles molluscum contagiosum. All patients with cutaneous manifestations have systemic disease.

Coccidoidomycosis

Coccidioidomycosis occurs almost exclusively in severely ill HIV patients. Clinically, the lesions are hemorrhagic but are otherwise non-specific.

Histoplasmosis

Histoplasmosis can present with a wide variety of patterns, including hemorrhagic, papular, and ulceronecrotic.

Diagnosis

In the context of sufficient clinical suspicion, prompt initiation of treatment should not be delayed. Biopsy of the lesion for fungal culture and histopathologic examination is necessary for definitive diagnosis. PCR/probe amplification tests for invasive fungal organisms are commercially available and are particularly useful, as fungal cultures can take days to weeks. On histopathologic examination, Cryptococcus is a 4–7 µm encapsulated budding yeast; Coccidioides immitis consists of 30–60 µm spherules containing 2–5 µm endospores; and Histoplasma typically shows 2–4 µm yeast forms packed within macrophages. Grocott Methenamine Silver (GMS) and Periodic Acid Schiff (PAS) stains are useful to highlight the fungal organisms. Mayer's mucicarmine is also useful in highlighting Cryptococcus. Additionally, Cryptococcal antigen testing and India ink stained wet mounts of cerebrospinal fluid is useful in identifying this organism.

Management

As cutaneous lesions should be considered indicative of systemic disease, single agent or systemic chemotherapy with Amphotericin B, Flucytosine, Fluconazole or itraconazole is warranted.

Bacterial Infections

Syphilis

Coinfection with *Treponema pallidum* and HIV can alter the course of either disease. The presence

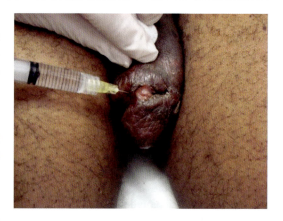

Fig. 2.10 A chancre of syphilis in an AIDS patient. This ulcer just proximal to the glans of the penis did not respond to ample doses of therapy, so a biopsy was done to make sure the patient did not have a squamous cell cancer (more common on the genitalia in AIDS patients). However, there was no malignancy on biopsy and the pathology confirmed a syphilitic chancre. The patient finally responded to repeat therapy. He gave no history of re-exposure when the ulcer was resistant to treatment

of a syphilitic chancre increases the likelihood of contracting HIV following exposure to an HIV-positive sexual partner. For this reason, these two diseases have a tendency to coexist in the same individual, and the diagnosis of either should prompt evaluation for the other disease.

Clinical Features

With advanced immunosuppression, the typically painless chancre may be particularly painful due to secondary bacterial infection. The course of syphilis may be altered in that there can be (1) a shorter latency period between primary infection and development of meningovascular syphilis; (2) rapid progression to tertiary disease within the first year of infection; (3) lack of response to penicillin therapy; (4) a tendency for relapse in the absence of reexposure despite adequate treatment, as seen in Fig. 2.10; and (5) increased frequency of Lues maligna (pleomorphic skin lesions consisting of pustular nodules, ulcers, and necrotizing vasculitis).

Diagnosis

Immunosuppression may lead to limited or absent antibody mediated responses to infection. This means the reactive plasma reagin (RPR) and fluorescent treponemal antibody (FTA) tests may not be as sensitive as they are in immunocompetent individuals. Examination of skin lesions via dark-field microscopy (seldom done today in most laboratories), immunohistochemical staining of a biopsy, and direct fluorescent antibody staining of the exudate are useful adjuncts in establishing the diagnosis.

Treatment

Aggressive treatment with close follow-up should be pursued in all cases of syphilis. The CDC recommends penicillin regimens for all stages of syphilis. Some authorities recommend CSF evaluation for all cases, regardless of clinical stage, and a treatment regimen appropriate for neurosyphilis. At the very least, the threshold for evaluation of CSF involvement should be considerably lower in the context of HIV. All patients should be followed clinically and with quantitative VDRL and RPR tests at 1, 2, 3, 6, 9, and 12 months. An increase in titers or a failure to decrease within 6 months should prompt examination of CSF and retreatment.

Bacillary Angiomatosis

Bacillary angiomatosis is caused by Bartonella henselae and Bartonella quintana. In the case of B. henselae, contact with a cat is a significant risk factor, as the domestic cat (Felis domesticus) is a reservoir for the organism, with the cat flea Ctenocephalides felis acting as a vector for transmission. It was first described in 1983 among HIV patients with cutaneous and subcutaneous vascular lesions mimicking Kaposi's sarcoma. It is typically seen in patients with CD4 counts of less than 100 cells/mm^2. While it can involve the liver or spleen, skin lesions are most frequently reported.

Clinical Features

Bacillary angiomatosis typically presents as small, erythematous vascular papules, which may enlarge to form exophytic, friable nodules surrounded by a collarete of scale with or without erythema. Subcutaneous lesions may have the appearance of flesh-colored cystic nodules or epidermal inclusion cysts. Deeper soft tissue masses may also be seen.

Diagnosis

An incisional biopsy to evaluate for characteristic histologic findings is usually required. Histologically, biopsy shows a lobular proliferation of small capillary sized blood vessels. Endothelial cells are enlarged and have abundant cytoplasm. The vascular proliferation is surrounded by an inflammatory infiltrate with neutrophils, focal necrosis, and purple granular material scattered throughout. The presence of bacillary organisms distinguishes this lesion from lobular capillary hemangioma, Kaposi sarcoma, angiosarcoma, epithelioid hemangioma, and epithelioid hemangioendothelioma. Additionally, bacterial cultures, PCR, and serologic testing may be useful in establishing a definitive diagnosis.

Management

Treatment for bacillary angiomatosis has not been systematically evaluated, although anecdotal evidence suggests erythromycin and doxycycline are the agents of choice. In the absence of osseous or parenchymal disease, an 8- to 12-week regiment of oral antimicrobial treatment is typically effective.

Staphylococcal Skin Disease

Staphylococcus aureus is the most common cutaneous and systemic bacterial pathogen in HIV patients. The nares are typically colonized, with 50 % of HIV-infected homosexual men harboring the organism in their nares. The combination of frequent nasal carriage, impaired cutaneous barriers, and decreased numbers of neutrophils favors frequent infections. The presence of indwelling venous catheters, and the presence of pruritus and the scratching that ensues are both risk factors for developing the disease.

Clinical Features

In AIDS patients S. aureus can cause infections similar to those in immunocompetent patients, including bullous impetigo, ecthyma, folliculitis, and abscesses. Bullous impetigo in the groin, especially when recurrent, can be an AIDS marker. More unusual presentations of staphylococcal infection may be seen as well, including botryomycosis, atypical platelike lesions of the scalp, axilla or groin, and pyomyositis. These more unusual infections may be refractory to treatment.

Diagnosis

Gram stain and culture are always helpful in the diagnosis of staphylococcal infection. For common superficial infections, a gram stain of purulent material is adequate. In the case of deeper infections and recurrent disease, culture and susceptibility testing is warranted, particularly since both resistance and drug reactions are common in this patient population.

Treatment

Where clinical findings are present, and the gram stain is consistent, empiric treatment is reasonable. The choice of antibiotics and the treatment strategy should be no different than with HIV-negative patients: abscesses should be drained and therapy should continue until infection is cleared. If an infection fails to improve, the choice of antibiotics and/or dosage may need to be reevaluated. In general, treatment will usually take longer than with immunocompetent patients. Staphylococcus species have proved adept in developing antibiotic resistance, so mention of any specific antibiotic and or dosage risks obsolescence and should be cross-referenced with a regional antibiogram. The relatively higher incidence of drug reactions in this patient population, discussed below, should be taken into consideration when selecting an effective antibiotic regimen.

Mycobacterial Infection

Cutaneous mycobacterial infections are associated with AIDS. In the immunocompromised host, cutaneous inoculation with *M. tuberculosis* results in a tuberculous chancre. Occasionally, cutaneous tuberculosis manifests as tuberculosis verrucosa cutis. Disseminated tuberculosis may involve the skin as well. *M. hemophilum* and *M. avium-intracellulare*, seen in Fig. 2.11, have also been reported to cause skin lesions.

Clinical Features

A tuberculous chancre presents as a painless ulceration at the exposure site with under-mined margins and associated lymphadenopathy. Tuberculosis verrucosa cutis consists of a hyperkeratotic plaque with no lymphadenopathy. Disseminated tuberculosis can involve the skin as scrofuloderma, lupus vulgaris, and

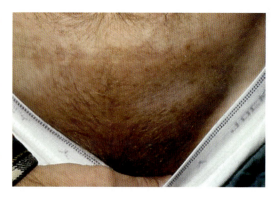

Fig. 2.11 A dull red/brown, slightly indurated pubic plaque in an AIDS patient, which on biopsy showed mycobacterium intercellulare

metastatic tuberculous abscesses. Cutaneous military tuberculosis presents as a diffuse maculopapular skin eruption. Tuberculous lymphadenitis has been associated with IV drug abuse.

Non-tuberculous, disseminated mycobacterial infections produce an acute pustular eruption. In the case of *M. haemophilum*, soft tissue swelling, skin nodules, and ulcerating skin lesions may be present.

Diagnosis

Biopsy of involved skin lesions shows ill-formed granulomas with extensive necrosis and acid fast bacilli.

Management

Lesions limited to the skin may not require systemic therapy. With disseminated mycobacterial infections, treatment with pyrazinamide, ethambutol, rifampin, isoniazid, and streptomycin is indicated. Multidrug resistant strains are more common in AIDS patients.

Parasites and Infestations

Scabies

Pruritus is one of the most common dermatologic complaints in AIDS patients, and may be attributable to a variety of possible causes. In addition to molluscum, discussed earlier, common causes that can be ruled out easily are xerosis due

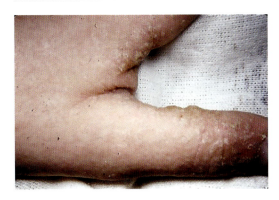

Fig. 2.12 Myriads of burrows between the finger webs in a child with AIDS. These burrows are much more numerous than would be expected in a patient with a normal immune system

to excessive bathing and use of harsh soaps, *S. aureus* infection, and scabies.

Clinical Features

Scabies can follow two possible clinical patterns. Most patients show scabetic burrows at the wrist and finger web spaces, as seen in Fig. 2.12. In AIDS patients with altered peripheral or central nervous systems, crusted or "Norwegian scabies" may be seen.

Diagnosis

Suspicious lesions scraped with a sterile scalpel blade allow for identification of scabetic mites, mite ova, or feces. Characteristic clinical features, including linear or serpiginous scabetic burrows measuring 0.3–1.0 cm in length, and papulovesicular lesions located on the volar aspect of the wrists or in finger web spaces, are sufficient for a presumptive clinical diagnosis. Pruritic, crusted penile or scrotal papules are highly suggestive of scabies as well.

Treatment

First-choice treatment consists of lindane and permethrin antiscabetic agents. It should be applied to the entire body, including the head and neck and under the fingernails, for a minimum of 8 h. Repeated applications may be required for patients with crusted scabies. Asymptomatic close household contacts should be treated. In children under 6 years of age, permethrin is preferred.

Neoplastic Lesions

Kaposi's Sarcoma

Kaposi's sarcoma (KS) is an endothelially derived multifocal tumor first described by Moritz Kaposi in 1872 as an "idiopathic pigmented sarcoma of the skin." Several variants of KS have been described with varying degrees of behavior ranging from indolent to aggressive. Epidemic KS is the most common AIDS-associated cancer in the U.S. and Africa. Ninety-five percent of lesions are associated with human herpesvirus 8 (HHV-8). HHV-8 appears to be sexually transmitted, and homosexual sex seems to be a significant risk factor in its transmission. In the San Francisco Men's Health Study, a direct correlation was found between homosexuality and HHV-8 seroprevalence, as well as the number of intercourse partners and HHV-8 seroprevalence. There is some speculation regarding receptive anal intercourse as the primary mode of transmission, which would certainly explain why it is far less common in the heterosexual population. Pathogenesis appears to involve induced proliferation of mesenchymal cells by HIV infected T-lymphocytes and tumor cells. Eventual formation of vascular channels leads to clinical appearance of Kaposi's sarcoma.

Clinical Features

In the AIDS population, Kaposi's sarcoma presents initially as multifocal asymptomatic reddish purple patches and macules. They then develop a yellow-green bruiselike discoloration at the periphery, and then finally progress to raised violaceous to brown plaques or nodules. It is typically distributed over the face, trunk, and arms. Early lesions can be easily mistaken for a bruise, insect bite, or benign nevus, as shown in Fig. 2.13. Exophytic nodules or tumors may also occur, as shown in Fig. 2.14. One-third of patients experience oral cavity lesions associated with red to purple plaques or nodules of the hard and soft palate, gums, tongue, and oropharynx. Periorbital, genital, and lower extremity lesions may become edematous. Ulceration, bleeding, and pain may complicate lesions.

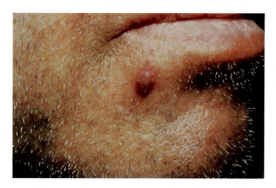

Fig. 2.13 An AIDS patient with biopsy-proven Kaposi's sarcoma on the chin. The dome-shaped, well-demarcated, reddish-brown tumor mimics a benign compound nevus

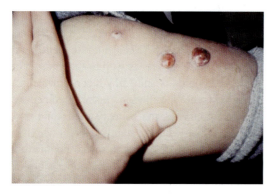

Fig. 2.14 Reddish-brown, ozzing, exophytic tumors over the lower anterior leg of an AIDS patient

Diagnosis

Biopsy for definitive pathologic diagnosis is necessary. Histopathologic features, consisting of a proliferation of atypical spindle cells, vascular channels, and hemosiderin laden macrophages, are diagnostic. Immunoperoxidase stains for HHV-8 can be particularly helpful in equivocal cases.

Therapy

HAART is the principal treatment for Kaposi's sarcoma, as lesions tend to regress with recovery of immune function. The outcome of patients with AIDS and KS is variable and appears related to the degree of immunosuppression rather than the KS. Radiation, interferon alpha, and angiogenesis inhibitors may be necessary for persistent lesions.

Cutaneous Lymphomas

HIV-infected patients have approximately a 200-fold higher risk of developing a malignant lymphoma than normal individuals. In addition to the cutaneous lymphomas described below, there is a wide spectrum of extracutaneous lymphomas that are prone to develop in HIV-infected individuals, including diffuse large B-cell lymphoma, Burkitt lymphoma, and primary effusion lymphoma. This section will focus on cutaneous lymphomas associated with AIDS.

Clinical Features

Cutaneous lymphomas affecting adults with HIV may in fact represent the first AIDS-defining illness. In contrast to their immunocompetent counterparts, mycosis fungoides is less common than cutaneous B-cell lymphomas. Plasmablastic lymphoma of the oral cavity is mostly restricted to AIDS. Association with EBV has been documented in plasmablastic lymphoma, other cutaneous B-cell lymphomas, and cutaneous CD30-positive anaplastic large cell lymphoma.

Plasmablastic lymphoma typically presents with nodules and tumors arising in the oral mucosa or at other mucosal sites. Cutaneous lesions in other lymphomas generally resemble those observed on non-HIV infected individuals.

Diagnosis

Definitive diagnosis requires a biopsy and comprehensive evaluation of histopathologic, immunophenotypical, and molecular genetic features by a pathologist. Plasmablastic lymphoma can present with a spectrum of morphologic features, including plasmablasts, and mature-looking plasma cells. Neoplastic cells are positive for CD38, CD138, and multiple-myeloma oncogene 1 (MUM-1). In AIDS patients, diffuse large B cell lymphomas have a greater tendency to show plasmablastic differentiation and an association with EBV.

Treatment and Prognosis

Plasmablastic lymphoma is extremely aggressive with a survival of less than 1 year. Better management of the underlying HIV infection is likely to improve prognosis. A combination of antiviral therapy and chemotherapy is ideal in these patients. With other cutaneous lymphomas, death often ensues from complications of AIDS rather than from direct lymphoma spread, stressing the importance of treating the underlying

immunodeficiency rather than the lymphoproliferative disorder.

Squamous Cell Carcinoma and Basal Cell Carcinoma

Cloacogenic carcinoma of the anal canal shows
increased incidence in homosexual males at risk
for HIV infection, and is specifically associated
with receptive anal intercourse. Since herpesvirus and papillomavirus have been implicated in
the pathogenesis of this carcinoma, with progressive immunosuppression the carcinogenicity of
condylomata and herpes ulcers increases. For a
more detailed description of HPV-related anal
carcinoma see the corresponding section under
Viral Infections.

Cutaneous malignancies also show increased
incidence in the immunocompromised patient.
Multiple squamous cell carcinomas, multiple
warts with evolving squamous cell carcinomas,
and metastatic basal cell carcinoma have all been
reported in AIDS patients.

Inflammatory Disorders

Eosinophilic Pustulosis (Ofuji Disease)

In the HIV-negative population, Ofuji's disease typically affects young Japanese adults.
Classically, it consists of sterile pruritic papules
and pustules on the face, trunk, and extremities with associated peripheral leukocytosis and
eosinophilia. Similar findings have been reported
in AIDS patients, with some distinguishing clinical and laboratory features, to the extent that
HIV-associated eosinophilic folliculitis, seen in
Fig. 2.15, is considered by some as a separate
entity from Ofuji's disease.

Clinical Features

In AIDS patients, the eruption can include non-
follicular pustules, coalescing plaques, and urticarial lesions. Lesions tend to be pruritic and
increase in severity with advanced immunosuppression. The majority of cases show elevated
serum eosinophil counts without leukocytosis
and increased IgE levels. In some cases, the
NRTI Didanosine has been associated with this
eruption.

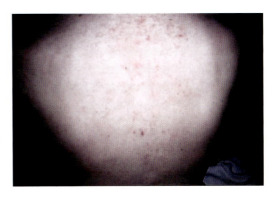

Fig. 2.15 Unbearable pruritic papules scattered over the
upper back in an AIDS patient. A skin biopsy confirmed
the diagnosis of eosinophilic pustular folliculitis

Treatment

A combination of Ultraviolet B phototherapy,
potent topical corticosteroids, and astemizole have
proven effective in ameliorating pruritus and clearing the eruption. Prolonged systemic corticosteroids are often necessary due to the extreme pruritis.

Drug Reactions

The incidence of drug reactions is eight to ten
times higher in HIV-positive individuals compared to the general population.

Severe bullous eruptions appear to be more
frequent in AIDS patients, including an increased
incidence of Stevens-Johnsons syndrome and toxic
epidermal necrolysis, most commonly related to
sulfonamides, although the NRTI Didanosine,
the NNRTI Nevirapine, and the protease inhibitor
Indinavir have been implicated as well.

Antiretroviral therapy can result in a wide
variety of mucocutaneous reactions, including
immune reconstitution inflammatory syndrome,
described below.

NRTI

Zidovudine is associated with nail and mucocutaneous hyperpigmentation (shown in Fig. 2.16),
hypertrichosis, paronychia, leukocytoclastic vasculitis, and hypersensitivity to mosquito bites.
Didanosine is associated with leukocytoclastic
vasculitis, SJS, and Ofuji's disease. Lamivudine is

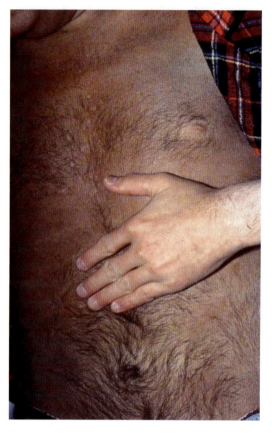

Fig. 2.16 Dramatic hyperpigmentation over the anterior trunk of an AIDS patient on prolonged zidovudine therapy

associated with paronychia with lateral nail-fold pyogenic granuloma like lesions, as well as allergic contact dermatitis and alopecia. Zalcitabine is associated with a morbilliform eruption and DRESS syndrome. Abacavir is associated with hypersensitivity syndrome.

NNRTI

Nevirapine is associated with a non-specific nevirapine rash and hypersensitivity syndrome as well as SJS.

Protease Inhibitors

In general, protease inhibitors can induce lipodystrophy, hypersensitivity reaction, and acute

generalized exanthematous pustulosis (AGEP). Additionally, Indinavir is associated with alopecia, paronychia, SJS, and hypersensitivity syndrome. Ritonavir is associated with various drug eruptions, IgA-mediated hypersensitivity reactions, and spontaneous bleeding and hematomas. Nelfinavir is associated with a morbilliform eruption and urticaria. Saquinavir is associated with a fixed drug eruption and urticaria.

Immune Reconstitution Inflammatory Syndrome (IRIS)

This usually occurs within the first 12 weeks of initiation of HAART therapy and usually indicates successful therapy, with a concurrent log decline in viral load and an increase in CD4 counts. Cutaneous manifestations are by far the most prevalent, constituting 54–78 % of all reported IRIS. They often consist of the common cutaneous infections associated with HIV, including warts, molluscum, HSV, and VZV. HAART should be continued while providing adequate treatment for these infections.

Inflammatory Skin Diseases

Seborrheic Dermatitis

In certain cohorts, seborrheic dermatitis is the most common dermatologic diagnosis in AIDS patients, and tends to be more severe and resistant to therapy. In adults, it is more common in men and is frequently localized to the genital areas. In children aged 2 years and above, the distribution favors flexural areas and the trunk. Severity of the disease correlates with CD4 count. Seborrheic dermatitis is associated with tuberculosis, Pneumocystis pneumonia, and CMV infection, as well as toxoplasmosis involving the central nervous system. Superinfection of untreated lesions with S. aureus and HSV-1 is common. Pityrosporum orbiculare colonies have been associated with the disease, although in some cohorts they have been entirely absent.

Treatment

Treatment with a combination of low-dose corticosteroids and topical antifungals is usually effective, although in AIDS patients it tends to recur with cessation of therapy.

Psoriasis

The prevalence of psoriasis is no higher in HIV-positive individuals than in the general population. Psoriatic arthritis, on the other hand, does show a higher prevalence (2–10 % versus 0.10 %) among HIV-positive individuals. With the onset of AIDS, however, psoriasis undergoes severe exacerbation, and treatment options become limited.

The clinical lesions are no different than in usual psoriasis, and include guttate, small or large plaque, inverse, palmoplantar, pustular, and erythrodermic. The appearance of severe psoriasis in an individual at risk for HIV may indicate both HIV infection and progression to AIDS. In one report, 70 % of HIV-positive patients with severe psoriasis died of AIDS.

Treatment

Methotrexate (this is controversial and some authors, including editor JH, think this is safe and efficacious in AIDS patients) and other immunosuppressives are contraindicated in AIDS-associated psoriasis because of the risk for further immunosuppression, leukopenia, and infection. Etretinate is a useful adjunct in this setting. Psoriasis has been shown to respond to HAART.

Pruritic Papular Dermatitis of AIDS

This is probably the most common skin eruption in AIDS patients, occurring in up to 40 % of AIDS patients. In up to 50 % of cases it can be the presenting sign. It can be disfiguring and stigmatizing. The cause remains unknown. Lichenoid and granulomatous dermatitis and prurigo of AIDS may be a variants of this disease.

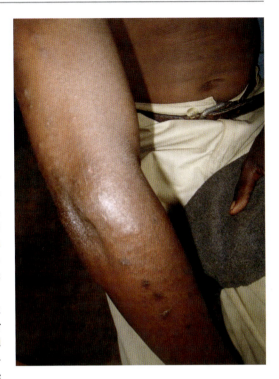

Fig. 2.17 Pruritic papular dermatitis of HIV in a patient in Kenya who had persistent pruritic papules even though HAART therapy had been instituted for over 1 year (Thanks to Scott Stanley for photographs)

Clinical Manifestation

Very pruritic excoriated papules and nodules scattered widely over the extremities (seen in Fig. 2.17), and trunk with sparing of face, mucous membranes, mucous membranes genetalia, and palms and soles.

Treatment

Topical antihistamines, emollients, and corticosteroids are used but often without success. Narrowband UVB and PUVA may be helpful. Pentoxyphylline has been tried also. HAART usually, but not always, is beneficial.

Other Inflammatory Skin Diseases

Acquired icthyosis, generalized xerosis, pitytriasis-like eruption, and erythroderma are also described in AIDS patients.

Conclusion

Since the discovery and elucidation of the AIDS epidemic, the skin has been the primary harbinger of the disease. HAART has changed the control of these cutaneous disorders but has not eliminated them as important early markers of the crippling of the immune system. Dermatology will continue to be an important contributor to the diagnosis and control of the plague that has characterized a major part of the culture for the last part of the previous two decades of the twentieth century and into the first part of the twenty-first.

Suggested Reading

Aly R, Berger T. Common superficial fungal infections in patients with AIDS. Clin Infect Dis. 1996;22 Suppl 2:s128–32.

Anglaret X, Minga A, Gabillard D, Ouassa T, Messou E, Morris B, et al. AIDS and non-AIDS morbidity and mortality across the spectrum of CD4 cell counts in HIV-infected adults before starting antiretroviral therapy in Cote d'Ivoire. Clin Infect Dis. 2012;54(5):714–23.

Cedeno-Laurent F, Gomez-Flores M, Mendez N, Ancer-Rodriguez J, Bryant JL, Gaspari AA, et al. New insights into HIV-1 primary skin disorders. J Int AIDS Soc. 2011;14:5.

Centers for Disease Control (CDC). Kaposi's sarcoma and pneumocystis pneumonia among homosexual men—New York City and California. Morb Mortal Wkly Rep. 1981;30:305–8.

Cerroni L, Gatter K, Kerl H. Cutaneous lymphomas in immunosuppressed individuals. In: Skin lymphoma: the illustrated guide. 3rd ed. Oxford: Wiley-Blackwell; 2009.

Chatis PA, Miller CH, Schrager LE, Crumpacker CS. Successful treatment with foscarnet of an acyclovir-resistent mucocutaneous infections with herpes simplex in a patient with AIDS. N Engl J Med. 1989;320:279.

Chilek K, Routhouska S, Tamburro J. Disseminated varicella zoster virus as the acquired immunodeficiency syndrome-defining illness. Pediatr Dermatol. 2010;27(2):192–4.

Cockerell CJ. Human immunodeficiency virus infection and the skin: a crucial interface. Arch Intern Med. 1991;151:1295–303.

Coopman SA, Johnson RA, Platt R, Stern RS. Cutaneous disease and drug reactions in HIV infection. N Engl J Med. 1993;328(23):1670–4.

Doni SN, Mitchell AL, Bogale Y, Walker SL. Skin disorders affecting human immunodeficiency virus-infected children living in an orphanage in Ethiopia. Clin Exp Dermatol. 2011;37:15–9.

Dover JS, Johnson RA. Cutaneous manifestations of human immunodeficiency virus infection. Arch Dermatol. 1991;127(1383–91):1549–58.

Garman ME, Tyring SK. The cutaneous manifestations of HIV infection. Dermatol Clin. 2002;20:193–208.

Gershon AA. Prevention and treatment of VZV in patients with HIV. Herpes. 2001;8(2):32–6.

Horn CK, Scott GR, Benton EC. Resolution of severe molluscum contagiosum on effective antiretroviral therapy. Br J Dermatol. 1998;138(4):715–7.

Johnson TM, Duvic M, Rapini RP, Rios A. AIDS exacerbates psoriasis. N Engl J Med. 1985;313:1415.

Kaplan MH, Sadick N, Mcnutt NS, Meltzer M, Sarngadharan MG, Pahwa S. Dermatologic findings and manifestations of acquired immunodeficiency syndrome (AIDS). J Am Acad Dermatol. 1987;16:485–506.

Kreuter A, Potthoff A, Brockmeyer NH, Gambichler T, Swoboda J, Stucker M, et al. Anal carcinoma in human immunodeficiency virus-positive men: results of a prospective study from Germany. Br J Dermatol. 2010;162:1269–77.

Mankahla A, Mosam A. Common skin conditions in children with HIV/AIDS. Am J Clin Dermatol. 2012;13(3):153–66.

Marcoux D, Jafarian F, Joncas V, Buteau C, Kokta V, Moghrabi A. Deep cutaneous fungal infections in immunocompromised children. J Am Acad Dermatol. 2009;61(5):857–64.

Martin JN, Ganem DE, Osmond DH, Page-Shafer KA, Macrae D, Kedes DH. Sexual transmission and the natural history of human herpesvirus 8 infection. N Engl J Med. 1998;338(14):948–54.

Munoz-Perez MA, Rodriguez-Pichardo A, Camacho F, Colmenero MA. Dermatological findings correlated with CD4 lymphocyte counts in a prospective 3 year study of 1161 patients with human immunodeficiency virus predominantly acquired through intravenous drug abuse. Br J Dermatol. 1998;139:33–9.

Singh F, Rudikoff D. HIV-associated pruritus: etiology and management. Am J Clin Dermatol. 2003;4(3):177–88.

Soeprono FF, Schinella RA, Cockerel CJ, Comite SL. Seborrheic-like dermatitis of acquired immunodeficiency syndrome. J Am Acad Dermatol. 1986;14:242–8.

Tappero JW, Perkins BA, Wenger JD, Berger TG. Cutaneous manifestations of opportunistic infections in patients infected with human immunodeficiency virus. Clin Microbiol Rev. 1995;8(3):440–50.

Skin Disorders in Patients with Primary Immunodeficiencies

3

Natasha Klimas and Travis W. Vandergriff

Abstract

Primary immunodeficiencies (PIDs) are conditions caused by molecular defects in the genes required for normal immune function. PIDs are rare, with a prevalence of approximately 1 in 25,000. Though much remains to be explored in the field of PIDs, over 185 distinct defects have been described. Infections are generally the most pronounced feature of PIDs. However, PIDs have many non-infectious sequelae also. Cutaneous involvement, infectious and non-infectious, is prominent in many cases. In fact, cutaneous manifestations precede immunologic diagnosis in 79 % of PID patients.

PIDs are subject to wide clinical, immunological, and genetic heterogeneity. Different mutations in the same gene may yield variable phenotypes. This chapter will detail the clinical manifestations, genetics and pathophysiology, diagnosis, and management of selected PIDs with a special focus on those with historically prominent cutaneous findings.

Keywords

Granuloma • Agammaglobunemia • Combined immunodeficiencies • Autoimmunity • Phagocytic defects • Complement deficiencies • Autosomal recessive • IgA deficiency

Introduction

Primary immunodeficiencies (PIDs) are conditions caused by molecular defects in the genes required for normal immune function. PIDs are rare, with a prevalence of approximately 1 in 25,000. Though much remains to be explored in the field of PIDs, over 185 distinct defects have been described. Infections are generally the most pronounced feature of PIDs. However, PIDs have many non-infectious sequelae also. Cutaneous

N. Klimas, BS
Department of Dermatology,
UT Southwestern Medical Center, Dallas, TX, USA

T.W. Vandergriff, MD (✉)
Department of Dermatology,
UT Southwestern Medical Center,
5323 Harry Hines Blvd., NL8.120DA,
Dallas, TX 75390-9069, USA
e-mail: travis.vandergriff@utsouthwestern.edu

J.C. Hall (ed.), *Skin Diseases in the Immunocompromised*,
DOI 10.1007/978-1-4471-6479-1_3, © Springer-Verlag London 2014

involvement, infectious and non-infectious, is prominent in many cases. In fact, cutaneous manifestations precede immunologic diagnosis in 79 % of PID patients.

Chronic or recurrent skin infections are often the initial manifestation of a PID. Various other non-infectious skin disorders, including erythroderma and severe, recalcitrant dermatitis are also common in PIDs. In addition, autoimmune conditions and granulomata are seen. Dermatologic manifestations may lead to early suspicion and prompt intervention. Thus, practitioners should be familiar with the cutaneous warning signs of PIDs.

The International Union of Immunological Societies (IUIS) Expert Committee on Primary Immunodeficiency classifies PIDs into the following groups based on various immunopathogenic defects of the diseases and the cell types involved:

   I. combined immunodeficiencies
   II. well-defined   syndromes   with immunodeficiency
   III. predominantly antibody defects
   IV. defects of immune dysregulation
   V. phagocytic defects
   VI. defects of innate immunity, including VII and VIII, below
   VII. autoinflammatory conditions
VIII. complement

PIDs are subject to wide clinical, immunological, and genetic heterogeneity. Different mutations in the same gene may yield variable phenotypes. This chapter will detail the clinical manifestations, genetics and pathophysiology, diagnosis, and management of selected PIDs with a special focus on those with historically prominent cutaneous findings.

Combined Immunodeficiencies

Severe Combined Immunodeficiency (SCID)

Genetics and Pathophysiology

SCID is caused by mutations in genes required for the development and function of both T and B lymphocytes. In certain cases, the molecular defect impairs only T cell-mediated cellular immunity, while B cell function is normal. However, T cell signaling is necessary for B cells to produce antibodies; thus T cell dysfunction prevents effective B cell-mediated humoral immunity also. The most frequently mutated genes in SCID are the common cytokine receptor gamma chain gene (IL2RG), interleukin-7 receptor alpha (IL7RA), Janus kinase 3 (JAK3), Artemis, adenosine deaminase (ADA), and recombinase activating genes 1 and 2 (RAG1, RAG2). Common gamma chain deficiency, inherited as an X-linked trait, is the most common SCID subtype. Autosomal recessive RAG1 and RAG2 defects are responsible for most cases of Omenn Syndrome.

Clinical Manifestations

Chronic mucocutaneous candidiasis, seen in Fig. 3.1, is a common early manifestation. Eczematous morbilliform exanthems are also seen. Patients may exhibit erythroderma, seen in Fig. 3.2, defined as diffuse erythema with scale involving ≥90 % skin surface area. In Omenn syndrome, erythroderma, often with alopecia, is the most commonly described initial cutaneous presentation. Erythroderma in SCID may range from transient morbilliform eruptions to graft-versus-host disease (GVHD). GVHD occurs due to transplacental engraftment of maternal lymphocytes or transfusions and may be rapidly fatal. Microsatellite analysis helps exclude maternal engraftment as a cause of GVHD. Epitheliod and noncaseating granulomata are also seen in Omenn Syndrome.

Severe viral infections with pathogens including influenza, adenovirus, rotavirus, norovirus, parainfluenza, respiratory syncytial virus (RSV), herpesviridae (seen in Fig. 3.3), and measles are often fatal. Vaccination with attenuated organisms (e.g., oral polio, rotavirus, or varicella) may result in fulminant or fatal infections. Patients are also susceptible to opportunistic infections by organisms such as *Pneumocystis jirovecii*.

Tonsillar buds and palpable lymphoid tissue are generally absent in patients with SCID.

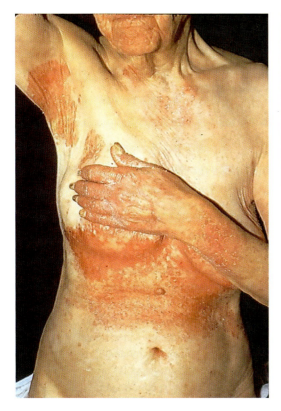

Fig. 3.1 Generalized candidiasis with diffuse erythema, satellite lesions, and worsening in intertriginous areas (axillae). Usually seen in SCID and the hallmark of muccocutaneous candidiasis

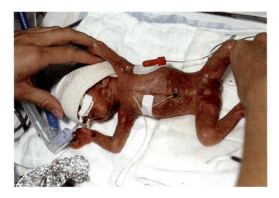

Fig. 3.2 Generalized erythroderma with some adherent fine scale in a newborn. Skin biopsy, genetic, and metabolic studies are indicated. It is the most common skin condition in Omenn Syndrome

Diagnosis

Failure to thrive, recurrent severe infections, and chronic diarrhea should raise suspicion for SCID. Peripheral T lymphocytes are absent or

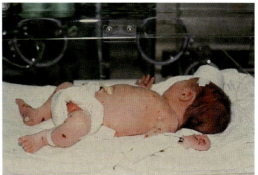

Fig. 3.3 Generalized cutaneous herpes simplex infection in a newborn. Widely scattered vesicles (some are hemorrhagic) showed a positive culture for herpes simplex. It can be seen in SCID and other primary immunodeficiency syndromes

profoundly low and a decreased absolute lymphocyte count is typical. Eosinophilia is characteristic for Omenn Syndrome. Hypogammaglobulinemia is common, though the presence of maternal IgG may mask this finding in early infancy. T cell mitogen responses are ineffectual or absent and cutaneous anergy is frequent. Fluorescent activated cell sorter (FACS) use allows patients to be distinguished based on the presence or absence of B cells and NK cells. Direct genetic analysis and flow cytometry with assays for aberrant or absent cell surface proteins (for example, JAK3) of mononuclear cells confirm a specific genetic diagnosis. Assays for carrier states and prenatal diagnosis are possible in certain SCID subtypes.

Management

HLA-matched hematopoietic stem cell transplantation (HSCT) is the definitive therapy. Retrovirally mediated gene transfer and enzyme replacement have been successful in X-linked SCID (ADA deficiency). Within the first 2 years of life, death from infection usually occurs without intervention. Thus prompt diagnosis and treatment are critical. Patients should undergo frequent surveillance for infection, and antimicrobial therapy should be started at the earliest sign of infection. In the hospital, SCID patients should be kept in protective isolation, and at home patients should avoid sick contacts and young children. Immunoglobulin replacement via IVIG and *Pneumocystis jirovecii* pneumonia

(PCP) prophylaxis are also recommended. Live vaccines are contraindicated for SCID patients and their family or caregivers.

Hyper IgM, Hyper Immunoglobulin M Syndrome

Genetics and Pathophysiology

Hyper IgM syndrome is a family of diseases defined by impaired immunoglobulin class-switch recombination, most often due to auto-somal recessive mutations in the CD40 ligand (CD40L) of TH2 cells. B cells initially produce IgM prior to class-switch recombination follow-ing antigen exposure. In Hyper IgM syndrome, however, B cells continually produce IgM, result-ing in low serum levels of of IgG, IgA, and IgE with normal or increased levels of IgM. CD40 is also expressed on dendritic cells and monocytes/macrophages, thus defective signaling through the CD40 receptor also results in impaired responses to opportunistic agents.

Clinical Manifestations

Patients manifest skin infections, particularly pyodermas and early-onset, recalcitrant HPV-induced verrucae. Large, painful, recurrent oral ulcers are also seen. These ulcers are usually non-infectious and involve the inside of the cheeks and tongue. Though the lesions may take months to heal, they typically resolve without scarring. In many cases, oral ulcers are associated with peri-ods of neutropenia. In addition, thrombocytope-nic purpura may be observed.

Patients have recurrent sinopulmonary infec-tions, frequently by encapsulated organisms or opportunistic pathogens. Gingivitis and stoma-titis are also common features of Hyper IgM syndrome. Patients may have failure to thrive due to chronic diarrhea. Lymphadenopathy and hepatosplenomegaly may be found on physical examination. In addition, cirrhosis and cholangiocarcinoma as a complication of cytomegalovirus or *Cryptosporidium* infec-tion are seen. Autoimmune conditions such as hemolytic anemia and inflammatory bowel dis-ease are also associated with Hyper IgM syn-drome. In addition, patients are at increased risk for malignancies, particularly pancreatic and gastrointestinal peripheral neuroectoder-mal tumors, hepatocellular carcinoma, and cholangiocarcinoma.

Diagnosis

Flow cytometry assays for CD40L expression on the surface CD4 lymphocytes are the first step in diagnosis. The diagnosis is confirmed by muta-tion analysis. Platelet and neutrophil-deficiencies are also associated.

Management

Replacement of immunoglobulins and prophy-laxis for PCP are necessary. HSCT provides definitive treatment when successful. Hygiene practices to prevent gastrointestinal infec-tion with pathogens such as *Cryptosporidium*, including avoidance of water that has not been filtered or boiled; avoidance of swimming in ponds, lakes, and pools; and prophylactic azithromycin are recommended. Surveillance for *Cryptosporidium* infection through stool polymerase chain reaction (PCR), liver ultra-sound, and liver function tests are also suggested every 6–12 months.

Well-Defined Syndromes with Immunodeficiency

Wiskott–Aldrich Syndrome (WAS)

Genetics and Pathophysiology

WAS results from absence or truncation of the WAS protein, which produces dysfunctional remodeling of the actin cytoskeleton of hemato-poietic cells. This impairs interactions between T lymphocytes and antigen-presenting cells, including macrophages and dendritic cells. On the basis of clinical features and molecular aberran-cies, patients may be classified into three major groups: (i) classic WAS (ii) X-linked thrombo-cytopenia (XLT) which results from "loss of function" mutations in the WAS gene, and (iii) X-linked neutropenia (XLN) which results from "gain of function" mutations.

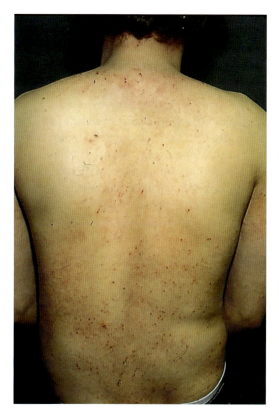

Fig. 3.4 Generalized excoriations and and lichenification over the back in a patient who has had eczema all of his life. Approximately 80 % of WAS patients have eczema

Clinical Manifestations

Petechiae and epistaxis secondary to thrombocytopenia are often initial signs of WAS. Eighty percent of WAS patients are affected by eczematous dermatitis, seen in Fig. 3.4. WAS-associated dermatitis is recalcitrant and generally develops during the neonatal period. The scalp, face, and flexural surfaces are preferentially involved. Patients may experience progressive lichenification. The hemorrhagic component of WAS-associated dermatitis distinguishes it from atopic dermatitis. Secondary infection by bacteria and viruses resulting in molluscum contagiosum and eczema herpeticum is common. Twenty percent of patients with WAS also develop cutaneous small vessel vasculitis within the first 15 years of life.

By 3 months of age, recurrent bacterial infections are seen in conjunction with decreasing maternal antibody levels. Common infections include pneumonia, sinusitis, conjunctivitis, and meningitis. Patients are highly susceptible to encapsulated organisms such as *Streptococcus pneumoniae, Haemophilus influenzae* and *Neisseria meningitides*. Viral infections become more common with advancing age.

Hepatosplenomegaly and lymphadenopathy may be noted on physical exam. Three major clinical features characterize classical WAS: dermatitis, thrombocytopenia, and recurrent pyogenic infections. XLT, a milder phenotype, presents with thrombocytopenia and mild or intermittent eczema. XLN presents with infections linked with both lymphocyte deficits and neutropenia. The XLN subpopulation is also at increased risk for myelodysplasia.

Diagnosis

Petechiae or bruises with early-onset thrombocytopenia associated with low mean platelet volume in males should raise suspicion for WAS/XLT. Flow cytometry with anti-WAS protein antibody may be used to screen for WAS mutations. *WAS* gene sequence analysis confirms the diagnosis.

Management

HSCT represents a curative treatment approach, resulting in reconstitution of immunity and resolution of platelet deficiency and dermatitis. IVIG and prophylactic trimethoprim/sulfamethoxazole or penicillin are widely used. Conventional therapy also includes acyclovir for herpes simplex prophylaxis. Platelet transfusions are given to prevent major blood loss during surgery or to treat major episodes such as central nervous system hemorrhage or gastrointestinal bleeding. Patients with recurrent hemorrhage may benefit from splenectomy. Autoimmune cytopenias often respond to B cell antibodies targeting CD20 (rituximab). Topical corticosteroids are a treatment of choice for WAS-associated dermatitis.

Ataxia-Telangiectasia (AT)

Genetics and Pathophysiology

AT results from mutations in the ataxia telangiectasia mutated (ATM) gene, a key regulator of cell-cycle and apoptotic responses to DNA damage, particularly double-stranded breaks. Double stranded breaks are induced by ionizing radiation and also physiologic events such as meiosis, V(D)J recombination in lymphocytes, and telomere maintenance.

Clinical Manifestations

Telangiectasias develop on exposed areas, particularly the face, ears, and neck/upper back at around 6 years of age. Sterile granulomata resembling granuloma annulare, which may be ulcerative and/or painful, are observed in 8 % of patients. These lesions may precede diagnosis. Granulomata in AT involve the limbs; facial and truncal lesions are also seen. Ninety percent of patients develop progeric changes of the skin and hair. Young children develop gray hair and are often diffusely gray at adolescence. Facial atrophy and sclerosis due to subcutaneous fat loss are also observed. Children often present with pigmentary mosaicism in the form of hyper and/or hypopigmentation, for example, café-au-lait lesions. Poikiloderma, eczematous dermatitis, seborrheic dermatitis, recurrent impetigo, keratosis pilaris, vitiligo, warts, hirsutism, and acanthosis nigricans have also been described in AT.

Progressive neurodegeneration in the form of cerebellar ataxia begins at a median age of 15 months. AT is also associated with thymic aplasia or hypoplasia. Up to 20 % develop malignancies, particularly acute leukemias and lymphomas.

Diagnosis

Elevated serum carcinoembryonic antigen (CEA) and alpha-fetoprotein (AFP) levels are consistently seen. In patients older than 2 years, serum AFP levels and cerebellar atrophy on MRI may aid in establishing a diagnosis. Deficient or absent serum IgA (in 70 %), IgE (in up to 80 %), lymphopenia (in 70 %), deficient in vitro antigen and mitogen responses, and relative CD4 T cell deficiencies are observed in AT. Immunoblotting assays for the ATM protein deficient in ATM may also help confirm the diagnosis.

Management

Therapy for AT is supportive. Vigilant sun protection, screening for malignancies, and antibiotics and/or IVIG aid in controlling infections.

Hyper Immunoglobulin E Syndrome (HIES)

Genetics and Pathophysiology

Mutations in the dedicator of cytokinesis 8 (DOCK8) and signal transducer and activator of transcription 3 (STAT3) genes generate the autosomal recessive and autosomal dominant forms of HIES, respectively. Autosomal dominant HIES is also known as Job's syndrome. STAT3 is integral to the signal transduction pathways of a broad range of cytokines and the subsequent development of TH17 cells. DOCK8 mutations impede cytoskeletal remodeling required for processes such as T cell polarization and activation.

Clinical Manifestations

Within the first few weeks of life, many Job's syndrome patients develop a follicular-based papulopustular eruption on the face and scalp which progresses to involve the buttocks, shoulders, and upper trunk. This newborn rash is present in 65–80 % of Job's syndrome cases and 24 % of autosomal recessive HIES cases. In many patients, it may resemble neonatal acne. This rash progresses to an intensely pruritic, diffuse dermatitis resembling eczema. The eczematous lesions of HIES, unlike those of atopic dermatitis, frequently involve the retroauricular and intertriginous regions. Patients with autosomal recessive HIES also manifest eczematous dermatitis. In patients with autosomal recessive HIES the dermatitis is more severe than in Job's syndrome, with a distribution more typical for atopic dermatitis. Dermatitis in autosomal recessive HIES often coincides with food allergy, in contrast to Job's syndrome. Unique features of autosomal recessive HIES also include a higher incidence of severe, recurrent, or chronic viral infections. Molluscum contagiosum and verrucae are common. Herpes zoster and herpes simplex also affect patients with autosomal recessive HIES. In addition, patients with autosomal recessive HIES have an increased risk of mucocutaneous squamous cell carcinomas linked with HPV.

Bacterial skin infections, particularly furuncles, cellulitis, and abscesses which may be cold (i.e., devoid of cardinal signs of inflammation) in classical cases or warm and erythematous are prevalent. Folliculitis, often involving the back and shoulders, is also seen. Chronic candidiasis of the nail beds and mucosa affects 83 % of HIES patients.

Elevated serum IgE levels, dermatitis, recurrent sinopulmonary infections, and cutaneous staphylococcal abscesses are shared in autosomal recessive HIES and Job's syndrome.

Patients with Job's syndrome may be distinguished from autosomal recessive HIES by the development of "leonine" facies and coarse facial skin, typically at adolescence. In this subpopulation, musculoskeletal disorders including scoliosis, osteopenia, and early-onset degenerative joint disease are seen. Primary teeth are often retained. Patients may also have vaulted or high arched palates. Additionally, vascular aneurysms and recurrent pulmonary infections leading to bronchiectasis or pneumatoceoles are observed. HIES also confers an increased risk of malignancy, especially lymphoma.

Diagnosis

A scoring system based on clinical and laboratory findings may aid in the diagnosis of HIES. This scoring system encompasses recurrent skin infections (mainly abscesses), sinopulmonary infections, and IgE levels above 2,000 IU. Another set of guidelines stratifies the diagnosis of STAT3 deficiency as follows:

- **possible:** IgE > 1,000 IU/mL plus a weighted score of clinical features over 30 (based on characteristic facies, recurrent pneumonia, newborn rash, pathologic fractures, and high palate)
- **probable:** the characteristics above plus a lack of TH17 cells or a family history of definitive HIES
- **definitive:** probable characteristics plus a dominant-negative heterozygous mutation in STAT3.

Management

Emollient use and hydration are key for management of HIES-associated dermatitis. Corticosteroids may also be applied to uninfected regions. Antihistamines can be used for control of pruritus.

Prompt treatment of infections that develop is paramount, and prophylactic trimethoprim-sulfamethoxazole can be used to prevent infections. Interferon (IFN) gamma therapy may regulate immunoglobulin production in HIES and is recommended in patients with severe infections such as pulmonary aspergillosis.

Predominantly Antibody Deficiencies

Bruton's Agammaglobulinemia (XLA)

Genetics and Pathophysiology

Plasma cells, which develop from the B cell lineage, are responsible for immunoglobulin production. Thus, defects of B cell development or function yield hypogammaglobulinemia, or alternatively, agammaglobulinemia. XLA, also known as Bruton's agammaglobulinemia, results from mutations in the Bruton's tyrosine kinase (BTK) gene, an essential regulator of the pro-B to pre-B cell transition. Autosomal recessive mutations in multiple other genes necessary for normal B cell development and function leading to agammaglobulinemia/hypogammaglobulinemia have also been identified.

Clinical Manifestations

Patients with XLA manifest skin infections such as cellulitis and furuncles. In addition, patients are predisposed to develop ecthyma gangrenosum as seen in Fig. 3.5, a cutaneous infection typically caused by *Pseudomonas* characterized by hemorrhagic pustules which progress to necrotic ulcers. Lymphocytic infiltration results in a papular dermatitis, and eczematous dermatitis is also observed. Non-infectious granulomata are seen as well. Rare cases of a rapidly fatal syndrome resembling dermatomyositis in patients with echoviral central nervous system infections have also been described.

Patients with agammaglobulinemia present with infections of the sinopulmonary and gastrointestinal tracts, often by *Haemophilus* and *Streptococcal*, *Staphylococcal*, and *Pseudomonal*

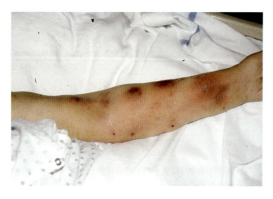

Fig. 3.5 Ecthyma gangrenosum with necrotic bruised-appearing tumors over the upper extremities in a patient with pseudomonas sepsis. This can be seen in XLA

species. An arthritis similar to rheumatoid arthritis is also seen in one-third of patients.

Diagnosis
Low immunoglobulin levels paired with absent or deficient B cells on flow cytometry for lymphocytes raises suspicion for XLA. Mutations in the BTK gene or aberrant BTK expression may be assessed by DNA, mRNA, or protein analysis. XLA may be diagnosed prenatally through direct gene or restriction fragment length polymorphism analysis. Detection of female carriers may occur through evaluation of X chromosome inactivation patterns in B cells.

Management
Immunoglobulin repletion with IVIG is paramount in XLA. Early, aggressive antimicrobial therapy should be initiated for suspected infections. Live viral vaccines are contraindicated.

Selective Immunoglobulin (IgA) Deficiencies

Genetics and Pathophysiology
Selective IgA deficiency, the most common immunodeficiency state, is an isolated deficiency of serum IgA within the context of normal IgG and IgM levels in whom other immunodeficiencies have been excluded. Selective IgA deficiency

is thought to be a heterogeneous disorder generated by multiple distinct genetic mechanisms, most of which have yet to be elucidated.

Clinical Manifestations
Most patients with isolated IgA deficiency are asymptomatic. However, patients are at increased risk for atopic dermatitis and mucocutaneous candidiasis. Associations with autoimmune disorders including vitiligo, alopecia areata, dermatomyositis, systemic lupus erythematosus (SLE), scleroderma, lipodystrophia centrifugalis abdominalis, and dermatitis herpetiformis have been described.

Autoimmunity in IgA deficiency may also present as thyroiditis, rheumatoid arthritis, and a necrotizing vasculitis similar to polyarteritis nodosa. Gastrointestinal associations with IgA deficiency include celiac disease and inflammatory bowel disease.

Diagnosis
Evaluation of serum IgA, IgG, and IgM levels is necessary. Serum IgG and IgM levels must be within normal limits for a diagnosis of selective IgA deficiency. Other causes of immunodeficiency must also be excluded. Partial deficiency and severe deficiency are distinguished by serum IgA levels of above or below 7 mg/dL, respectively.

Management
Infections should be controlled with prompt antimicrobial therapy. IVIG is contraindicated in selective IgA deficiency, as the small quantities of IgA contained in IVIG may trigger anaphylaxis.

Common Variable Immunodeficiency (CVID)

Genetics and Pathophysiology
CVID is a family of hypogammaglobulinemia syndromes arising from heterogeneous genetic defects. In most cases, the specific molecular defect is unknown. However, major histocompatibility

linkage between CVID and selective IgA deficiency has been identified. CVID may develop from selective IgA deficiency.

Clinical Manifestations

Skin infections such as dermatophytosis, mucocutaneous candidiasis, and extensive verrucae are seen. Patients may have eczematous dermatitis. Granulomatous dermatitis presenting as inflammatory nodules which microscopically show non-caseating aseptic granulomata similar to sarcoidosis are seen. Cutaneous granulomata generally involve the extremities, but may also arise on the face or buttocks. Granulomata may be prognostic: CVID patients with granulomatous disease have higher rates of morbidity and mortality than the general CVID population. Patients with granulomata also have higher rates of autoimmune disorders. As in selective IgA deficiency, autoimmune associations include alopecia areata, vitiligo, and vasculitis.

In addition, granulomata may involve the eyes, lungs, liver, and lymphoid tissues. Antibody responses are limited or absent, and recurrent sinopulmonary infections are common. Patients are at increased risk for gastric carcinomas and lymphomas.

Diagnosis

Low levels of IgG and IgA may suggest CVID. One-half of patients also have low IgM levels. Patients with CVID generally have higher serum IgG levels than those with XLA. Patients demonstrate reduced antibody production in response to common antigens or immunization with polysaccharide or protein antigens.

Management

IVIG for immunoglobulin repletion reduces infections in CVID. Granulomata may be treated with topical, intralesional, or systemic corticosteroids. In patients with steroid-refractory cutaneous and extracutaneous aseptic granulomata, tumor necrosis factor (TNF) alpha inhibitors may be of benefit. Infections should be treated with early antimicrobial therapy.

Diseases of Immune Dysregulation

Chediak-Higashi Syndrome (CHS)

Genetics and Pathophysiology

CHS is characterized by impaired neutrophil chemotaxis and natural killer cell dysfunction. This results from mutations in lysosomal trafficking regulator (CHS1/LYST). The clinical manifestations of CHS are attributed to dysregulation of lysosome-related organelles, including the cytolytic granules of leukocytes, platelet-dense granules, and melanosomes.

Clinical Manifestations

Patients generally present with hypopigmentation. The extent of hypopigmentation is variable, but the majority of patients have amelanotic or hypomelanotic skin and hair, frequently with a metallic appearance. Ocular albinism is also common. Skin infections are another frequent manifestation. These range from superficial pyodermas to deep abscesses and ulcerations, many of which yield atrophic scars. Platelets in CHD are dysfunctional, yielding epistaxis, petechiae, and easy bruising.

Recurrent pyogenic sinopulmonary infections due to streptococcal and staphylococcal species are common. Patients who reach early adulthood experience progressive neurodegeneration in the form of peripheral neuropathy-induced motor and sensory deficits, ataxia, cranial nerve palsies, dementias, and seizures. Those who survive infections eventually enter the "accelerated phase" of CHD. The accelerated phase is characterized by multi-system hemophagocytic lymphohistiocytosis, which is generally lethal.

Diagnosis

Peripheral blood smear evaluation reveals characteristic giant azurophilic granules within granulocytes in CHD. Evaluation of cutaneous melanocytes similarly reveals giant melanosomes. Genetic testing for CHS1/LYST mutations confirms the diagnosis.

Management

Prophylactic antimicrobials and prompt, aggressive therapy for infections that develop are key. IFN gamma and granulocyte colony-stimulating factor (G-CSF) have also been used. IVIG, antivirals, and chemotherapy may slow the accelerated phase. Splenectomy and high-dose corticosteroids may also produce transient remissions of the accelerated phase. HSCT is the treatment of choice for the immunologic and hematologic complications of CHS. Transplantation is most successful with HLA-matched donors prior to the accelerated phase. HSCT, however, does not address the neurodegeneration or oculocutaneous albinism of CHS.

Congenital Defects of Phagocyte Number, Function, or Both

Leukocyte Adhesion Deficiency (LAD)

Genetics and Pathophysiology

In LAD, leukocyte trafficking into tissues from the vasculature in the setting of infection or inflammation is impaired. The most common and well-characterized of the three LAD syndromes is LADI. LADI results from defects in CD18, the common beta chain of the beta 2-integrin family of cell adhesion molecules. LADII is caused by defects in fucosylated ligands for selectins (another integral group of cell adhesion molecules), and LADIII results from impaired activation of all beta–integrins (1, 2, and 3).

Clinical Manifestations

Omphalitis with delayed separation of the umbilical stump and poor wound healing are common in LAD. Cutaneous staphylococcal and pseudomonal infections resembling pyoderma gangrenosum may also be seen.

Severe periodontitis and gingivitis are common to all patients who reach early childhood. Patients are predisposed to bacterial sinopulmonary and gastrointestinal infections. Patients are also affected by frequent fungal infections, though viral infections are less common. In LADI, the extent of CD18 deficiency is directly related to the severity of infectious complications.

Diagnosis

Flow cytometry to establish the absence of CD18 and associated subunit molecules (CD11a, CD11b, and CD11c) on the surface of leukocytes aids in diagnosis. Further evaluation may consist of sequence analysis to delineate the specific beta 2-subunit defect. Leukocytosis with absent pus formation is seen during infections, and a moderate neutrophilia is present at baseline. On microscopic examination, pyoderma gangrenosum-like lesions are neutrophil deficient.

Management

Phenotypic severity directs management in LAD. Patients with severe disease require transplantation of bone marrow or HSCT; however, transplantation is often complicated by GVHD or fulminant infection. Those with mild disease require only antimicrobial therapy for intercurrent infection. Vigilant dental hygiene practices attenuate periodontitis in LAD. In patients with LADII, a trial of fucose supplementation is recommended.

Chronic Granulomatous Disease (CGD)

Genetics and Pathophysiology

CGD is a heterogeneous group of conditions characterized by granuloma formation and severe, recurrent, life-threatening bacterial and fungal infections. CGD results from the defective generation of superoxide by the NADPH oxidase (phox) system. Phagocytes, including neutrophils and monocytes/macrophages, are therefore unable to destroy intracellular pathogens through the "respiratory burst." Patients are exquisitely susceptible to infection by organisms that produce catalase, which catalyzes hydrogen peroxide decomposition.

Clinical Manifestations

In neonates, cutaneous staphylococcal infections are common, particularly near the nose and ears. These infections may later progress to purulent dermatitis. In 15 % of patients with CGD, pyoderma is the initial manifestation. Regional lymphadenopathy, especially suppurative adenitis, is often seen as a complication of skin infections.

CGD patients are predisposed to granuloma formation from which organisms are difficult to isolate. Histologically, granulomata show macrophages with yellow-brown pigment. Other non-infectious dermatologic manifestations include vasculitis, rashes resembling discoid lupus, and photosensitivity.

Granulomata may affect virtually any site. Granuloma development in the liver and GI tract may result in a clinical picture similar to inflammatory bowel disease. Patients also develop active tuberculosis in endemic areas with increased frequency. Patients are also affected by recurrent pulmonary infections and gingivostomatitis. CGD predisposes patients to develop *Aspergillus* infections, including pulmonary and disseminated aspergillosis.

Diagnosis

Assessment of neutrophil superoxide production confirms the diagnosis. The classical nitroblue tetrazolium (NBT) reduction test, cytochrome c reduction assay, chemiluminescence, dihydrorhodamine 123 (DHR) oxidation test, or direct measurement of superoxide production may be used to evaluate phox function.

Management

Antifungal and antimicrobial prophylaxis, typically with itraconazole and trimethoprim-sulfamethoxazole, are recommended. IFN gamma may also augment prophylaxis. In periods of infection, antimicrobial therapy should be directed by microbiologic findings with biopsies as necessary for identification of the specific pathogen. HSCT provides definitive management, particularly in patients with severe, recurrent infections and/or recalcitrant inflammatory disease. Retrovirally mediated gene therapy has restored phox function, though its long-term risks and benefits have yet to be defined.

Defects in Innate Immunity

Chronic Mucocutaneous Candidiasis (CMC)

Genetics and Pathophysiology

CMC describes a collection of disorders distinguished by recurrent infections of the skin, nails, and mucous membranes with *Candida albicans*. Patients with CMC share T cell impairment, which represses effective immune responses to *Candida* species. In some cases, T cell deficits impede handling of *Candida* only. In other CMC patients, immune dysfunction prevents effective handling of other organisms. Molecular defects involving the beta-glucan receptor (dectin-1, betaGR), signal transducer and activator of transcription 1 (STAT1), lymphoid phosphatase (Lyp), and others have been described. Mutations in the autoimmune regulator (*AIRE*) gene responsible for autoimmune polyendocrinopathy-candidiasis-ectodermal dystrophy (APECED) syndrome also produce the CMC phenotype.

Clinical Manifestations

The clinical spectrum in CMC is highly variable. Treatment-resistant thrush is common. Paronychia and/or candidal onychomycosis often result in in malformed nails secondary to involvement of the nail bed. Cutaneous lesions present as scaly erythematous plaques often localized to the intertriginous areas, hands, feets, and scalp. Crusted granulomatous plaques are also seen. Scarring alopecia may occur as a complication of scalp involvement. Vitiligo and alopecia areata are common in patients with APECED; alopecia affects nearly one-third of patients over age 20 and may progress to alopecia universalis.

CMC is associated with an autoimmune diathesis manifested as endocrinopathies (especially in patients with APECED), rheumatoid arthritis, immune thrombocytopenia purpura (ITP), autoimmune hemolytic anemia, and autoimmune neutropenia.

Diagnosis

CMC is generally a clinical diagnosis. Testing for specific genetic defects may be performed, particularly for AIRE, STAT1, Lyp, or Dectin-1 mutations. Patients may demonstrate cutaneous anergy to *Candida* or ineffective immune responses to *Candida* through T cell proliferation assays, particularly patients with AIRE deficiency. Screening for alternative primary or secondary immune deficiencies should occur via complete blood count with differential, B and T lymphocyte subsets and immunoglobulin levels at minimum. Patients with CMC should also be evaluated for associated endocrinopathies, such as hypoparathyroidism and adrenal insufficiency.

Management

Antifungal therapy is the cornerstone of CMC management. Azoles are preferred. Patients may benefit from chronic suppressive therapy to prevent recurrences. Hormone replacement should be administered as required for associated endocrinopathies. Associated autoimmune disorders should also be managed as indicated.

Autoinflammatory Disorders

Muckle-Wells Syndrome (MWS)

Genetics and Pathophysiology

MWS, also known as urticaria-deafness-amyloidosis (UDA) syndrome, results from abnormal function of cryopyrin, produced by the *NLRP3* gene. In most cases, *NLRP3* gene aberrancies are inherited in an autosomal dominant pattern. *NLRP3* gene expression predominately occurs in chondrocytes and leukocytes, particularly neutrophils.

Cryopyrin is a key component of an intracellular protein complex contributing to innate immunity known as the inflammasome. The aberrant function of the inflammasome results in uncontrolled activation of caspase-1, an enzyme which yields overproduction of interleukin-1 (IL-1) beta. In turn, uninhibited inflammatory responses are initiated due to the body's inability to suppress inflammation.

Clinical Manifestations

Early, progressive sensorineural hearing loss is a characteristic feature of MWS. Patients experience periodic acute attacks of MWS symptoms. Some patients have daily recurrent attacks, while others have only rare, intermittent symptoms. Patients may rarely report a temporal association of attacks with cold exposure or the evening hours. The duration of attacks is generally longer in MWS than those with the closely-related familial cold autoinflammatory syndrome (FCAS), lasting from several days to continuous symptomatology. Urticarial eruptions are frequent in MWS attacks. Urticaria are migratory and may evolve from maculopapular lesions. These wheals, typically 0.2–3 cm in diameter, are associated with pruritus or pain. Some patients may also have oral ulcers. Conjunctivitis is another frequent finding.

Patients may experience fever to 39–40 ° C, chills, and/or malaise in conjunction with attacks. Joint pathology ranging from brief arthralgias to destructive polyarticular arthritis is also seen. Severe headaches occur, and may indicate elevated intracranial pressure or meningitis. In one-fourth of patients, MWS is complicated by amyloidosis, often producing renal dysfunction.

Diagnosis

Laboratory studies reveal thrombocytosis and leukocytosis with neutrophilia, anemia of chronic inflammation, and elevated acute phase reactants such as erythrocyte sedimentation rate (ESR) and C-reactive protein (CRP). MWS may be differentiated from FCAS by its associated secondary amyloidosis.

In many cases, a clinical diagnosis is possible. However, the presence of germline mutations in *NLRP3* may be established by Sanger sequencing. Sensorineural hearing loss may be detected via audiogram. Urinalysis demonstrating proteinuria and/or kidney biopsy may confirm amyloidosis with renal involvement.

Management

Anti-IL-1 therapies, including anakinra, rilonacept, and canakinumab have been successful in many patients. Fever, urticaria, conjunctivitis, and acute phase reactants respond to anti-IL-1 treatment. Anti-IL-1 therapy has reversed sensorineural hearing loss in cases of early intervention. In some patients, anakinra has reversed amyloidosis.

Complement Deficiencies

C2 Deficiencies

Genetics and Pathophysiology

The complement system is a protein cascade that functions in inflammation, cell lysis, opsonization/phagocytosis, and immune complex removal. Deficiencies of complement generally follow autosomal recessive inheritance, though deficiency of C1 inhibitor responsible for hereditary angioedema is inherited as an autosomal dominant trait. In the United States and Europe, C2 deficiency is the most common complement deficiency. C2 deficiency results from defective pretranslational regulation of C2 gene expression rather than a major gene deletion or rearrangement.

Clinical Manifestations

Deficiencies in the early components of the classic complement pathway predispose patients to pyogenic infections caused by encapsulated pathogens and connective tissue disease. Associations between homozygous C2 deficiency and discoid lupus erythematosus, polymyositis, cold urticaria, and vasculitis (particularly IgA vasculitis, or Henoch-Schlonen purpura, seen in Fig. 3.6) have been described.

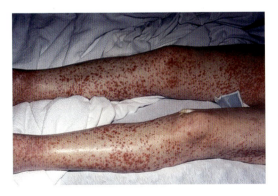

Fig. 3.6 Henoch-Schoenlein purpura with symmetric, palpable, petechial eruption over the legs. This represents an IgA vasculitis seen in several primary immunodeficiencies including complement deficiencies

SLE may affect up to 33 % of C2 deficient patients. Early onset disease, less renal disease, absent or low-titer ANA and anti-dsDNA antibodies, and pyogenic infections with encapsulated organisms may suggest SLE associated with C2 deficiency rather than classic SLE. Approximately two-thirds have Ro (SS-A) antibodies.

C2 deficiency is also linked with CVID, Hodgkin's lymphoma, and glomerulonephritis.

Diagnosis

Total hemolytic complement (CH50) levels are low or undetectable. ELISA or radial immunodiffusion assays may be used to quantify the levels of C2 and other specific complement components. Low titer antinuclear antibodies may be present, often with a speckled pattern. Double-stranded DNA antibodies are generally absent. IgG subclass deficiencies are also associated.

Management

Infection surveillance is a cornerstone of therapy. Patients may and should receive all routine vaccinations. Patients typically respond to standard antimicrobials, thus routine administration of plasma to replace C2 is not required.

Conclusion

Inherited immune diseases are at the forefront of modern medicine as genetics and immunology have given us new insights into the diagnosis and the holy grail of prevention. Dermatology as a marker of early disease, a stigma for those affected, and target for therapeutic intervention will continue to be an important science in the advancement of the care of these innocent patients.

Suggested Reading

Al-Herz W, Bousfiha A, Casanova JL, Chapel H, Conley ME, Cunningham-Rundles C, et al. Primary immunodeficiency diseases: an update on the classification from the International Union of Immunological Societies expert committee for primary immunodeficiency. Front Immunol. 2011;2:54.

Berron-Ruiz A, Berron-Perez R, Ruiz-Maldonado R. Cutaneous markers of primary immunodeficiency diseases in children. Pediatr Dermatol. 2000; 17(2):91–6.

Bolognia JL, Jorizzo JL, Rapini RP. Dermatology. Philadelphia: Elsevier; 2008.

Chiam LY, Verhagen MM, Haraldsson A, et al. Cutaneous granulomas in ataxia telangiectasia and other primary immunodeficiencies: reflection of inappropriate immune regulation? Dermatology. 2011;223(1):13–9.

Chu EY, Freeman AF, Jing H, Cowen EW, Davis J, Su HC, et al. Cutaneous manifestations of DOCK8 deficiency syndrome. Arch Dermatol. 2012;148(1):79–84.

Davies EG, Thrasher AJ. Update on the hyper immunoglobulin M syndromes. Br J Haematol. 2010;149(2):167–80.

Dohil M, Prendiville JS, Crawford RI, Speert DP. Cutaneous manifestations of chronic granulomatous disease: a report of four cases and review of the literature. J Am Acad Dermatol. 1997;36(6):899–907.

Dupuis-Girod S, Medioni J, Haddad E, Quartier P, Cavazzana-Calvo M, Le Deist F, et al. Autoimmunity in Wiskott-Aldrich syndrome: risk factors, clinical features, and outcome in a single-center cohort of 55 patients. Pediatrics. 2003;111(5 Pt 1):e622–7.

Gathmann B, Binder N, Ehl S, Kindle G, ESID Registry Working Party. The European internet-based patient and research database for primary immunodeficiencies: update 2011. Clin Exp Immunol. 2012;167(3):479–91.

Greenberger S, Berkun Y, Ben-Zeev B, Levi YB, Barziliai A, Nissenkorn A. Dermatologic manifestations of ataxia-telangiectasia syndrome. J Am Acad Dermatol. 2013;68(6):932–6.

Haas N, Kuster W, Zuberbier T, Henz BM. Muckle-Wells syndrome: clinical and histological skin findings compatible with cold air urticaria in a large kindred. Br J Dermatol. 2004;151(1):99–104.

Lehman H. Skin manifestations of primary immune deficiency. Clin Rev Allergy Immunol. 2014;46(2):112–9.

Neven B, Prieur A-M. Cryopyrinopathies: update on pathogenesis and treatment. Nat Clin Pract Rheum. 2008;4(9):481–9.

Olaiwan A, Chandesris MO, Fraitag S, Lortholary O, Hermine O, Fischer A, et al. Cutaneous findings in sporadic and familial autosomal dominant hyper-IgE syndrome: a retrospective, single-center study of 21 patients diagnosed using molecular analysis. J Am Acad Dermatol. 2011;65(6):1167–72.

Paradela S, Sacristan F, Almagro M, Prieto VG, Kantrow SM, Fonseca E. Necrotizing vasculitis with a polyarteritis nodosa-like pattern and selective immunoglobulin a deficiency: case report and review of the literature. J Cutan Pathol. 2008;35(9):871–5.

Shiflett SL, Kaplan J, Ward DM. Chediak-Higashi syndrome: a rare disorder of lysosomes and lysosome related organelles. Pigment Cell Res. 2002; 15(4):251–7.

Sullivan KE, Mullen CA, Blaese RM, Winkelstein JA. A multiinstitutional survey of the Wiskott-Aldrich syndrome. J Pediatr. 1994;125(6 Pt 1):876–85.

Thyss A, el Baze P, Lefebvre JC, Schneider M, Ortonne JP. Dermatomyositis-like syndrome in X-linked hypogammaglobulinemia. Case-report and review of the literature. Acta Derm Venereol. 1990;70(4):309–13.

Weary PE, Bender AS. Chediak-Higashi syndrome with severe cutaneous involvement: occurrence in two brothers 14 and 15 years of age. Arch Intern Med. 1967;119(4):381–6.

Cancer Patients and Skin Disease

4

John C. Hall

Abstract

Cancer patients are in the unique position for immune diseases. Their malignancy tends to be immunosuppressive and the therapies used to treat their cancer further compromises their immune systems. Newer therapies complicate the immunity further by acting to accentuate the immune response. The skin is not left out of these immunologic crises, and this chapter will review how the skin responds in a crucial way to lead the doctor to suspect underlying cancer.

Keywords

Paraneoplastic • Inflammatory • Immunity • Vasculitis • Pyoderma gangrenosum • Erythema nodosum • Herpes zoster • Candidiasis

Introduction

Skin findings in cancer patients can be related to the cancer or the treatment given for the cancer. The latter group of patients will be discussed in chapters later in this book. This chapter will emphasize skin conditions seen as a result of immune suppression caused by the cancer. Therefore, most examples are those seen as a sign that underlying malignancy is present but not yet diagnosed.

These can be mainly divided into infections and paraneoplastic syndromes. Other signs include interference with coagulation, metabolic dysregulation, and pigmentary abnormalities. These later signs will not be discussed here since they do not primarily involve the immune system.

Infections

Infections are either mild common infections that are (1) abnormally severe or extensive or (2) unusual infections not expected in the climate, anatomic location, or demographic in which they occur. The myeloproliferative diseases appear to be the most associated malignancies associated with skin infections and most likely related to importance of the hemolymphatic system in treating and preventing infection.

J.C. Hall, MD
St. Lukes's Hospital, University of Missouri Medical School, Kansas City Care Clinic (Free Health Clinic), 4400 Broadway Suite 416, Kansas City, MO 64111, USA

Truman Medical Center, Kansas City, MO, USA
e-mail: drjohnchall@att.net

J.C. Hall (ed.), *Skin Diseases in the Immunocompromised*,
DOI 10.1007/978-1-4471-6479-1_4, © Springer-Verlag London 2014

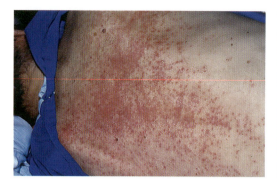

Fig. 4.1 Severe generalized candidiasis in a patient with lymphoma, showing generalized symmetric vesicles, pustules, and papules

Candidiasis

Candidiasis (we are referring here to *candida albicans*) is a ubiquitous, opportunistic organism present in the mouth and anogenital areas in healthy patients. When underlying cancer is present it is often more extensive and yet in its same morphology as in healthy patients. It can be present on the skin, as shown in Fig. 4.1 or on mucous membranes. On the skin it is often over a larger area and on skin that is not intertriginous, as is normally expected. On mucous membranes it is more extensive, and the not-uncommon thrush of infants is seen in adults. Candida can also present in a rare disseminated form, especially in patients with myeloproliferative diseases. Pink to purple macronodules are seen widely scattered over the trunk or extremities, as shown in Fig. 4.2.

Cellulitis

Bacterial infections of significance are most commonly illustrated by cellulitis. It mimics cellulitis in a healthy patient (see Fig. 4.3), but comes on more rapidly, spreads faster, and is more apt to be associated with sepsis. Staphylococcus aureus (this includes community acquired methicillin resistant and community acquired methicillin-resistant varieties) is the most common pathogen, but group A beta hemolytic streptococci can also be the cause.

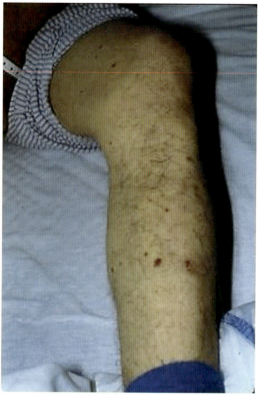

Fig. 4.2 Macronodules over the pretibial area indicating candida sepsis in a leukemia patient

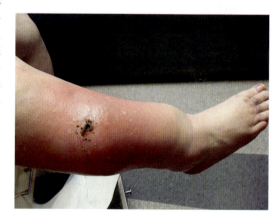

Fig. 4.3 Staphylococcal cellulitis in a lymphoma patient with well-demarcated erythema in a leg accompanied by tenderness, pain, induration in a febrile patient

Fungal infections with dermatophytes are not usually a sign of patients with underlying malignancy, but deep fungi—especially in patients in a temperate climate, where they are not expected—can alert the clinician to search for underlying malignancy.

Herpes Zoster and Herpes Simplex

Viral infections, most commonly herpes zoster and herpes simplex (see Fig. 4.4) tend to be much more severe and can often be used as an early sign that the patient may have an underlying cancer. Herpes zoster can be more severe locally and more widespread, as shown in Fig. 4.5. Herpes simplex in a similar fashion can be more severe locally and widespread. Culture, smear for polymerase chain reaction (PCR), biopsy with culture or PCR may be necessary to differentiate the two viruses. Both diseases may become more chronic, lasting months, or become deep, with ulcers and even gangrenous changes.

Paraneoplastic Skin Disease

The skin can be one of the organs involved in a paraneoplastic syndrome. Curth described paraneoplastic syndromes as having the following characteristics, which I have somewhat modified in the following list:

1. The cancer and the associated condition should appear at the same time but either can occur at variable intervals before the other.
2. The associated condition should be specific in definition and reproducibility to the same associated cancers.
3. The associated condition should be relatively uncommon compared to the cancer.
4. There should be a demonstrable association more significant than chance alone.

These can be divided into inflammatory, which probably are immunologic in origin, and tumors, which may be associated with cancer through embryologic or genetic mechanisms.

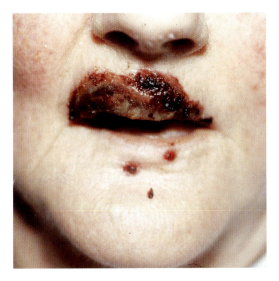

Fig. 4.4 Severe gangrenous localized herpes simplex infection of the upper lip in a chronic lymphocytic leukemia patient

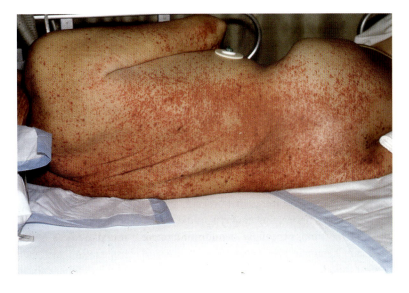

Fig. 4.5 Severe generalized herpes zoster (varicella) in a lymphoma patient with generalized symmetric vesicles. This patient was febrile and toxic

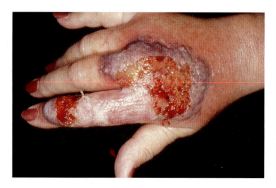

Fig. 4.6 Pyoderma gangrenosum over the dorsal hand with a fungating ulcer and a rolled border. The patient had myelodysplastic syndrome. She cleared with high-dose systemic corticosteroids

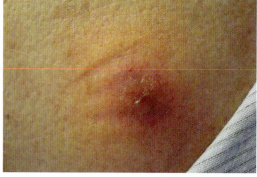

Fig. 4.7 Sweet's syndrome of the upper extremity mimicking a cellulitis. A search for underlying cancer was negative at the time of the photograph

Inflammatory Paraneoplastic Skin Disease

Inflammatory conditions include pyoderma gangrenosum, Sweet's syndrome, figurate erythemas, paraneoplastic pemphigus, vasculitis, erythema nodosum, dermatomyositis, and glucagonoma syndrome. These will be discussed in more detail since immune system abnormalities is a likely related to underlying cause.

Pyoderma Gangrenosum

Pyoderma gangrenosum is an initial papule or erosion that becomes a painful ulcerative disease that develops rapidly over weeks but heals slowly over months, even with aggressive immunosuppressive therapy. This therapy begins with high-dose systemic steroids and various steroid-sparing drugs including azathioprine, mycophenolate, avlosulfone, cyclosporine, and biologics. The lower extremities is the most common location but the deep ulcers with rolled borders and deep purulent ulcers can occur on trunk and upper extremities as well. The surface can be a hemorrhagic crust or serous debris and rarely is bullous. The histopathology is not specific but is filled with neutrophils that often invade under the apparent edge of the irregular border. It can be associated with underlying cancer approximately 20 % of the time, especially myeloproliferative disease as shown in Fig. 4.6, more often when it is most inflammatory or bullous. Approximately

50 % of cases are associated with ulcerative colitis or Crohn's disease. Ulcerative colitis is in turn associated with colon cancer. The underlying immunology is not well understood but an Arthrus-like reaction and cellular cross-reacting antigens have been suggested. Aberrant integrin oscillations on neutrophils and aberrant neutrophil tracking have bee noted.

Sweet's Syndrome

Sweet's syndrome looks histologically similar to pyoderma gangrenosum with a dramatic infiltration of neutrophils and clinically mimics most closely a cellulitis, as seen in Fig. 4.7. Treatment is similar to pyoderma gangrenosum with a more dramatic and rapid response to systemic corticosteroids. Approximately 20 % of patients have an underlying malignancy and 80 % of these are reticuloendothelial in origin. Theories of pathogenesis include increases cytokines (interleukin 6, granulocyte stimulating factor),

Figurate Erythemas

Figurate erythemas are annular erythematous plaques with elevated advancing borders that have a trailing, fine, adherent scale. The two of these associated are erythema annulare centrifugum, where a few plaques are rarely associated with underlying cancer, and erythema gyratum repens, where numerous plaques have an 80 % association with cancer—most commonly renal, lung, esophageal, and breast. It has a dramatic

Erythema Gyratum
Repens

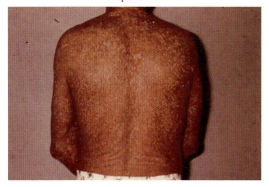

Fig. 4.8 Erythema gyratum repens with a wood-grain appearance over the trunk in a patient with brain cancer

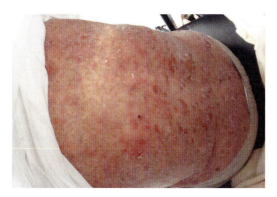

Fig. 4.9 Erosions on the trunk where superficial blisters have ruptured in a patient with underlying lymphoma. Direct immunofluorescence aided in the diagnosis of paraneoplastic pemphigus

clinical appearance as seen Fig. 4.8, with confluent waves giving a wood-grain appearance.

Paraneoplastic Pemphigus

Antibodies produced against the underlying cancer may cross-react against skin proteins. Paraneoplastic pemphigus consists of intractable oral mucous membrane ulcers and polymorphic skin lesions that include erosions (see Fig. 4.9), bullae, iris lesions, redness, and papules. Histologically it is also polymorphic with intraepidermal acantholysis with dyskeratosis and intraepidermal vacuolar degeneration. Intraepidermal IgG and complement as well as derm/epidermal junction complement may be present. In two-thirds of the patients they will

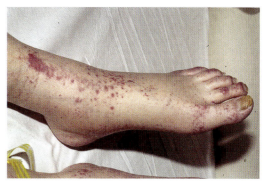

Fig. 4.10 Palpable purpura over the ankles that was probably due to an antibiotic allergy, but a search was made for an underlying malignancy. Variations in color and a splotchy look as well as induration on palpation help may the diagnosis clinically. However, a biopsy was done to confirm the diagnosis

already have the underlying cancer. The most common underlying cancer is B cell lymphoma non-Hodgkins lymphoma. Numerous immunosuppressive regimens have shown little benefit. The prognosis is poor with only 10 % survival over 2 years. Natural killer T-cells, CD8 cells, and macrophages may cause the cytotoxic reaction that causes the muccocutaneous findings.

Vasculitis

There are many types of vasculitis, but we will only consider immune complex leukocytoclastic vasculitis. These immune complexes are considered the underlying pathology in vasculitis associated with underlying cancer. Both solid tumors and hematologic cancers have been associated with vasculitis. It is a rare association but should be considered if no other cause of the vasculitis is apparent and the patient is over age 50. It presents as palpable purpura (seen in Fig. 4.10) especially over lower extremities or at sites of pressure. The histopathology shows polymorphonuclear lymphocytes invading vessel walls and disintegrating into polychrome bodies. Vessels may be clotted and fibrin deposits in their walls. Occasionally the immune complexes may be seen with direct immunofluorescence but it is very much dependent on the timing of the biopsy.

Erythema Nodosum

Erythema nodosum can rarely be associated with leukemias, lymphomas, or other cancers.

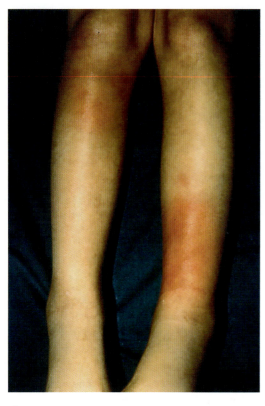

It presents most commonly in the pretibial areas as tender red subcutaneous self-limited nodules (seen in Fig. 4.11) or tumors that can be treated with bed rest, aspirin, nonsteriodal anti-inflammatory drugs and, if severe, systemic corticosteroids. Histologically it is a septal panniculitis with neutrophils and histiocytes that may form a granuloma. Capillary proliferation may be present but there is no vasculitis. The immunology is felt to be a type IV reaction to various antigens, the most common of which is streptococci and medications.

Dermatomyositis

Dermatomyositis is an autoimmune collagen vascular disease that most often involves the skin and muscle. In patients over age 50, up to 25 % may have underlying cancer; the most common are breast and gynecologic in women and lung cancer in men. Gastrointestinal malignancy can be seen in both sexes. The skin manifestations are protean but most commonly show a heliotrope (purple) dermatitis over eyelids; Gottron purplish papules over joints of hands, knees, and elbows; photosensitivity; alopecia; and a shawl-like erythema over the shoulders. Changes over the proximal nail folds is common with purple-red discoloration, desauamation, and clotted capillaries (Hueck-Gottron's sign, as seen in Fig. 4.12).

Fig. 4.11 Deep pink nodule on the pretibial area that was painful and tender in a patient with biopsy-proved erythema nodosum. The underlying etiology was not determined but signs looking for an underlying cancer continue to be monitored

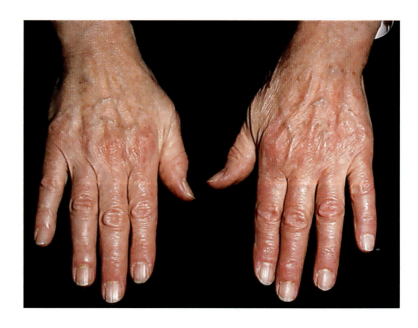

Fig. 4.12 Erythema, desquamtion, and clotted capillary loops over the proximal nail folds in a dermatomyositis patient

Dermatomyositis sine myositis or amyotrophic dermatomyositis is skin disease without muscle disease lasting for 2 or more years. This type may be more closely associated with underlying cancer. When cancer occurs with dermatomyositis it tends to be a malignancy more recalcitrant to therapy. The reason for the association may be an underlying trigger such as a virus, chemical, or drug that causes both the cancer and dermatomyositis in a victim with a genetic predisposition. Abnormalities of cellular or humoral immunity may allow for malignant clones to become tolerant and control mechanisms over inflammation in both the skin and muscle to be unleashed at the same time. Another immune-related problem is anti-cancer therapy, causing a depression of the immune system and more rapid spread of the underlying cancer.

Glucagonoma Syndrome

The skin manifestation of the glucagonoma syndrome is necrolytic migratory erythema. It consists of polycylic, migratory plaques with pustules, erosions, crusts, vesicles or bullae seen most commonly in the intertriginous areas, abdomen, and proximal lower extremities. Histopathology is characteristic. The diagnosis of underlying cancer is usually made years after the onset of the skin eruption and up to half already have metastatic disease. Almost 100 % are associated with a glucacon-secreting alpha-cell tumor of the pancreas. Lower levels of aminoacids due to increased liver uptake and direct toxicity of glucagon may be implicated in etiology of the skin disease.

Paraneoplastic Tumors of the Skin

Tumors will only be listed here since the immune system is not likely to be related to these syndromes. These include lentigo, Muir Torre Syndrome (sebaceous gland tumors and keratoacanthomas associated with colorectal cancer with usually good prognosis), tripe palms with velvety rugose hypertrophy of dermatoglyphics (90 % associated with malignancy especially gastrointestinal and lung), sign of Lesar Trelat (multiple eruptive seborrheic keratoses associated especially with stomach and lung cancer), Cowden's syndrome (multiple hamaratoma PTEN syndrome with tricelemomas, acrokeratosis, papillomatous papules, and mucosal lesions associated with breast, thyroid, and uterine cancer), Bazex's syndrome (acrokeratosis paraneoplastica [hyperkeratotic palms and soles] is associated almost 100 % with cancer especially squamous cell cancer of the upper aerodigestive tract), mammary paget's diseases (eczematous patch on the nipple of the breast associated with underlying ductal cancer), extramammary paget's (vulvar, rectal or penile mucosa associated with underlying adenocancer including endocervical, bladder, prostate, rectum, squamous cell cancer of the skin and melanoma), multicentric reticulohistiocytosis (reddish-brown widespread nodules with one third associated with underlying cancer), Birt-Hogg-Dubbe syndrome (trichodiscomas, trichofolliculomas, and skin tags associated with chromophobe renal cell carcinoma and renal oncocytoma), leiomyomas and piloleiomyomas associated with renal cell cancer.

Pigmentary Changes

Pigmentary changes are also not apt to be immune in nature so they are only listed in this chapter. Acanthosis nigricans has hyperpigmented velvety plaques in intertriginous areas associated mainly with gastrointestinal malignancy. Peutz Jeghers syndrome or hereditary polyposis syndrome has hyperpigmented macules on lip or oral mucosa with polyposis of the gastrointestinal tract and 50 % change of developing a gastrointestinal cancer.

Hypercoagulability Syndromes

Hypercoagulability syndromes include petechiae when the underlying cancer causes thrombocytopedia, purpura in syndromes such as purpura fulminans with disseminated intravascular coagulopathy that may be caused by underlying cancer, and the rare Trousseau syndrome with migratory thrombophelibitis. Multiple myeloma is associated with a specific type of purpura called "pinch purpura."

Metabolic Paraneoplastic Skin Disease

Metabolic abnormalities include carcinoid syndrome and calcinosis cutis. Calcinosis cutis can be seen in metastatic diseases to bone, such as breast cancer, with calcium abnormalities.

Nonspecific Inflammatory Paraneoplastic Skin Disease

The skin also has the ability to respond to malignancy in a nonspecific inflammatory pattern indistinguishable clinically or histologically from eczema. Clinically it can present as dry desquamative skin, papular "id-type" reaction, or eczematous oozing dermatitis among many other variants. Remember that psoriasis as well as eczema can mimic cutaneous T cell lymphoma and its variants. It may be diagnosed late because it is not suspected, has not developed into a malignancy yet, or sampling error has been caused by biopising the site where the malignancy is revealed most definitively.

Remember if the infection is unexpected, the inflammation has a pattern that can be associated with malignancy, or there is simply no other explanation for the skin disease, then think of alterations of the immune system associated with underlying cancer.

Conclusion

Most immunosuppressive diseases are a setup for infections. Cancer patients are no exception. Not only is their cancer an invitation to immunologic disaster (most notably reticuloendothelial malignancies), but the therapy used in these patients adds to this invitation to skin infections. Staphylococci, herpes simplex, herpes zoster/varicella, and candidiasis are the main culprits. Rare infections in patients who are assumed to be cancer-free makes looking for underlying cancer a must. Cutaneous T cell lymphoma (CTCL) is the most notable skin cancer to follow another underlying cancer.

Suggested Reading

Hall JC, Hall BJ. Hall's manual of skin as a marker of underlying disease. Shelton: PMPH-USA, Ltd.; 2011.
New Zealand Dermatological Society, DermNet NZ: The Dermatology Resource. 1996-2012. http://www.dermnetnz.org.
WebMD LLC. Medscape Today. 1994-2012. http://www.medscape.com.

Part II

Transplant Patients

Skin Disease in Solid Organ Transplant Patients

5

John C. Hall

Abstract

This chapter discusses the different types of skin diseases seen in solid organ transplants, which includes renal, heart, pancreas, and lung. It discusses infections, malignancies, and inflammatory skin diseases. We, as dermatologists and nondermatologists, need to address the needs of these patients by identifying the diseases associated with this increasing group of patients.

Keywords

Transplantation • Allogenic • Calciphylaxis • Actinic keratosis • Molluscum contagiosum • Porokeratosis • Human papilloma virus

Introduction

The number of solid organ transplant patients is increasingly dramatically worldwide for three main reasons. More transplantations are possible due to new immunosuppressive regimens that allow less perfect matches to be used as transplant donors. Transplant patients are living for longer periods of time as medical care of these individuals improves. More patients can be recruited as transplant recipients as older age groups and more advanced stage-illness patients are considered as possible transplant recipients.

We are discussing in this chapter allogenic transplants, only meaning the donor is separate from the recipient. Hopefully, in the not-too-distant future, all solid organ transplant patients with be autologous, in which the transplanted organ will be derived from the patient's own stem cells. This will eliminate the side effects, including cutaneous, that occur due to immunosuppression.

An important pre-transplant group of patients that will always be with us are dialysis patients, including hemodialysis and peritoneal dialysis. The number of these patients is also on the increase and they are also immunosuppressed but not to the same degree as transplant patients. The largest group of these patients are renal but there are an increasing number of especially heart and also lung and pancreas transplantations being done.

J.C. Hall, MD
St. Lukes's Hospital, University of Missouri Medical School, Kansas City Care Clinic (Free Health Clinic), 4400 Broadway Suite 416, Kansas City, MO 64111, USA

Truman Medical Center, Kansas City, MO, USA
e-mail: drjohnchall@att.net

J.C. Hall (ed.), *Skin Diseases in the Immunocompromised*,
DOI 10.1007/978-1-4471-6479-1_5, © Springer-Verlag London 2014

55

Table 5.1 Transplant patients and skin tumors

Tumor	Co-factors	Treatment
Squamous cell	Sun exposure	Protective clothing
Basal cell	Genetics	Limit sun
Melanoma	Phenotype	Sunscreen
Actinic keratosis	HIV	Surgery
Porokeratosis	Amount of suppression	PDT (photodynamic therapy)
Keratoacanthoma	Change immunosuppression drug	5-FU (fluorouracil)
	Switch to rapamune (sirolimus)	Imiquimod
		Solareze
		Cryosurgery
		Electrosurgery
		Laser
		Retinoids
		Green tea (Veregen)
Sebaceous hyperplasia	Cyclosporine	Retinoids
Increase size and number		Decrease cyclosporine

Most of the topics discussed in this chapter are also more common in other immune-compromised states. We will divide the topics into tumors, infections, and inflammatory skin conditions.

Tumors

The tumors associated with transplant patients are related to the co-factors of sun exposure, genetic predisposition, phenotype, and—in the case of squamous cell cancer—exposure to the human papilloma virus.

Sun exposure is the most intense after 10:00 AM and before 4:00 PM for UVB, which causes burning and increases the risk of all the tumors discussed in Table 5.1. UVA, which accentuates the carcinogenic effect of UVB, is constant throughout daylight and goes through window glass. Window glass can be treated to block both UVA and UVB. Newer sunscreens with Helioplex, titanium dioxide, zinc oxide, and combinations of light absorbers screen out both UVA and UVB. Photoprotective hats and clothing are a mainstay in prevention and are crucial in transplant patients.

Phenotypic predisposing factors are blonde or red hair, blue eyes, and fair skin. Genotypic disposing factors that cannot be seen in the phenotype but require genetic testing is illustrated by the p53 suppressor gene, which helps prevent carcinogenic transformation. Treatments include those shown in Table 5.1. For more information on these tumors, see the chapter on Skin Cancer in Transplant Patients.

Infections

Warts and molluscum contagiosum on common viral infections in transplant patients and can be very widespread and difficult to treat. The carcinogenic effect of human papilloma virus in rectal, cervical, genital, and subungual cancer is well documented and should be carefully monitored and treated aggressively (see Table 5.2).

Common infections such as herpes simplex, varicella/zoster, and candida can be more severe and often need more aggressive and prolonged therapy in these patients.

Uncommon infections in the skin are more common in transplant patients, most notably deep fungal infections, as seen in Fig. 5.1. Higher, more prolonged medicine dosages may be necessary for successful treatment. A history of visits to other countries such India and Africa for tuberculosis or South America for maduromycosis or deep fungi is an important part of the history.

Table 5.2 Transplant patients and infections

Infections	Co-factors	Treatment
Mollescum	Exposure, sexual contact	Cryosurgery
Warts		Laser
		Electrosurgery
		Retinoids
		Green tea (Veregen)
		Inerferon
		Immunotherapy (Candida Ag)
		Vaccine
Common severe		
HSV	Exposure, sexual contact	Vaccine, antivirals, episodic prophylactic
Varicella/Zoster	History	Antivirals, vaccine
Candida		
Topical	Bedridden, incontinence, antibiotics	Imidazoles, mycostatin
Systemic		Amphotericin B, fluconazole
Rare		
Deep fungi	Climate, amount of suppression	Amphotericin B, ketaconazole, fluconazole, flucytosine, voriconazole
Saprophytes		
Aspergillosis	Amount of suppression	Amphotericin B
Mucormycosis		

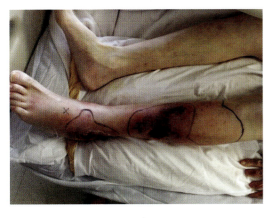

Fig. 5.1 Cryptococcal necrotizing cellulitis in a renal transplant patient. Large areas of gangrene on the lower extremities with surrounding erythema. Amputation was performed

Inflammatory Skin Diseases

Table 5.3 provides an overview of inflammatory skin diseases, co-factors, and treatments. Xerotic or dry skin can be associated with dialysis patients as well as renal transplant patients. Ichthyosis, shown in Fig. 5.2, differs from xerosis by the appearance of plate-like or fish-like scaling, and can be severe and difficult to treat. Both conditions can be treated with emollients (Vaseline, Aquaphor, Cerave), alpha hydroxy acids (Lachydrin, Amlactin), urea (Carmol) or combinations of the above (Eucerin Professional Repair Maximum Strength Lotion). Many other similar topicals are available.

Calciphylaxis, shown in Fig. 5.3, is a poorly understood calcification of vessels and subcutaneous tissue seen in dialysis and renal transplant patients. Extraordinarily painful areas of gangrene lead progressively to amputations and death. Sodium thiosulfate intravenously has been the best therapy (author's opinion) among many other treatment modalities. It does not respond to immunosuppressive treatment (including corticosteroids) which can actually make the disease worse. Cases have been reported at the time of transplantation.

The perforating skin disorders are associated with renal transplant patients who also often have diabetes. The diseases include elastosis perforans serpiginosa, reactive perforating collagenosis, Kyrle's disease, and most commonly and characteristically, perforating folliculitis.

Table 5.3 Transplant patients and inflammatory skin disease

Illness	Co-factors	Treatment
Xerosis	Drying soaps	Carmol
Ichthyosis	Cold, dry climate	Topical urea
	Change in temperature	Ceramide
		Cera Ve
		Lubricants
		Vaseline
		Aquaphor
		Eucerin
		Alpha hydroxy acids
		AmLactin
		Lac-Hydrin
Calciphylaxis	Renal transplant	Sodium thiosulfate, surgery, hyperbaric 02
Perforating folliculitis	Renal transplant	Urea, retinoids (oral and topical)
Pruritus	Especially renal	Narrowband UVB
		Topical and oral antihistamine
		Treat dry skin
		SSRIs
		Tricyclics
		PUVA
		Treat electrolyte and Fe abnormalities

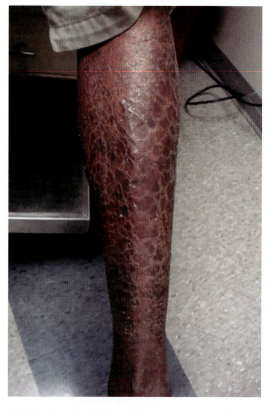

Fig. 5.2 Acquired ichthyosis in a renal patient. Plate-like scaling over the lower extremities is characteristic

Perforating folliculitis, shown in Fig. 5.4, consists of widely scattered perfollicular papules and nodules that are often crusted, pruritic, circular, firm, and sometimes painful. The hair and hair follicle are usually obliterated by the disease. Treatment is difficult but topical retinoids (tretinoin) and oral retinoids (Soriatane and Accutane) are often helpful. Intralesional corticosteriods or cryosurgery can be used for particularly troublesome or recalcitrant lesions. In dialysis patients, transplantation can alleviate these diseases.

Pruritis is another common ailment in dialysis patients that can be relieved with transplantation in some patients. It can be severe and recalcitrant to most therapies. Narrowband UVB, selective

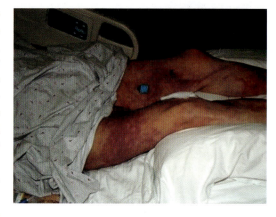

Fig. 5.3 Calciphylaxis showing large areas of hemorrhagic necrosis over the lower extremities. The patient died as a result of the disease. This was before sodium thiosulfate was a known therapy

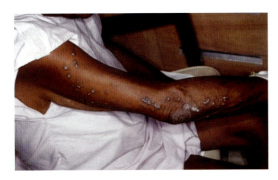

Fig. 5.4 Perforating folliculitis of the arm. Lesions are indurated crusted papules and nodules in a renal patient

serotonin reuptake inhibitors (most notably doxepin), tricyclic antidepressants, neurontin, and topical or systemic antihistamines have all had some success.

Conclusion

A completely new group of patients has emerged in the last 50 years with their own unique medical challenges. These are the transplant patients who have created special problems and opportunities for all of medicine, including dermatology. The scientific knowledge gained in the care of these ever-inspiring people has changed dermatology and medicine forever.

Suggested Reading

Lindelof B, Sigurgeirsson B, Gäbel H, Stern RS. Incidence of skin cancer in 5356 patients following organ transplantation. Br J Dermatol. 2000;143(3):513–9.

Ottley CC, Stasko T. Skin disease in organ transplantation. New York: Cambridge University Press; 2008.

Saray Y, Seçkin D, Bilezikçi B. Acquired perforating dermatosis: clinicopathological features in twenty-two cases. J Eur Acad Dermatol Venereol. 2006;20(6):679–88.

Wisgerhof HC, Edelbroek JR, de Fijter JW, Feltkamp MC, Willemze R, Bouwes Bavinck JN. Trends in skin diseases in organ-transplant recipients transplanted between 1966 and 2006: a cohort study with follow-up between 1944 and 2006. Br J Dermatol. 2010;162(2):390–6.

Graft vs Host Disease and Skin Manifestations

Min Kin Derek Ho and Noah Scheinfeld

Abstract

Graft-versus-host disease (GVHD) has a multitude of manifestations, but the most common organ involved is the skin. There are two main forms of the GVHD are acute GVHD and chronic GVHD: acute and chronic. We discuss the immunology of this fascinating syndrome seen in bone marrow transplant patients, and the skin disease that accompanies them.

Keywords

Allogenic • Lichen planus • Wickham's striae • Scleroderma • Extracorporeal photophoresis • Sicca syndrome • Poikiloderma

Introduction

Graft-versus-host disease (GVHD) is the primary cause of morbidity and mortality after a hematopoietic cell transplantation (HCT). GVHD occurs in approximately 75 % of patients with HCT and may be responsible for up to two-thirds of deaths. HCT is needed for hematologic malignancies, bone marrow failures, and various immunodeficiency syndromes due to ablation of the host's bone marrow and replacement with donor's mar-

M.K.D. Ho, BS
Department of Dermatology,
SUNY Downstate College of Medicine,
Brooklyn, NY, USA

N. Scheinfeld, MD, JD (✉)
Department of Dermatology,
Weil Cornell Medical College,
150 West 55th Street, New York, NY 10019, USA
e-mail: scheinfeld@earthlink.net

row and T cells. Although HCT is a life-saving procedure for many end-stage patients, all patients receiving HCT should be aware of the GVHD complications such that early interventions and targeted therapy can be implemented.

Bone marrow transplants are now basically allogenic transplants, which means the transplant is made from a non-self donor to a recipient. With advances in the science of immunobiology, the bone marrow cells may eventually be derived from stem cells of the patient himself and thus be autogenic transplants. This will eliminate GVHD. Until this great scientific achievement occurs, the number of GVHD patients will be increasing as older patients (with non-ablative or reduced conditioning regiments) and less well matched patients allow an increase in the population made eligible for allogenic bone marrow transplantation. In GVHD a state of immunosuppression as well as autoimmunity resembling autoimmune diseases such lupus erythematosus, lichen planus, and scleroderma develop.

J.C. Hall (ed.), *Skin Diseases in the Immunocompromised*,
DOI 10.1007/978-1-4471-6479-1_6, © Springer-Verlag London 2014

The risk of GVHD is related to prior history of GVHD, use of a non-T cell-depleted graft, and older donor and older recipient.

When a host accepts the donor's marrow, he/she will also be accepting the donor's T cells. T cells are part of our immune response system and help fight off infections and foreign microbes in our body. Normally, T cells recognize a specific group of proteins named human leukocyte antigens (HLA) to distinguish between self versus foreign. Each person inherits a copy of HLA from his/her mother and father, and no two people's HLA are the same except for identical twins. An autologous transplantation uses the patient's own hematopoietic stem cells (HSC) which he/she harvested before marrow ablation, while an allogeneic transplantation uses HSC from a non-identical relative or unrelated donor. A special phenomenon known as the graft-versus-tumor effect occurs in allogeneic HCTs when the donor T-cells can help attack the malignant cells. The advantage of an autologous transplant is that the patient is not at risk of immunologic rejections, and he/she would lose the graft-versus-tumor effect. Before a HCT is initiated, the host will often receive radio- or chemotherapy to reduce the activities of the bone marrow and malignant cells. The donor's marrow will be injected to the host's body and slowly reconstitute the immune system. A problem arises because there are usually some residual cells remaining in the host that will be seen by the donor's T cells. The donor T cells will attack host cells in various organs and cause an inflammatory response. Many organs, including the gastrointestinal tract, liver, and lungs, are involved, but the most prevalent manifestation is in the skin.

Classification

The original system for typing GVHD is split into two categories. Acute GVHD was defined as any manifestations within 100 days after HCT, and chronic GVHD as manifestations more than 100 days after HCT. This classification has been in place for a long time but has provided little value for clinicians in terms of patient management.

In 2005, the National Institutes of Health (NIH) reclassified the system to focus more on the patient's clinical presentations after HCT. A new group, late-onset acute GVHD and overlap syndrome, was coined to describe patients who had features of both acute and chronic GVHD and when the exact manifestation do not coincide with the original 100 days division. This change caused many chronic GVHD patients to be reclassified as late acute GVHD or overlap syndrome and this group was shown to have poorer outcomes and survival rates compared with other groups. Acute GVHD seems to be Th1 mediated, whereas chronic GVHD is Th2 mediated associated with eosinophilia, increase in IL-5, and IL-4.

Acute GVHD

The incidence of acute GVHD depends primarily on the degree of HLA compatibility between the donor and host. Common presenting symptoms include skin rashes (classically stated to be pruritic or painful rash), bilirubin elevations, and diarrhea. Skin manifestations are often the earliest signs of acute GVHD, usually within 2–4 weeks, but can present at any time after HCT. A staging system is used to describe the extent of the cutaneous findings: Stage 1 – less than 25 % of total body surface area (BSA) involvement; Stage 2 – 25–50 % BSA involvement; Stage 3 – greater than 50 % BSA involvement; Stage 4 – erythroderma with bullae. The skin lesions typically begin with erythematous macules on the palms and soles. Other common sites include the lateral neck, upper chest, and back. Follicular lesions may follow and the presentation becomes generalized, taking on a morbilliform appearance. Hyperkeratotic papules and hyperpigmentation may occur and, in more severe cases, patients develop generalized erythroderma, bullae, or extensive skin sloughing.

When acute GVHD is suspected after HCT, a 4 mm punch biopsy of the affected skin is sent for pathology readings. Common histopathological changes include vacuolization of the basal layer of epidermis, lymphocytic infiltrate in the superficial dermis, and epidermal apoptotic keratinocytes. The sensitivity and specificity of skin biopsy for acute GVHD has not been well established in the literature. Clinicians often rely on the onset of consistent cutaneous changes within a reasonable time frame after HCT and always have the suspicion of acute GVHD. Although skin biopsies do not necessarily rule in acute GVHD, they are still valuable because many other skin diseases can be explained well on histology and offer an alternative diagnosis. Along with the minimal complications including scarring, minor bleeding, and infection, skin biopsies are still performed routinely when post HCT patients present with skin eruptions that parallels with acute GVHD manifestations.

The pathophysiology of acute GVHD contains three phases. Initially, the deconditioning chemo- and radiotherapy for the host results in tissue damage, leading to the release of many inflammatory cytokines. With HCT and the introduction of mature donor T cells into this pro-inflammatory environment, the donor T cells get activated and self-proliferate in order to attack the "foreign" host cells. The expansion of these donor T cells into cytotoxic effector T cells causes additional tissue injury and results in a vicious cycle of cell attacks between competent donor T cells and immuno-compromised host cells.

Many other skin disorders may present similar to acute GVHD, both on a macroscopic and histopathological level. A skilled physician must consider all the possibilities before proceeding with treatment, including:

- Drug eruptions (Fig. 6.1). Present as erythematous papules in a morbilliform fashion and typically appears on the trunk, spreading to the lower extremities compared with head, neck, and acral areas in acute GVHD. Skin biopsies may demonstrate eosinophils for drug eruptions, but the presence of them does not rule out GVHD. Antibiotics such as beta-lactams and sulfonamides are common causes of drug eruptions, and voriconazole may cause phototoxic drug eruption mimicking acute GVHD.
- Viral exanthems. Viral infections from HHV-6, HHV-7, cytomegalovirus (CMV), and others may also cause maculopapular eruptions.

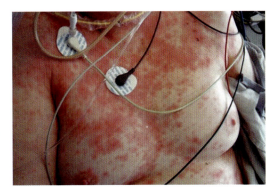

Fig. 6.1 Morbilliform drug eruption due to Tegretol. This can mimic a case of acute or chronic drug eruption. Skin biopsy can be helpful but can also be confusing. The difference is crucial, since stopping an important drug can be dangerous and initiating immunosuppressive therapy for GVHD is a major medical decision

Skin biopsies often show perivascular lymphocytic infiltrates, and specific pathopneumonic findings such as intranuclear inclusions in CMV may be useful for distinguishing viral causes from GVHD.

- Lymphocyte recovery. The return of lymphocytes to the circulation following marrow ablative procedures in the host may cause a self-limited skin exanthem with transient fevers. The lack of gastrointestinal and hepatic involvements distinguishes this entity from GVHD. Histopathology may show superficial perivascular mononuclear cell infiltrate.
- Acral erythema (Fig. 6.2). Usually a complication of chemotherapy when used for marrow ablation before HCT. The palms and soles are affected with painful symmetrical edema and erythema.
- Toxic epidermal necrolysis (Fig. 6.3). A severe skin reaction classically induced by medication, but shares a similar clinical and histopathological presentation with high-grade acute GVHD. Dark, erythematous macules that rapidly progress to extensive blistering and desquamation. Biopsies show subepidermal bullae and full thickness epidermal necrosis.
- Engraftment syndrome. Cutaneous eruptions and signs of capillary leak syndrome with fever, but no identifiable infectious causes. It commonly occurs after autologous HCT.

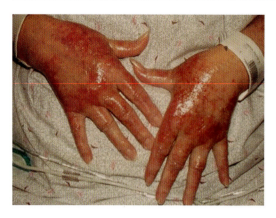

Fig. 6.2 Acral erythema due to doxyrubricin. This can also occur in acute GVHD

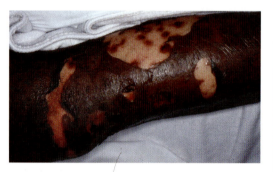

Fig. 6.3 Toxic epidermal necrolysis on the knee and pretibial with erosive blisters and positive Nikolsky's sign, which is denudation of the epidermis with digital pressure on the skin. This patient probably had the condition as a drug reaction to doxycycline, but a indentical reaction occurs in acute GVHD at its worse. It is life-threatening

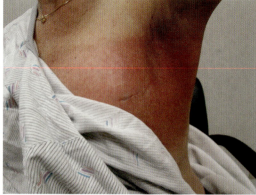

Fig. 6.4 This woman has acute radiation dermatitis on her chest from breast cancer radiotherapy. An identical generalized reaction is the commonest cutaneous reaction in acute GVHD (Photo courtesy of James Coster, MD)

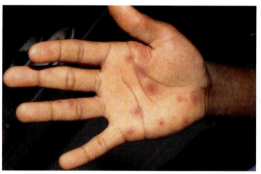

Fig. 6.5 Erythema multiform secondary to herpes simplex, which is the commonest cause. Acute GVHD in the skin often has palmar involvement but it is usually diffuse erythema and not the characteristic target lesions of erythema multiforme

- Radiation Dermatitis (Fig. 6.4). Presents with cutaneous erythema, desquamation, blistering, and necrosis. Histopathology demonstrates vacuolization of basal layer, apoptotic keratinocytes, and a superficial perivascular lymphocytic infiltrate
- Erythema multiforme (Fig. 6.5). Targetoid lesions that most often occur with herpes simplex virus infection.

Chronic GVHD

The classic triad for chronic GVHC is skin, liver, and gastrointestinal involvement with the skin and mucous membranes being the most common. Other organ systems involved are peripheral nerves, muscles, central nervous system, eyes, lungs, and heart. Chronic GVHD occurs within 3 years of transplantation and often in patients who have had acute GVHD. The most severe manifestations include end-stage lung disease, contractures, blindness, and severe immunosuppression leading to generalized and life-threatening varicella/zoster, pneumocystis carinii, herpes simplex, CMV (cytomegalovirus infection), and, more rarely, deep fungal, candida, and saprophyte infections.

The pathophysiology behind chronic GVHD is not well understood, but recent research suggests that it might parallel autoimmune disorders. There is a high incidence of detectable

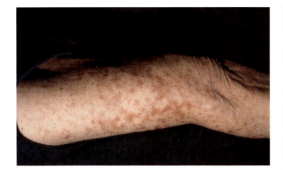

Fig. 6.6 Mottled, net-like alternating hyperpigmentation and hypopigmentation with telangiectasiasis. Epidermal atrophy is seen in the center of the forearm with a shiny area that also has cigarette paper wrinkling. This is poikiloderma in a patient who had severe cutaneous GVHD

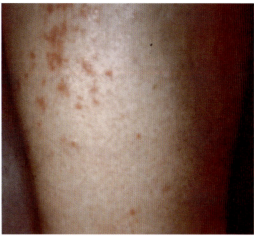

Fig. 6.7 Polygonal, pruritic papules on the pretibial area mimicking lichen planus in a patients with chronic cutaneous GVHD

autoimmune antibodies in chronic GVHD patients, including antinuclear, double-stranded DNA, and smooth muscle antibodies. Compared with classic autoimmune diseases, the antibodies in chronic GVHD do not correlate with specific organ manifestations. Animal models have shown that the regulatory T-cells (Tregs), natural inhibitors of T cells, are successful in treating acute and chronic GVHD.

The recently updated classification for chronic GVHD includes lichen planus-like lesions, sclerotic skin manifestations, and poikilodermatous (reticulate hypopigmented alternating with hyperpigmented changes, fine cigarette-paper wrinkling atrophy, and telangictasias) skin, as seen in Fig. 6.6.

- Lichen planus-like lesions (Fig. 6.7). Erythematous/violaceous plaques often on the dorsal hands and feet, forearms, and trunk. Patient may complain of associated pruritus. These can also occur in a dermatome distribution following previous herpes zoster scars or Blaschko's lines. Lichen planus-like lesions are considered an earlier form of chronic GVHD, but it is not required for sclerotic skin changes.
- Sclerotic manifestations. Scleroderma of morphea-like changes involve the dermis and presents with firm, hyper- or hypopigmented plaques, as seen in Fig. 6.8. The affected area is shiny and demonstrates hair loss. Lichen sclerosis-like changes occur in the superficial dermis and presents with epidermal atrophy (Fig. 6.9) and superficial dermal fibrosis. They

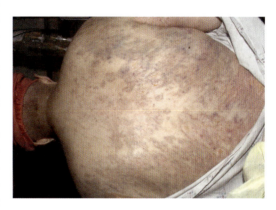

Fig. 6.8 Chronic cutaneous GVHD mimicking generalized morphea over the back. Some areas have a lilac color with pokilodermatous skin that is very indurated on palpation

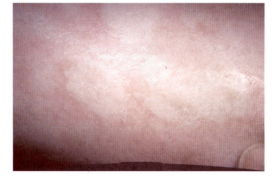

Fig. 6.9 White areas on the inner calf with fine wrinkling indicating atrophy. These areas are compatible with nongenital LSetA but in this case are due to chronic GVHD

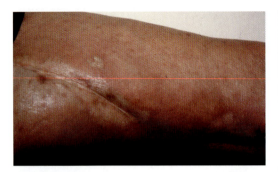

Fig. 6.10 The "groove sign" in chronic cutaneous GVHD that looks like "coup de saber" type of linear morphea. The surrounding skin exhibits induration and poikilodermatous changes

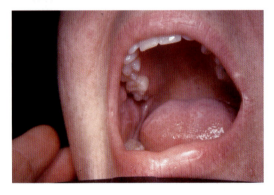

Fig. 6.11 Milky-white linear (Wickham's striae) and papular areas over the tongue and buccal mucosa that appear just as they would in a patient with lichen planus, but this is a patient with chronic cutaneous GVHD

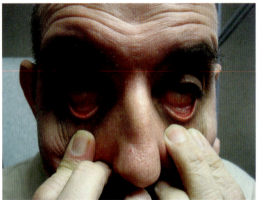

Fig. 6.12 Keratoconjunctivitis sicca with dry and inflamed bulbar and eyelid conjuctiva in a patient with severe muccocutaneous GVHD

tissicca], seen in Fig. 6.12) and dry skin forming which mimics Sjogren's syndrome may occur in some patients.
- Hair disorders. Alopecia and scaly papules on the scalp have been documented in the literature.
- Nail disorders. Abnormalities from mild nail dystrophy to total nail loss have been described.

Management

are often located on the upper back as gray-white plaques. Deep sclerosis involving the fascia may lead to prominent linear demarcations known as the "groove sign" seen in Fig. 6.10. Sclerodermatous thickening of the skin, which sometimes causes contractures and limits joint mobility—which is debilitating and difficult to treat—can also occur.
- Oral lesions. Reticulated white plaques resembling Wickham's striae (milky white papules or striations in a reticulate distribution seen over the surface of skin or mucous membrane, better viewed on wiping with alcohol swab or oil) may occur on the tongue (seen in Fig. 6.11), buccal mucosa, or palate. Pain and perioral sclerosis limits the oral aperture, leading to poor hygiene and nutritional intake. Sicca (dry mouth, dry eyes [keratoconjuntivi-

For acute GVHD patients, high-potency topical corticosteroids may provide improvements for those with limited skin changes. Phototherapy is an additional alternative to help control disease manifestations when they are refractory to corticosteroids. Previous retrospective studies have shown improvements with psoralen plus UVA (PUVA) and narrowband UVB phototherapy, but the precise pharmacokinetics and safety profiles have yet to be determined. Extracorporeal photophoresis (the patient takes oral psoralen and through plasmaphoresis, the plasma is exposed to UVA) has been very helpful for skin and mucous membrane disease in my patients (editor JH). Systemic corticosteroids are the mainstay of severe disease with cyclosporine and tacrolimus are used alone or often in combination with systemic corticosteroids. Ertritinate, hydroxychloroquine, and thalidomide have also been tried.

Chronic GVHD patients are recommended to undergo preventative skin care recommendations including skin cancer screening, monitoring of side effects from corticosteroids or immunosuppressant, management of pruritus, and wound care. Cutaneous squamous cell carcinoma (SCC) is a long-term complication of HCT due to the natural disease process of HCT and the targeted therapies for GVHD, which increase the risk of developing SCC. Patients are encouraged to use broad-spectrum sunscreen, broad-brimmed hats, and practice sun avoidance between 10 a.m. and 4 p.m. Daily use of emollients helps reduce pruritus and, if severe, an oral antipruritic such as diphenhydramine maybe be used. Patients should also follow up with a wound care specialist routinely due to possible spontaneous ulcerations. These wounds may be difficult to heal and require special medical care.

Prophylaxis for CMV, peumocystis carinii, and HSV is usually given for the paradoxical state of immune suppression in the milieu of the hyperimmune condition of GVHD.

Conclusion

One of the most fascinating and often most frustrating recent illnesses is GVHD. It is a result of the perfection of the lifesaving bone marrow transplantation procedure. The skin manifestations of this syndrome will continue to be a challenge for these patients and a major part of their morbidity.

Suggested Reading

Filopovich AH, Weisdorf D, Pavletic S, Socie G, Wingard JR, Lee SJ, et al. National Institutes of Health consensus development project on criteria for clinical trials in chronic graft-versus-host disease: I. diagnosis and staging working group. Biol Blood Marrow Transplant. 2005;11(12):945–56.

Hymes SR, Turner ML, Champlin RE, Couriel DR. Cutaneous manifestations of chronic graft-versus-host disease. Biol Blood Marrow Transplant. 2006;12(11):1101–13.

Ratanatharathorn V, Ayash L, Lazarus HM, Fu J, Uberti JP. Chronic graft-versus-host disease: clinical manifestation and therapy. Bone Marrow Transplant. 2001;28(2):121–9.

Scheinfeld NS. Dermatological manifestations of graft-versus-host disease. Medscape. 2013;92(3):151–3.

Part III

Drug Related

Cutaneous Reactions to the Biologics

7

David J. Chandler and Anthony P. Bewley

Abstract

Biological therapies have been associated with a wide variety of cutaneous adverse events. The increasing use of biologics in clinical practice has meant that physicians are encountering these adverse events more frequently. In this chapter we review skin conditions that are known to be caused or exacerbated by the use of biological therapies. Safety data are limited and much of the presented evidence is taken from case reports and case series. Infections with bacteria, viruses, fungi, and parasites have been described in patients treated with biologics, including reactivation of latent infection. Cutaneous malignancies have been reported during treatment with biological therapies, however, strong evidence of an association is lacking. The relationship between biologics and inflammatory skin disease is complex and poorly understood, and clinical features may be atypical. It is important that clinicians understand how to recognise and manage these complications.

Keywords

Biologics • Biological therapies • Anti-TNF • Cutaneous adverse events • Infection • Malignancy • Cutaneous immunology

D.J. Chandler, MB, ChB, DTM&H, MSc (✉)
Department of Dermatology, Human Immunology Unit,
Weatherall Institute of Molecular Medicine,
University of Oxford, Oxford OX3 9DS, England, UK
e-mail: david@queenspoint.com

A.P. Bewley, MB, ChB, FRCP
Department of Dermatology, Barts Health NHS Trust,
London, UK

J.C. Hall (ed.), *Skin Diseases in the Immunocompromised*,
DOI 10.1007/978-1-4471-6479-1_7, © Springer-Verlag London 2014

Introduction

Biological response modifiers, or biologics, are a class of protein-based drugs engineered using recombinant DNA technology. Biologics target specific mediators of immune and inflammatory disease pathways, and are becoming increasingly used in the treatment of many cutaneous and systemic inflammatory diseases. Biologics represent an established therapeutic option for diseases such as psoriasis and rheumatoid arthritis (RA); however this field is rapidly expanding, with the identification of immune dysfunction in other diseases driving the development of novel therapeutic agents. Biologics can target a multitude of key signalling molecules including cytokines (tumor necrosis factor (TNF)-α and interleukins), enzymes and growth factors, while other biologics act directly on specific subpopulations of B cells and T cells. Concerns have been raised regarding the adverse effects of long-term treatment with immunosuppressive agents. The most comprehensive safety data available are related to the use of anti-TNF-α therapies in patients with RA, however it can be difficult to draw reliable conclusions. The use of biological therapies has been associated with a wide variety of skin disease, including exacerbation of existing skin conditions and the development of new skin disease.

Infection

The use of biologics has been associated with a wide range of bacterial infections affecting the skin and subcutaneous tissues. In a retrospective study of patients receiving anti-TNF therapy for rheumatic diseases, more than one-third of patients developed infectious events. Skin and skin-associated tissues were the most frequently involved sites of serious infection, and these were caused mainly by bacteria. Factors identified as conferring increased risk of infection in those receiving anti-TNF therapy include increasing age, male sex, disease duration, diabetes, and use of corticosteroids. The inhibition of immune cell subpopulations and key cytokines such as TNF-α

increases host susceptibility to infection, putting patients at increased risk of infection with opportunistic pathogens and reactivation of latent infection. It is important that physicians using biological treatments understand the risks of skin infections and are well equipped to manage these complications. Impairment of the immune system by biological therapies may significantly alter the host response to infection; the physical signs of infection such as fever may be diminished or absent, necessitating a high index of suspicion to detect infectious complications.

Bacterial Infection

Mycobacterial Infection
Tuberculosis

Anti-TNF therapy is associated with an increased risk of mycobacterial infection. The relative risk of tuberculosis (TB) ranges from 1.6 to 25 depending on various clinical factors including the drug used and the patient's country of origin. TNF-α is a proinflammatory cytokine produced by activated macrophages and other immune cells. TNF-α exists in soluble (sTNF) and transmembrane (tmTNF) forms and has various biological effects including the formation and maintenance of granulomas. Experimental data have shown that the binding of soluble TNF-α to TNF receptor 1 (TNFR1, p55) is important for granuloma formation in *M. tuberculosis* infection and in the immune response to intracellular pathogens. TNF-α improves the ability of macrophages to phagocytose and kill mycobacteria, and is important for the formation of granulomas which contain the mycobacteria and prevent their dissemination. Thus TNF-α occupies a central role in the cellular immune response to *Mycobacterium tuberculosis* infection, and the use of anti-TNF agents can be expected to contribute to the progression of recently acquired infection and the reactivation of latent infection.

The majority of reported cases of TB associated with anti-TNF therapy are extrapulmonary and can present with disseminated disease. Cutaneous TB has been described in a patient treated with infliximab for RA. Twelve weeks after treatment was started an indurated lesion appeared on the forearm. Infliximab was discontinued, and after 5 months of anti-tuberculous therapy the cutaneous lesion resolved. The clinical features of this case were consistent with the results of a study by Keane and colleagues in which 70 patients treated with infliximab developed TB on average 12 weeks after starting treatment. Infliximab is a widely used chimeric human-murine anti-TNF monoclonal antibody. Infliximab forms stable complexes with the monomeric and trimeric forms of sTNF and tmTNF, and is able to cross-link TNF molecules, thus preventing TNFR-mediated signalling.

Leprosy

Several case reports describe an association between anti-TNF therapy and the development of leprosy. Scollard and colleagues reported two cases of confirmed borderline lepromatous (BL) leprosy in the United States following 1–2 years of treatment with infliximab for inflammatory arthritis. After discontinuation of infliximab and initiation of multidrug therapy (MDT) for leprosy, both patients developed type 1 or reversal reactions. Oberstein and others described a patient from the Amazon region of Brazil who presented with a symmetrical polyarthritis unresponsive to corticosteroids and methotrexate. Four weeks after starting adalimumab (a fully human anti-TNF monoclonal antibody) the patient developed a widespread macular erythematous rash with some surface scaling which was presumed to be a psoriasiform epidermal reaction; however histological findings were consistent with tuberculoid leprosy. It was thought that this patient presented with an inflammatory arthritis of leprosy and subsequently developed a type 1 reaction following treatment with adalimumab. These and other similar cases highlight the importance of distinguishing between RA and the musculoskeletal manifestations of leprosy, particularly in areas endemic for leprosy. Anti-TNF therapy may increase the risk of developing clinical disease in those infected with *M. leprae* and may lead to more rapid disease progression.

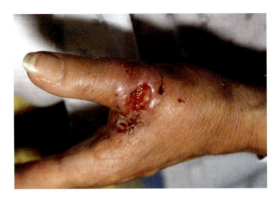

Fig. 7.1 Atypical mycobacterium infection with ulceration and surrounding induration. Not in a patient on biologics, but certainly could be

Furthermore, discontinuation of anti-TNF therapy may precipitate immune-mediated complications of leprosy such as type 1 reactions.

Other Mycobacterial Infections

The atypical or nontuberculous mycobacteria (NTM) are a large, diverse group of environmental bacteria that can cause skin and soft tissue infections, pulmonary disease, lymphadenitis and disseminated disease in the immunocompromised (see Fig. 7.1). In patients receiving biological therapies, NTM infections are reported approximately twice as frequently as TB. *Mycobacterium kansasii* primarily causes lung disease, however the potential for dissemination to other body sites is increased in patients receiving biological therapies as highlighted in a case of bilateral olecranon bursitis caused by *M. kansasii* in a patient receiving infliximab for Behçet's disease. Disseminated *Mycobacterium marinum* infection has been reported in patients treated with infliximab and etanercept for various inflammatory diseases. Cutaneous lesions demonstrate extensive sporotrichoid distribution, and systemic dissemination has been observed. Severe cutaneous and subcutaneous disease has also been reported due to infection with other NTM including *M. chelonae* and *M. poriferae* in patients treated with anti-TNF agents. Lutt and colleagues reported a case of extensive soft tissue and bone infection caused by *M. kansasii* in a patient treated with rituximab for refractory inflammatory myopathy.

Rituximab is a human-murine IgG1 monoclonal antibody that targets CD20 on the surface of mature B cells, causing depletion of circulating and tissue-based B cells. Clinical observations in addition to experimental data suggest a role for peripheral B cells in the host defence against mycobacteria and draw attention to the need to consider these complications in patients receiving treatment with rituximab.

Staphylococcal Infection

Large cohort studies have demonstrated an increased risk of serious skin and soft tissue infection (SSSI) in patients receiving anti-TNF therapy for RA compared with those receiving non-biologic disease-modifying anti-rheumatic drugs (nbDMARD). Staphylococci account for the majority of organisms identified in these cases and are responsible for a variety of skin infections, the most common of which is cellulitis. Severe cellulitis requiring hospitalization and intravenous antibiotics has been reported following treatment with the TNF-inhibitors etanercept and adalimumab. Hawryluk and colleagues described a case of acute pustular folliculitis caused by *Staphylococcus aureus* in a patient receiving infliximab for Crohn's disease. The skin eruption consisted of multiple erythematous papules and nodules involving the axillae, lateral breasts, abdomen, and medial thighs. Culture of these lesions grew methicillin-sensitive *Staphylococcus aureus* (MSSA). Other cases of pustular folliculitis have been described in association with anti-TNF therapy although microbiological cultures were negative. Although not of infectious aetiology, cases of perforating folliculitis have been described in patients receiving treatment with the TNF-α inhibitors infliximab and etanercept and the multi-kinase inhibitor sorafenib. De Simone and colleagues report a case of recurrent cutaneous abscesses following infusions of infliximab in a patient with psoriasis and psoriatic arthropathy. Three days after the first three infusions the patient developed multiple painful, suppurative nodules on her lower abdomen. On each occasion methicillin-sensitive *S. aureus* was cultured and oral treatment with amoxicillin and clavulanic acid was effective. Prophlyactic antibiotic therapy was administered for 5 days prior to all subsequent infusions and this successfully prevented the recurrence of abscesses.

Orbital cellulitis and various ophthalmic infections have been described in patients treated with biologics. Roos and Ostor describe a case of severe unilateral orbital cellulitis in a patient treated with infliximab for ankylosing spondylitis. Culture grew flucloxacillin-sensitive S. aureus and full recovery was made following treatment with appropriate antibiotics. In a retrospective analysis of 430 patients treated with anti-TNF agents for inflammatory arthritis Akhmed and Lichtenstein showed that infections with both MSSA and methicillin-resistant *Staphylococcus aureus* (MRSA) occurred more commonly that any other infection, causing a multitude of severe infections, most common of which was cellulitis. The majority of these patients required hospitalization and treatment with intravenous antibiotics. Wegscheider and others describe a case of impetigo contagiosa caused by penicillin-resistant *Staphylococcus aureus* occurring after the fifth infusion of infliximab in a patient with chronic uveitis. This responded well to treatment with an oral cephalosporin and subsequent infusions of infliximab were well tolerated.

Streptococcal Infection

The use of anti-TNF agents has been associated with the development of streptococcal skin infections including erysipelas, cellulitis, and necrotising fasciitis (NF). Roos and others describe a severe unilateral necrotising periorbital infection occurring during treatment with adalimumab for RA. Cultures grew β-haemolytic *Streptococcus* (Lancefield group A). The patient became systemically unwell, requiring admission to the intensive care unit and parenteral treatment with benzylpenicillin, ciprofloxacin, and clindamycin. Other anti-TNF agents including etanercept and infliximab have been associated with necrotizing fasciitis. Indeed Chan and colleagues report a case of fatal necrotising fasciitis in a patient treated with infliximab for RA. The patient presented with an acute widespread, erythematous, pustular dermatitis involving the trunk and limbs following treatment with infliximab and later developed necrosis of subcutaneous tissue and systemic group A β-haemolytic streptococcal infection.

Less-Common Bacterial Infections

Nocardiosis is a rare opportunistic bacterial infection. *Nocardia* is a genus of aerobic, nonmotile, filamentous, gram-positive bacteria belonging to the order Actenomycetales. Infection is usually by inhalation, causing pulmonary disease. Primary cutaneous and subcutaneous infection (actinomycetoma) results from direct inoculation of these ubiquitous soil organisms into the skin, for example by thorn, splinter, or insect bite. Cutaneous nocardiosis is frequently caused by *Nocardia brasiliensis* and *Nocardia otitidiscaviarum*. Haematogenous dissemination is associated with immunocompromised states, and common sites include the skin and subcutaneous tissues. Experimental data suggest a role for TNF-α in resistance to *N. brasiliensis* infection and this is supported by reports of nocardiosis occurring in patients treated with anti-TNF agents. Fabre and colleagues describe a case of primary cutaneous nocardiosis in a patient treated with infliximab for 3 years. Two weeks after sustaining a penetrating injury to the right hand while gardening, the patient developed a painless ulcer on the right forearm. *N. otitidiscaviarum* was isolated and treatment with oxfloxacin and clindamycin for 3 months was successful. Singh and others describe a case of cutaneous nocardiosis presenting with multiple erythematous papulopustular lesions on the leg following traumatic injury in a patient receiving infliximab for Crohn's disease. Systemic nocardiosis with cutaneous involvement has been reported in a patient treated with etanercept and adalimumab for RA. The patient developed subcutaneous nodules on the trunk, and imaging confirmed the presence of nodular lesions in the lungs and brain. Surgical brain biopsy confirmed the presence of *N. farcinica*. A fatal case of disseminated *N. farcinica* infection has been described in a patient treated with alefacept and infliximab for psoriasis.

The use of biologic agents has been associated with various infections caused by gram-negative bacteria. Pseudomonal skin infection has been observed more frequently in patients receiving anti-TNF therapy. Lazzeri and others report a case of periorbital necrotizing fasciitis caused by *Pseudomonas aeruginosa* in a patient treated for CLL with a chemotherapy regimen that included the anti-CD20 monoclonal antibody rituximab. Reactivation of brucellosis has been described in a patient treated with infliximab for RA. The patient presented with a febrile illness 3 weeks after the third infusion of infliximab, and examination of the skin and mucous membranes revealed pallor, aphthous ulceration, and ecchymotic lesions on the abdomen. Gerster and Dudler note a case of cellulitis with localized skin necrosis at the site of a recent cat bite on the lower leg. The patient had received treatment with etanercept for RA. *Capnocytophaga cynodegmi* was cultured from microbiological specimens and treatment with clarithromycin was successful. Nguyen and colleagues report a case of extensive recurrent cellulitis affecting the left lower leg followed by the right leg in a patient receiving intravenous rituximab every 3 months as maintenance treatment for diffuse large B-cell lymphoma. *Bordetella holmesii* was isolated from blood cultures on both occasions and the infection responded to interruption of rituximab treatment.

Viral Infection

Hepatitis Viruses
Hepatitis C Virus
Anti-TNF therapy has been used in hepatitis C virus (HCV)-positive patients with no increase in hepatotoxicity or viral replication. The use of etanercept as adjuvant therapy to ribavirin and interferon improved viral clearance rates with no significant increase in adverse events. The use of anti-TNF agents in patients with chronic HCV infection may be associated with emergence of mixed cryogloobulinaemia. In a small prospective study, cryoglobulinaemia appeared in two out of six patients with chronic active HCV

infection treated with anti-TNF therapy for RA. Cutaneous manifestations of cryoglobulinaemia were not present in these patients, but include purupuric skin lesions, diffuse vasculitis, and skin ulcers. The long-term safety of anti-TNF therapy in patients with chronic HCV infection is not known, however HCV infection should not be an absolute contraindication to treatment with anti-TNF agents.

Hepatitis B Virus

In contrast to HCV infection, TNF-α may play a role in the control and clearance of hepatitis B virus (HBV) through synergistic action with interferons to reduce viral replication. Thus treatment with anti-TNF agents may lead to increased viral replication and worsening of disease. Cases of severe HBV reactivation and fulminant hepatitis have been reported in patients treated with the anti-TNF agents infliximab and etanercept. The risk of reactivation seems to be greater in hepatitis B surface antigen (HBsAg)-positive patients compared with HBsAg-negative and hepatitis B core antibody (HBcAb)-positive patients. Adalimumab was well tolerated in a small study of patients with psoriatic arthritis and chronic inactive HBV infection. HBsAg-positive carriers requiring anti-TNF therapy should receive anti-HBV treatment or prophylaxis, whereas HBsAg-negative and HBcAb positive patients can be monitored only.

Human Herpes Virus Infections
Herpes Simplex Viruses (HHV-1 and HHV-2)

Primary infection with herpes simplex virus (HSV) is often mild or asymptomatic. Reactivation of the virus in the sensory nerve ganglia in immunocompromised people can lead to severe disseminated disease. This has been observed in those with haematological malignancies and following bone marrow and organ transplants. Disseminated disease including encephalitis has been described in patients receiving immunosuppressive treatment with biologics. Justice et al. describe a case of disseminated cutaneous HSV-1 infection following sequential treatment with the anti-TNF agents etanercept and infliximab. After the third infusion of infliximab the patient developed fever and a widespread pruritic vesicular rash. HSV-1 was detected by polymerase chain reaction (PCR) in skin vesicle fluid.

Varicella Zoster Virus (HHV-3)

Primary infection with varicella zoster virus (VZV) causes chickenpox. Subsequent impairment of VZV-specific cell-mediated immunity can lead to reactivation of latent VZV infection causing herpes zoster or shingles. In the immunocompromised host atypical and severe disseminated infections are more likely. Leung and colleagues report a case of primary varicella infection that developed 9 days after treatment with infliximab was started for Crohn's disease. Skin examination revealed multiple non-pruritic pustules on the chest and back. The patient developed fulminant hepatic failure and disseminated intravascular coagulation, ultimately leading to multiple organ failure and death. Several cases of VZV infection have been previously reported following treatment with infliximab. Experimental studies suggest a role for Th1-type cytokines including TNF-α in immune protection against VZV infection, and data from two large retrospective cohorts in the United States and the United Kingdom suggest that patients treated with biological DMARDs (infliximab, etanercept, and anakinra) are at increased risk of herpes zoster; however the evidence is conflicting with other studies showing no additional risk compared with patients receiving conventional (nonbiologic) treatments. Anakinra is. Data from the German biologics register RABBIT showed an increased risk of herpes zoster in patients treated with anti-TNF monoclonal antibodies but not etanercept. This finding could reflect the different mechanisms of action of these drugs. A study by García-Doval and others demonstrated a tenfold increase in the rate of hospitalization due to VZV infections in patients treated with anti-TNF agents compared with the general population. Further studies are needed to determine the role of prophylactic vaccination.

Cytomegalovirus (HHV-5)

Several cases of cytomegalovirus (CMV) infection complicating anti-TNF therapy have been described. Prior to commencing anti-TNF therapy, a careful physical examination should be performed to identify end-organ manifestations of CMV infection, and serological tests can be used to confirm suspected infection. Immuno-suppression can lead to severe and disseminated infection and this usually involves the gastrointestinal tract. Helbling and colleagues reported a case of disseminated CMV infection with cutaneous involvement in a 63-year-old woman following treatment with a single dose of infliximab for Crohn's disease. Shortly after treatment with infliximab the patient developed multiple widespread painful skin ulcers and a dermatomal papular eruption characteristic of herpes zoster. Skin biopsy revealed numerous endothelial CMV inclusions with local inflammation and necrosis. Interruption of immunosuppressive treatment together with anti-viral therapy produced a satisfactory response.

Kaposi's Sarcoma-Associated Herpes Virus (HHV-8)

Infection with Kaposi's sarcoma-associated herpes virus or human herpes virus 8 (HHV-8) is needed for Kaposi's sarcoma (KS) to develop, however other contributing factors are important. KS has been reported in patients receiving long-term treatment with various immunosuppressive medications including biologics. Cohen described a case of KS associated with the use of infliximab for severe RA. The patient developed multiple firm, purple plaques and nodules over the left lower leg a few weeks after treatment was initiated. The development of KS has been associated with the use of infliximab in subsequent case reports. Further evidence of an association between KS and anti-TNF therapy is provided in two case reports describing the development of KS in patients with adalimumab for RA. Iatrogenic immunosuppression is a common cause of KS and biologics represent an increasing component of this risk.

Other Viral Infections

Several published case reports describe an association between the use of biologic agents and the development of clinical infection with human papilloma virus (HPV) and molluscum contagiosum virus (MCV). Somasekar and others report of case of profuse genital and perianal condylomata, commonly caused by HPV types 6 and 11, in a patient treated with infliximab for refractory Crohn's disease. Genital condylomata have also been reported following treatment with etanercept. Adams and colleagues describe a case of extensive bilateral plantar warts, commonly caused by HPV types 1, 2, and 4, in a patient treated with etanercept and concomitant methotrexate. Antoniou and colleagues describe the development of widespread molluscum contagiosum and the exacerbation of pre-existing genital condylomata in a 29-year-old patient 2 weeks after the first infusion of infliximab for chronic plaque psoriasis. Other case reports describe severe presentations of molluscum contagiosum, including bilateral eyelid lesions following treatment with infliximab and disseminated eruptive giant mollusca (umbilicated papules and nodules up to 1 cm diameter) in a patient treated with efalizumab. Hartmann and colleagues describe a patient with relapsed grade II follicular lymphoma who developed a persistent parvovirus B19 infection following treatment with rituximab, fludarabine, and cyclophosphamide. The patient presented with a febrile illness and a widespread maculopapular rash and subsequently developed progressive anaemia.

Fungal Infection

Superficial Mycoses

The clinical and microscopic features of dermatophyte infection may be atypical in the immuno-compromised host. Infection may be widespread and can invade into the dermis and subcutaneous tissue causing a nodular granulomatous perifolliculitis or Majocchi's granuloma. Lowther and colleagues describe a 64-year-old woman who presented with erythematous plaques and nodules on both legs and the dorsum of the right hand following long-term treatment with infliximab and corticosteroids. Skin biopsy revealed inflammation and necrosis in the dermis and the presence of multinucleated giant cells containing fungal spores. *Trichophyton rubrum* was cultured. Bardazzi and others report the occurrence of severe dermatophytosis caused by *Trichophyton* species in two patients treated with anti-TNF agents. The first patient presented 1 month after starting treatment with adalimumab with large well-demarcated erythematous lesions affecting the trunk and limbs. *Trichophyton rubrum* was isolated. The second patient presented with a diffuse nodular perifolliculitis following the fourth infusion of infliximab for chronic psoriasis. Treatment for bacterial folliculitis was commenced, however the patient did not respond. Skin biopsy demonstrated the presence of granulomatous perifolliculitis and fungal elements. Trichophyton mentagrophytes was grown on culture. Treatment in both cases involved discontinuation of anti-TNF therapy and systemic therapy with fluconazole for 21 days.

Use of biologics has been associated with superficial mycoses caused by non-dermatophyte molds and yeasts. In a study by Lee et al., 35 of 150 patients developed new skin eruptions during treatment with an anti-TNF agent. Thirteen of these patients had an infectious complication, including three cases of pityriasis versicolor and three cases of dermatophyte infection. Wallis and others observed an increased rate of candidiasis in patients treated with infliximab compared with than those treated with etanercept.

Subcutaneous and Systemic Mycoses

Case reports describe the occurrence of various subcutaneous mycoses in patients receiving anti-TNF therapy. Gottlieb and colleagues describe a case of disseminated sporotrichosis in a patient treated with etanercept and infliximab. Mazzurco and others report a case of subcutaneous phaeohyphomycosis in an elderly patient treated with infliximab for severe RA. Clinical presentation was with a slowly enlarging nodule on the left leg that appeared 1 month after being pricked by a thorn from a pyracantha bush. Deep fungal culture was positive for *Phaeoacremonium* species.

The increasing use of biologic agents has led to a rise in cases of endemic mycoses, with histoplasmosis identified as the most common cause of invasive fungal infection among patients receiving anti-TNF therapy. The cutaneous features of histoplasmosis are variable and include ulcers, erythematous and keratotic papules, exudative nodulo-pustular lesions, and lesions resembling molluscum contagiosum. Rogan and Thomas describe a case of fatal disseminated coccidioidomycosis in an elderly patient receiving immunosuppressive treatment with infliximab and methotrexate. The initial presentation was with an ulcerated papule on the right cheek and treatment consisted of empirical antibiotics for presumed cellulitis. His condition deteriorated, leading to progressive respiratory failure and death. A retrospective study by Bergstrom et al. identified an increased risk of developing symptomatic coccidioidomycosis in patients with inflammatory arthritis receiving treatment with infliximab, compared with those not receiving infliximab. A meta-analysis of the anti-TNF agents infliximab and adalimumab in 3,493 patients with RA demonstrated an increased risk of serious infection; however of the 126 serious infections reported there was 1 case of histoplasmosis and 1 case of coccidioidomycosis. A case of paracoccidioidomycosis was reported in a patient treated with methotrexate, leflunomide, and adalimumab for RA. The use of anti-TNF agents has been associated with an increased risk of infection with opportunistic pathogens, including invasive (systemic) fungal infections with *Candida* and *Aspergillus* species. These fungi have low innate virulence; however they can cause fatal infections in immunocompromised patients. Invasive cryptococcosis has been reported in association with the anti-TNF agent adalimumab. The patient presented with an acutely inflamed left second finger approximately 1 year after starting treatment with adalimumab. Clinical examination was notable for tenosynovitis of the digital flexor tendon and subsequent surgical decompression revealed extensive cellulitis. *Cryptococcus neoformans* was cultured. Hoang and Burruss describe a case of localized scalp infection with *Cryptococcus albidus* in a 14-year-old boy receiving etanercept for psoriasis.

Parasitic Infection

Leishmaniasis

The high prevalence of latent leishmaniasis in Europe together with the increasing use of anti-TNF agents has led to an increase in the number of reported cases of opportunistic leishmaniasis associated with anti-TNF therapy. Visceral, cutaneous, and mucocutaneous forms of leishmaniasis have been described in association with anti-TNF treatment. The available data suggest that the risk of opportunistic leishmaniasis is greater in patients receiving anti-TNF monoclonal antibodies compared with those receiving etanercept. Cases of severe and relapsing cutaneous leishmaniasis have been reported in patients treated with anti-TNF monoclonal antibodies. Cutaneous leishmaniasis is often self-limiting; however it can progress to involve the mucous membranes causing destructive changes. Three cases of mucocutaneous leishmaniasis have been reported in patients treated with adalimumab.

Malignant Disease

Cutaneous Lymphoma

Chronic inflammation and previous use of immunosuppressive therapies are known to increase the risk of lymphoproliferative disorders, particularly non-Hodgkin's lymphoma. It is less clear from the available evidence whether anti-TNF therapy confers additional risk of lymphoma; however several case reports describe an association between anti-TNF therapy and cutaneous lymphoma. Mahe et al. report a case of cutaneous CD30+ T-cell lymphoma following combination treatment with infliximab and ciclosporin for erythrodermic psoriasis. The patient developed painless, purple nodular lesions affecting the limbs associated with inguinal lymphadenopathy. Discontinuation of these treatments resulted in regression of the lymphoma. Adams and colleagues describe a case of rapidly progressive cutaneous T-cell lymphoma (CTCL) in an elderly man following treatment for 18 months with etanercept. Cases of mycosis fungoides and Sézary syndrome have been reported in patients receiving treatment with infliximab for ankylosing spondylitis. Dalle and others report a case of mycosis fungoides with follicular mucinosis in a 49-year-old man treated with adalimumab for ankylosing spondylitis. On examination there were infiltrated plaques and follicular papules with alopecia affecting the trunk and limbs. Histology was remarkable for a perifollicular and perivascular inflammatory cell infiltrate with infiltration of the follicular epithelium by atypical T-cells and mucinous degeneration of the hair follicles. The patient responded to discontinuation of adalimumab and treatment with retinoids and PUVA. Data from clinical trials suggest that lymphoma accounts for approximately 20 % of malignancies occurring in patients treated with adalimumab. Two cases of atypical CD8+ CTCL have been reported in patients treated with efalizumab and/or infliximab.

Non-melanoma Skin Cancer

Immunosuppression is known to increase the risk of skin cancer, and high-quality evidence suggests that the use of biologics may be associated with an increased risk of non-melanoma skin cancer (NMSC). Patients with psoriasis, in particular, may be at increased risk from treatment modalities known to increase the risk of skin cancer, such as PUVA and ciclosporin. In a prospective study of patients receiving anti-TNF therapy, Flendrie and others noted the occurrence of basal cell carcinoma (BCC), squamous cell carcinoma (SCC) and pre-malignant lesions including actinic keratosis and Bowen's disease. Smith et al. report the development of multiple rapidly progressive squamous cell carcinomas in seven patients treated with etanercept, and cases of SCC with fatal outcome have been described in patients treated with etanercept for psoriasis. Esser and colleagues describe the development of multiple SCCs and keratoacanthomas in a 76-year-old woman four months after infliximab was commenced for refractory RA. Of note, the patient had a history of extensive sun exposure and previous NMSC. These data highlight the need for close surveillance of patients receiving anti-TNF therapies, especially in those with a history of sun exposure or previous treatment with immunosuppressive agents. The use of anti-T-cell agents including alefacept and efalizumab has been associated with the development of NMSC. Among 1,869 patients treated with alefacept in clinical trials, 46 cases of NMSC (20 BCC, 26 SCC) were diagnosed in 27 patients. However, safety data presented by Krell and colleagues failed to demonstrate an increased risk of malignancies in 1,174 patients treated with alefacept compared with the background rate in patients with psoriasis. Treatment with efalizumab at any dose in 2,980 patients with psoriasis across 14 clinical trials was not found to increase the risk of NMSC compared with placebo. Ustekinumab is a fully human IgG1κ monoclonal antibody that binds with high affinity and specificity to the p40 subunit common to interleukin (IL)-12 and IL-23.

Pooled data from four clinical trials of ustekinumab for psoriasis suggest that the rate of NMSC is comparable with that of the general population. Rates of NMSC were comparable for up to 5 years in patients treated with ustekinumab at doses of 45 mg (0.64 per 100 patient-years) and 90 mg (0.44 per 100 patient-years). The proportion of patients with NMSC was 2.9 % in those with previous PUVA exposure compared with 1.0 % in those with no prior PUVA exposure. In the placebo-controlled period of clinical trials, the frequency of NMSC was 0.2 % in ustekinumab-treated subjects compared with 0.3 % in placebo-treated subjects.

Melanoma

A large observational study conducted by Wolfe and Michaud in the United States demonstrated an increased risk of melanoma in patients treated with infliximab and etanercept, with odds ratios of 2.6 (1.0–6.7) and 2.4 (1.0–5.8) respectively. No increased risk was detected in patients treated with adalimumab. The results of a meta-analysis by Leombruno and colleagues suggest that anti-TNF therapy is not associated with an increased

risk of skin malignancies. No increased risk was observed in the composite endpoint of non-cutaneous cancer and melanoma in patients treated with recommended doses of anti-TNF, however the use of infliximab and adalimumab at doses higher than recommended could be important. A recent analysis by Gottlieb and others failed to demonstrate any increased risk of melanoma in approximately 14,000 patients treated with etanercept in 49 clinical trials. Gordon et al. reported the development of malignant melanoma following treatment with adalimumab 40 mg every other week for 60 weeks in a patient with psoriasis and previous exposure to PUVA. Anti-TNF agents should be used with caution in patients with a history of treated melanoma. Fulchiero and colleagues describe the reactivation of metastatic melanoma in two patients within 90 days of starting treatment with etanercept and adalimumab. The patients had received surgical treatment 4 and 9 years previously for stage IB and IA melanoma, respectively. The occurrence of eruptive melanocytic naevi is associated with immunosuppression and has been reported in patients treated with biological therapies. Bovenschen et al. describe the development of eruptive naevi in patients treated with biologics including infliximab, etanercept, and alefacept. The nature of these naevi and their potential for malignant transformation is not fully understood, thus it is important to screen for dysplastic naevi and melanoma.

Inflammatory and Autoimmune Disorders

Psoriasis and Psoriasiform Eruptions

Biological therapies targeting TNF-α are effective in the treatment of psoriasis; however a significant literature describes the worsening of pre-existing psoriasis or the development of psoriasiform skin eruptions during anti-TNF therapy (see Fig. 7.2). The occurrence of these paradoxical reactions serves to highlight the complex nature of the immune dysfunction underlying psoriasis. Wollina and colleagues

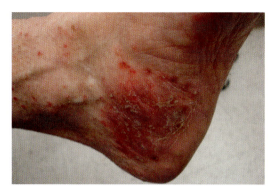

Fig. 7.2 Papulosquamous dermatitis with silvery white scale on the heel in a patient that developed after etanercept given for rheumatoid arthritis

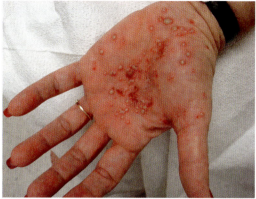

Fig. 7.3 Pustular eruption of the palms that developed after etanercept started for arthritis. Resolved when etanercept was discontinued

discuss 120 published cases of psoriasis developing in the context of anti-TNF therapy. New onset of psoriasis was reported by 74 patients and exacerbation of pre-existing psoriasis was observed in 25 patients. The authors described various clinical forms of psoriasis including palmoplantar pustular psoriasis in 37 patients. Associated clinical data including baseline disease characteristics, family history of psoriasis, duration of anti-TNF therapy, and type of anti-TNF agent used varied widely between patients. Data from the British Society for Rheumatology Biologics Register suggest that these reactions do not occur in patients treated with traditional (non-biologic) disease-modifying anti-rheumatic drugs. Further, the rate of new-onset psoriasis was significantly higher in patients treated with adalimumab, compared with etanercept and infliximab. A pustular eruption localized to the palms, as seen in Fig. 7.3, and soles resembling palmoplantar pustulosis is the most frequently observed pattern of psoriasis associated with anti-TNF therapy. This is often accompanied by other psoriatic skin lesions including erythematous, scaly plaques and guttate lesions, as seen in Fig. 7.4. Localized scalp involvement has been described and presentation can involve psoriatic nail changes including pitting, onycholysis, discoloration, and subungual hyperkeratosis. Widespread pustular psoriasis has been described in patients treated with anti-TNF therapy, particularly with infliximab. It has been suggested that the reactivation of silent streptococcal infection by anti-TNF

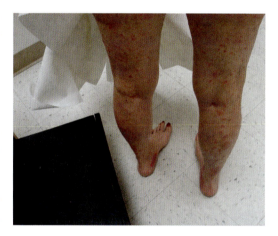

Fig. 7.4 Symmetric oval papulosquamous dermatitis of sudden onset after etanercept was started. Patient had no personal or family history of psoriasis

agents could induce psoriatic eruptions in persons predisposed to developing psoriasis (positive family history).

Ettler and colleagues reported a case of new-onset psoriasis presenting as pityriasis amiantacea (PA) during treatment with infliximab and adalimumab for Crohn's disease. The patient described a pruritic scalp eruption that progressed over years to involve the face, trunk, and limbs. Examination of the scalp revealed erythema with hyperkeratotic scaly plaques and clumping together of the hair shafts. Thin scaling plaques were seen on the face and guttate lesions were noted on the lower limbs. There was no personal or family history of psoriasis. Significant improvement was seen following discontinuation of anti-TNF therapy and treatment with topical corticosteroids, tar, and keratolytic shampoo. Seneschal et al. describe the onset of psoriasiform drug eruptions in eight patients treated with anti-TNF agents. All patients developed small plaque-type psoriasis and three patients had a pustular eruption affecting the palms and soles. Histologic findings in six patients included epidermal hyperplasia, parakeratosis, and spongiosis; however a lichenoid pattern was observed in three samples with evidence of a CD8+ cytotoxic T-cell inflammatory infiltrate. True psoriasis can occur in the context of anti-TNF therapy, although Seneschal and colleagues suggest that most psoriasiform eruptions represent a "class effect" of biological therapies targeting TNF-α that are compatible histologically with lichenoid or spongiotic psoriasiform drug eruptions. The pathogenesis of these reactions is poorly understood. Werner de Castro and others describe the resolution of adalimumab-induced psoriasiform lesions following correction of vitamin D deficiency. Skin lesions often respond to discontinuation of the responsible anti-TNF agent and use of topical treatments for psoriasis.

these histologic features are seen in conditions where TNF-α is thought to be responsible for skin lesions, such as toxic epidermal necrolysis and cutaneous graft-versus-host disease (GVHD). Several cases of lichen planus (LP) or LP-like eruptions of varying clinical morphology have been described in patients treated with anti-TNF agents. Battistella and colleagues report a case of extensive LP in a 38-year-old woman 4 months after initiation of etanercept for severe RA. The appearance of a pruritic papular eruption on the right lower leg was rapidly followed by spread to the trunk and limbs, resulting in widespread coalescent violaceous lichenoid papules. Skin biopsy findings were consistent with LP.

Etanercept has been associated with the development of other lichenoid disorders, including lichen planopilaris. Utsu and others reported a case of LP-like eruptions following the lines of Blaschko in a 56-year-old female with RA and Sjögren syndrome. Erythematous papules occurred in several bands on the left side of the body. It has been suggested that the clonal keratinocytes on the lines of Blaschko are more sensitive to the cytokine imbalance, between TNF-α and interferon (IFN)-α, that is thought to play a major role in the pathogenesis of LP-like eruptions.

Lichenoid Disorders

Various lichenoid disorders, with histological features in keeping with an interface dermatitis pattern, have been described in patients treated with biological therapies. Cutaneous eruptions consistent with erythema multiforme (EM) and lichenoid drug reaction have been described in patients treated with infliximab. Histologic features involved the dermoepidermal junction and included vacuolar degeneration of the basal epidermis, necrotic keratinocytes, satellite lymphocytes, and a band-like infiltrate. Cases of severe EM-like skin reactions have been reported in patients treated with other anti-TNF agents including adalimumab and etanercept, suggesting that inhibition of TNF-α may be important in the pathogenesis of these reactions. Interestingly,

Eczema

Flendrie et al. described the occurrence of various types of eczema in patients treated with anti-TNF agents for RA. These included dyshidrotic eczema, contact dermatitis, nummular eczema, atopic dermatitis, and papular eruptions. Skin lesions resolved on discontinuation of anti-TNF therapy in three cases, and others patients responded well to treatment with topical corticosteroids. In a prospective study by Lee and others, eczematous skin lesions and atopic dermatitis (AD)-like eruptions were observed in patients treated with etanercept, infliximab and adalimumab, accounting for 23 % of all cutaneous adverse events associated with anti-TNF therapy. AD-like conditions have been associated with anti-TNF therapy in several case reports, including severe eruptions requiring hospitalization. Vestergaard and colleagues described a 46-year-old Caucasian man treated with infliximab for severe psoriasis and psoriatic arthritis. The patient had a history of atopy and hand eczema. After the seventh infusion of infliximab the patient developed severe impetigo. After the eighth infusion widespread eczematous lesions were noted and the patient was admitted to hospital with severe erythroderma. Interruption of infliximab therapy and treatment with antibiotics and topical steroids produced a satisfactory response.

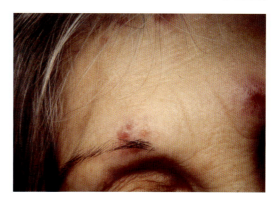

Fig. 7.5 Apple-jelly colored nodules above eyebrow. Sarcoidosis, just like psoriasis, may respond to biologics, but biologics can also cause and flare sarcoidosis as a paradoxical response

Acne

Case reports have described the development of acneiform eruptions in patients receiving anti-TNF therapy, however data from controlled clinical trials is lacking. Bassi and colleagues reported the appearance of inflammatory and non-inflammatory acneiform lesions in two male patients, aged 30 and 32 years, with no previous history of acne. Data from placebo-controlled trials suggest that there is an increased rate of acne among those treated with efalizumab.

Granulomatous Disorders

Non-infectious cutaneous granulomatous disease has been well described in patients treated with biologics. Anti-TNF therapies, in particular infliximab, have been used successfully in the treatment of sarcoidosis, shown in Fig. 7.5; however there are several reports of paradoxical worsening of disease and cases of new-onset sarcoidosis developing during treatment with various anti-TNF agents. Two case reports describe the development of pulmonary and cutaneous sarcoidosis in patients treated with etanercept for rheumatic diseases. Firm, non-tender, red-brown skin nodules were present, and biopsy revealed multiple non-caseating granuloma. In addition, Dhaille and colleagues describe two cases of cutaneous sarcoidosis, without systemic involvement, associated with infliximab and

adalimumab. Deng and others describe five cases of interstitial granulomatous dermatitis (IGD) occurring during treatment with etanercept, infliximab, and adalimumab. Clinical presentation was with multiple erythematous annular lesions including macules, papules, and indurated plaques. Pruritus was present in some cases and lesions involved the trunk and extremities. Voulgari and others reported the development of 9 cases of generalized granuloma annulare (GA) among 199 patients treated with anti-TNF agents for RA. All patients responded well to treatment with topical corticosteroids. The increased prevalence of GA in this cohort is suggestive of an association between TNF-α inhibition and the development of GA.

Vasculitis

Leukocytoclastic vasculitis (LCV), as shown in Fig. 7.6, has been reported frequently in patients treated with anti-TNF agents. Ramos-Casals and others identified 233 cases of autoimmune diseases secondary to anti-TNF therapy published between 1990 and 2006, of which 113 were vasculitis. LCV was the most common type of vasculitis, occurring in 70 % of cases (n=79); however, many other types of vasculitis were reported, including cutaneous necrotising vasculitis (n=8), cutaneous lymphocytic vasculitis (n=4), Henoch-Schönlein purpura (n=2), and

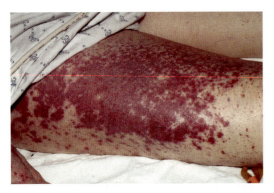

Fig. 7.6 Severe cutaneous vasculitis with hemorrhage that is indurated (palpable purpura) and surrounding petechiae on the anterior thigh. Systemic disease should be looked for. This patient had hematuria indicating renal vasculitis. A common underlying cause is a drug reaction, including reaction to biologics

urticarial vasculitis (n = 1). Vasculitis presented with cutaneous lesions in the majority of patients and these were most commonly purpura; others included ulcerative lesions, nodules, digital vasculitis, and maculopapular rash. Systemic features including renal impairment and peripheral neuropathy may also be present. Clinical improvement is seen in the majority of patients on cessation of anti-TNF therapy, although treatment with corticosteroids or immunosuppressive agents may be required. Serum sickness-like reactions have been reported in patients treated with rituximab and anti-TNF agents, including infliximab. Serum sickness is a type 3 (immune-complex) hypersensitivity reaction consisting of fever, rash (urticarial and vasculitic eruptions), and arthralgia. Severe systemic involvement may require hospitalization and treatment in an intensive care unit. In a study of 500 patients treated with infliximab for Crohn's disease, serum sickness-like disease was attributed to infliximab in 2.8 % of patients (n = 14). A previous severe serum sickness reaction to an anti-TNF agent should be considered a contraindication to further treatment with this class of drug.

Devos and others described two cases of perniosis affecting the hands and fingers in two patients treated with infliximab. Wang and colleagues describe a case of eczematid-like purpura of Doucas and Kapetenakis in a 40-year-old woman with Crohn's disease. One week after her fifth infusion of infliximab, the patient developed a pruritic eruption affecting the lower extremities, consisting of petechiae; papules; and scaly, erythematous macules. Spontaneous improvement was noted after 2 months, although re-challenge with a sixth dose of infliximab resulted in return of the rash.

Lupus Erythematosus

Drug-induced lupus erythematosus or drug-induced lupus-like syndromes have been reported in up to 1 % of patients treated with anti-TNF agents, most commonly in those treated with etanercept and infliximab. Clinically these reactions may manifest as systemic, subacute cutaneous, or discoid lupus erythematosus. Women in the fifth decade of life are most frequently affected. In a French national survey, 0.18 and 0.19 % of patients treated with etanercept and infliximab, respectively, developed systemic lupus erythematosus. Cutaneous manifestations included malar rash, photosensitivity, urticarial rash, purpura, alopecia, and perniosis. Drug-induced lupus usually responds to discontinuation of anti-TNF therapy, however cases of persistent disease have been described. The use of alternative anti-TNF agents without disease recurrence in patients with previous anti-TNF-associated lupus erythematosus has been described in a few cases, although the evidence base for this practice is limited.

Alopecia Areata

Cases of alopecia areata (AA) have been reported during treatment with various anti-TNF agents including etanercept, infliximab, adalimumab, and certolizumab pegol. The pathogenesis of AA is poorly understood and these paradoxical reactions raise further questions.

Other Adverse Effects

A vast number of cutaneous side effects have been reported in patients receiving biological therapies. Injection site reactions have been reported with the subcutaneous administration of etanercept, infliximab, adalimumab, and rituximab. Infusion reactions have been consistently described with the use of intravenous infliximab. Acute infusion reactions occur within the first 24 h following infusion, and have been observed in up to 6 % of patients treated with infliximab. The majority of acute reactions are non-immune-mediated, however a minority may represent an IgE-mediated immediate hypersensitivity reaction. Delayed infusion reactions occur 24 h to 14 days following infusion, and clinical presentation frequently includes a maculopapular rash or urticarial eruption. The pathogenesis involves the formation of antibodies to infliximab resulting in a type 3 (immune complex-mediated) hypersensitivity reaction. Pruritus has been reported frequently in patients treated with monoclonal antibodies, including rituximab and others used in the treatment of malignancies. Mutant BRAF inhibitors such as dabrafenib and vemurafenib have improved the treatment of metastatic malignant melanoma, but have been associated with a variety of cutaneous side effects. In a study by Anforth et al., dabrafenib was shown to cause verrucal keratotic squamoproliferative lesions (49 %), Grover's disease (27 %), and reactive hyperkeratotic lesions on the soles (22 %). Vemurafenib has been shown to cause folliculocentric and toxic erythema-like rashes, photosensitivity, and squamoproliferative eruptions. Hand–foot syndrome or palmar-plantar erythrodysesthesia has been associated with the use of the multiple tyrosine kinase inhibitor (multi-TKI) class of biologics, including sorafenib, sunitinib, and axitinib. Many other cutaneous toxicities have been described with this drug class; these include stomatitis, alopecia, skin discoloration, subungual splinter haemorrhage, facial swelling, erythema, and xerosis.

Conclusion

The use of biological therapies has been associated with a wide variety of cutaneous adverse events, not all of which could be considered in this chapter. A wealth of clinical trials demonstrate the efficacy of these interventions, however such trials are powered to detect efficacy and not adverse events. Therefore, uncommon adverse events may not be detected and reported, thus safety data must be interpreted with caution. In addition, safety data are lacking for many of the more recently developed biologics. The available data suggest that biological therapies can increase susceptibility to infection from a wide range of pathogens and increase the risk of reactivation of latent infection. Opportunistic and endemic infections can cause severe disease and must be considered where clinically relevant. Convincing evidence supports an association between biologics and non-melanoma skin cancer, and the risks of melanoma and cutaneous lymphoma may also be increased. Data from various sources suggest that biological therapies can interact with immune-mediated and inflammatory pathways, leading to the exacerbation of pre-existing skin conditions and/or the development of new inflammatory or autoimmune skin diseases. With the increasing use of biologics, rare dermatological conditions are becoming more frequently encountered.

Physicians must carefully consider the risks and benefits of targeting the immune system to treat disease and should be well equipped to deal with the potential complications. A high level of vigilance and prompt investigation of new or worsening skin lesions is critical in the management of these patients.

Suggested Reading

Antoniou C, Kosmadaki MG, Stratigos AJ, Katsambas AD. Genital HPV lesions and Molluscum contagiosum occurring in patients receiving anti-TNF-alpha therapy. Dermatology. 2008. http://www.ncbi.nlm.nih.gov/pubmed/18285688. Accessed 25 Sep 2013.

Asarch A, Gottlieb AB, Lee J, Masterpol KS, Scheinman PL, Stadecker MJ, et al. Lichen planus-like eruptions: an emerging side effect of tumor necrosis factor-alpha antagonists. J Am Acad Dermatol. 2009. http://www.ncbi.nlm.nih.gov/pubmed/19539844. Accessed 23 Oct 2013.

Beuthien W, Mellinghoff H-U, von Kempis J. Skin reaction to adalimumab. Arthritis Rheum. 2004. http://www.ncbi.nlm.nih.gov/pubmed/15146441. Accessed 23 Oct 2013.

Borrás-Blasco J, Navarro-Ruiz A, Borrás C, Casterá E. Adverse cutaneous reactions induced by TNF-alpha

antagonist therapy. South Med J. 2009. http://www.ncbi.
nlm.nih.gov/pubmed/19864977. Accessed 23 Oct 2013.

Chandler D, Bewley A. Biologics in dermatology.
Pharmaceuticals. 2013. http://www.mdpi.com/1424-
8247/6/4/557. Accessed 26 Oct 2013.

Filler SG, Yeaman MR, Sheppard DC. Tumor necrosis
factor inhibition and invasive fungal infections. Clin
Infect Dis. 2005. http://www.ncbi.nlm.nih.gov/
pubmed/15983902. Accessed 23 Oct 2013.

Flendrie M, Vissers WHPM, Creemers MCW, de Jong
EMGJ, van de Kerkhof PCM, van Riel
PLCM. Dermatological conditions during TNF-alpha-
blocking therapy in patients with rheumatoid arthritis:
a prospective study. Arthritis Res Ther. 2005. http://
www.pubmedcentral.nih.gov/articlerender.fcgi?artid=
1174960&tool=pmcentrez&rendertype=abstract.
Accessed 20 Oct 2013.

Fulchiero GJ, Salvaggio H, Drabick JJ, Staveley-O'Carroll
K, Billingsley EM, Marks JG, et al. Eruptive latent
metastatic melanomas after initiation of antitumor
necrosis factor therapies. J Am Acad Dermatol. 2007.
http://www.ncbi.nlm.nih.gov/pubmed/17434043.
Accessed 21 Oct 2013.

González-López MA, Blanco R, González-Vela MC,
Fernández-Llaca H, Rodríguez-Valverde V. Development of sarcoidosis during etanercept therapy. Arthritis
Rheum. 2006. http://www.ncbi.nlm.nih.gov/pubmed/
17013853. Accessed 26 Oct 2013.

Keane J, Gershon S, Wise RP, Mirabile-Levens E,
Kasznica J, Schwieterman WD, et al. Tuberculosis
associated with infliximab, a tumor necrosis factor
alpha-neutralizing agent. N Engl J Med. 2001. http://
www.ncbi.nlm.nih.gov/pubmed/11596589. Accessed
23 Sep 2013.

Mohan N, Edwards ET, Cupps TR, Slifman N, Lee J, Siegel
JN, et al. Leukocytoclastic vasculitis associated with
tumor necrosis factor-alpha blocking agents. J Rheumatol.
2004. http://www.ncbi.nlm.nih.gov/pubmed/15468359.
Accessed 26 Oct 2013.

Moustou A-E, Matekovits A, Dessinioti C, Antoniou C,
Sfikakis PP, Stratigos AJ. Cutaneous side effects of anti-
tumor necrosis factor biologic therapy: a clinical review.
J Am Acad Dermatol. 2009. http://www.ncbi.nlm.nih.
gov/pubmed/19628303. Accessed 10 Oct 2013.

Navarro R, Daudén E, Gallo E, Santiago Sánchez-Mateos
D, García-Diez A. Alopecia areata during treatment of

psoriasis with adalimumab and leflunomide: a case and
review of the literature. Skin Pharmacol Physiol. 2012.
http://www.ncbi.nlm.nih.gov/pubmed/22301842.
Accessed 10 Oct 2013.

Salmon-Ceron D, Tubach F, Lortholary O, Chosidow O,
Bretagne S, Nicolas N, et al. Drug-specific risk of non-
tuberculosis opportunistic infections in patients
receiving anti-TNF therapy reported to the 3-year
prospective French RATIO registry. Ann Rheum
Dis. 2011. http://www.ncbi.nlm.nih.gov/pubmed/
21177290. Accessed 18 Sep 2013.

Smith KJ, Skelton HG. Rapid onset of cutaneous squamous
cell carcinoma in patients with rheumatoid arthritis
after starting tumor necrosis factor alpha receptor
IgG1-Fc fusion complex therapy. J Am Acad Dermatol.
2001. http://www.ncbi.nlm.nih.gov/pubmed/11712048.
Accessed 20 Oct 2013.

Sun G, Wasko CA, Hsu S. Acneiform eruption following
anti-TNF-alpha treatment: a report of three cases.
J Drugs Dermatol. 2008. http://www.ncbi.nlm.nih.
gov/pubmed/18246701. Accessed 26 Oct 2013.

Thielen AM, Kuenzli S, Saurat J-H. Cutaneous adverse
events of biological therapy for psoriasis: review of
the literature. Dermatology. 2005. http://www.ncbi.
nlm.nih.gov/pubmed/16205065. Accessed 10 Oct
2013.

Winthrop KL, Yamashita S, Beekmann SE, Polgreen
PM. Mycobacterial and other serious infections in
patients receiving anti-tumor necrosis factor and other
newly approved biologic therapies: case finding
through the Emerging Infections Network. Clin Infect
Dis. 2008. http://www.ncbi.nlm.nih.gov/pubmed/
18419421. Accessed 6 Oct 2013.

Winthrop KL, Chang E, Yamashita S, Iademarco MF,
LoBue PA. Nontuberculous mycobacteria infections
and anti-tumor necrosis factor-alpha therapy. Emerg
Infect Dis. 2009. http://www.pubmedcentral.nih.gov/
articlerender.fcgi?artid=2866401&tool=pmcentrez&r
endertype=abstract. Accessed 2 Oct 2013.

Wollina U, Hansel G, Koch A, Schönlebe J, Köstler E,
Haroske G. Tumor necrosis factor-alpha
inhibitor-induced psoriasis or psoriasiform exanthe-
mata: first 120 cases from the literature including a
series of six new patients. Am J Clin Dermatol. 2008
http://www.ncbi.nlm.nih.gov/pubmed/18092839.
Accessed 22 Oct 2013.

Cutaneous Reactions to Chemotherapy

Jessica A. Savas and Reshma L. Mahtani

Abstract

Patients undergoing cancer chemotherapy are often challenging to physicians from a management standpoint due to an unfortunate combination of general poor health, immunosuppression, and multi-drug regimens. Several chemotherapeutic agents are associated with well-described mucocutaneous toxicities.

This chapter will address the commonly encountered adverse events associated with traditional chemotherapy medications such as chemotherapy-induced alopecia, mucositis, extravasation reactions, dyschromia, and acral erythema, among others. This will be followed by a discussion of the cutaneous toxicities associated with newer agents, namely, targeted therapies such as monoclonal antibodies and tyrosine kinase inhibitors. Finally, a brief discussion of radiation recall and enhancement is also included.

By addressing important considerations in the recognition, diagnosis, and management of the cutaneous effects of cancer treatment, additional morbidity and potential mortality can be avoided in this already at-risk patient population.

Keywords

Cancer • Chemotherapy • Immunosuppression • Mucocutaneous • Kinase inhibitors • Blocking antibodies • Alopecia • Mucositis

Introduction

Oncology patients represent a complicated demographic when it comes to management due to an unfortunate combination of general poor health, immunosuppression, and multi-drug regimens. Cutaneous toxicities complicate chemotherapeutic treatments in a significant number of patients and these adverse effects may be dose dose-limiting, often requiring alteration of the treatment plan.

The mucocutaneous side effects associated with chemotherapy may be localized or systemic and range in severity from completely benign to life threatening. It is important to quickly

J.A. Savas • R.L. Mahtani, DO (✉)
Division of Hematology/Oncology,
University of Miami, 1192 East Newport
Center Drive, Deerfield Beach, FL 33442, USA
e-mail: rmahtani@med.miami.edu

J.C. Hall (ed.), *Skin Diseases in the Immunocompromised*,
DOI 10.1007/978-1-4471-6479-1_8, © Springer-Verlag London 2014

recognize and treat these adverse reactions to prevent further morbidity as well as any excess emotional angst beyond that already experienced from simply carrying a diagnosis of cancer. This task is not always an easy one, as the potential etiology of cutaneous and mucosal eruptions in the immunosuppressed patient is nearly limitless. When diagnosing a chemotherapeutic drug reaction, one must consider and subsequently exclude other likely possibilities such as an opportunistic infection associated with immunosuppression, a nutritional deficiency, radiation reactions, non-chemotherapeutic drug-induced reactions, primary cutaneous malignancies, or metastatic spread of the primary tumor.

Mucocutaneous Side Effects of Systemic Chemotherapeutic Agents

Chemotherapy-Induced Alopecia (CIA)

Alopecia is the most common adverse cutaneous manifestation of chemotherapy treatment and may be observed in two distinctive patterns: anagen effluvium and telogen effluvium. Anagen effluvium is the pattern of hair loss that occurs most often and is secondary to the targeting of rapidly dividing follicular cells by antineoplastic agents. This exogenous insult results in either complete destruction of the hair follicle or growth of thin, brittle hairs that easily break. Anagen effluvium begins 7–10 days after the initiation of therapy but becomes most obvious at around 1–2 months. Telogen effluvium, while not the primary mechanism of alopecia in patients undergoing cancer chemotherapy, may contribute to global hair loss secondary to malnutrition, high fever, and the severe emotional distress that accompanies a cancer diagnosis.

The severity or degree of alopecia is dependent upon several factors, including the specific drug used, the dosage, duration of therapy, serum half-life, and duration of drug infusion. In general, CIA is more severe in patients on multi-agent regimens. The rapidly dividing terminal

hairs located on the scalp are the most commonly affected and the most prominent, however, axillary, eyebrow, eyelash, and pubic hair may be lost as well in patients undergoing long-term chemotherapy.

Hair loss caused by chemotherapy is almost always reversible, although there have been rare reports of permanent alopecia after treatment with cyclophosphamide and busulfan before bone marrow transplantation. While hair regrowth is generally the rule, it is important to counsel patients that the color and texture of their new hair may be different.

Several drugs are known to cause alopecia, as seen in the list below. The agents most often associated with CIA are shown in bold.

- Amsacrine
- Aminocamptothecin
- **Bleomycin**
- Busulfan
- Carmustine
- Chlorambucil
- **Cyclophosphamide**
- Cytarabine
- Dacarbazine
- **Dactinomycin**
- **Daunorubicin**
- **Docetaxel**
- **Doxorubicin**
- **Etoposide**
- Epirubicin
- 5-Fluorouracil
- Gemcitabine
- Granulocyte macrophage-colony stimulating factor
- Hydroxyurea
- **Idarubicin**
- **Ifosfamide**
- Interferon-alpha
- **Irinotecan**
- **Mechlorethamine**
- Melphalan
- **Methotrexate**
- Mitomycin
- **Mitoxantrone**
- Nitrogen mustard derivatives
- Nitrosources
- **Paclitaxel**

- Procarbazine
- Teniposide
- Thiotepa
- **Topotecan**
- **Vinblastine**
- **Vincristine**
- Vindesine
- Vinorelbine

With regard to prevention and management of CIA, several techniques have been employed, albeit with very limited success. The use of scalp hypothermia and tourniquets has been used in attempts to prevent or lessen the severity of CIA; however, due to a lack of safety and efficacy data, the use of these modalities is based largely on anecdotal success. Minoxidil has been shown to decrease the duration of CIA and be of some benefit in certain patients.

Mucositis/Stomatitis

Approximately 40 % of patients undergoing chemotherapeutic treatment will experience an oral complication. Stomatitis, or mucositis, is associated with a variety of chemotherapeutic agents, as listed below, and is most often observed due to either a direct effect from drug-related toxicity or indirectly via drug-induced bone marrow suppression. The agents most often associated with mucositis/stomatitis are shown in bold.

- Aminogluethimide
- Amsacrine
- **Bleomycin**
- Cyclophosphamide
- Cytarabine
- **Dactinomycin**
- **Daunorubicin**
- **Docetaxel**
- **Doxorubicin**
- Doxorubicin (liposomal)
- **Edatrexate**
- Epirubicin
- Floxuridine
- **Fluorouracil**
- Hydroxyurea (high dose)
- Idarubicin
- Interleukin-2

- Mechlorethamine
- 6-Mercaptopurine
- **Methotrexate**
- Mithramycin
- Mitomycin
- Nitrosoureas
- Paclitaxel
- Plicamycin
- Procarbazine
- Tegafur
- 6-Thioguanine
- **Tomudex**
- **Topotecan**
- Vinblastine
- Vincristine

The oral epithelium is characterized by a high mitotic rate and rapid cell turnover, making it highly susceptible to agents that target rapidly dividing cells. As a result, the oral mucosa may become atrophic, ultimately leading to unpleasant clinical manifestations such as pain, burning, and xerostomia, or dry mouth. Clinical examination may simply reveal an erythematous mucosa; however, ulceration may occur, and when present, creates a portal of entry for secondary infection, as shown in Fig. 8.1.

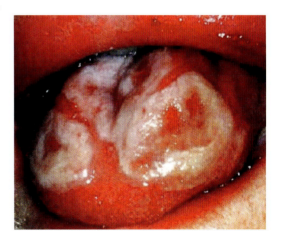

Fig. 8.1 Grade 4 mucositis with erythema, pain, and ulceration making oral alimentation impossible (Reprinted with kind permission from Springer Science + Business Media from Peterson DE, Keefe DM, Hutchins RD, Schubert MM. Alimentary tract mucositis in cancer patients: impact of terminology and assessment on research and clinical practice. *Support Care Cancer*. 2006;14:499–504

Patients at greatest risk for oral complications are those with hematologic malignancies, younger patients (<20 years), patients with poor dentition or hygiene practices, and patients with pre-existing oral disease.

Prevention is important largely because symptomatic mucositis or stomatitis may prevent oral intake in a patient population that is already undernourished. Increased risk for infection through ulcerations in the mucosa can greatly increase morbidity as well.

Good oral hygiene practices remain first line for primary prevention of mucosal complications; however, oral cooling through ice chips given 5 min prior to chemotherapy and maintained for a total of 30 min seems to be somewhat efficacious in reducing the incidence of mucositis. The vasoconstrictive response to cold may explain the potential benefit of oral cryotherapy, decreasing the exposure of the mucosal vasculature to the toxic agents.

Treatment, when needed, is largely supportive and is accomplished primarily through pain management. Frequent assessment of patients for early recognition of infection is paramount to prevent further complication.

Extravasation Reactions

Several chemotherapeutic agents may cause local irritation due to extravasation of the agent into the soft tissues during intravenous administration. Incidence estimates suggest that these cutaneous injuries occur in approximately 0.1–6 % of patients. Clinically, this may present with mild erythema, edema, and tenderness, which can potentially evolve into a chemical cellulitis, phlebitis, or in the most extreme cases, frank necrosis and/or ulceration.

Chemotherapeutic agents that cause extravasation reactions may be designated as either a vesicant or an irritant based on their potential to cause local injury. In the simplest terms, the feature that distinguishes the two is the severity of the reaction, namely, the presence or absence of necrosis. If the agent is an irritant, an inflammatory reaction characterized by pain, warmth, and erythema at the injection site or along the vein may be appreciated. Necrosis is highly unlikely with irritants and there is no associated long-term morbidity. Conversely, vesicant reactions tend to produce a more severe inflammatory response, with necrosis and ulceration often complicating the clinical picture. Permanent disfigurement or dysfunction has been reported after extravasation with vesicant agents.

If an extravasation reaction is identified, infusion of the agent should be stopped immediately and aggressive local control should ensue. Treatment options include ice and elevation of the limb as well as attempted aspiration of as much of the agent as possible and/or administration of an antidote if available. Local cryotherapy is recommended for all vesicant reactions save those involving the vinca alkaloids, as application of cold has been shown to increase the incidence of ulceration in animal models. If necrosis or ulceration occurs, possible debridement and appropriate wound care should be initiated.

Dyschromia

Hyperpigmentation of the skin, hair, mucous membranes, and nails is commonly reported in association with cancer chemotherapy treatment. The increased pigment may be local, such as at the site of drug infusion, or diffuse. Many agents produce selective discoloration of the nails, producing either longitudinal or horizontal bands of pigment. Mucosal surfaces commonly experience pigmentary alteration as well. The exact mechanism of hyperpigmentation secondary to chemotherapeutic agents has yet to be fully elucidated and while several theories have been postulated, the pathophysiology likely varies with the drug used.

The key to distinguishing chemotherapeutic agents as the etiology lies in documenting a temporal association between drug administration and symptom onset. Some drugs result in well-characterized patterns of hyperpigmentation such as the flagellate hyperpigmentation accompanied by intense pruritus unique to bleomycin use, as seen in Fig. 8.2. A more diffuse darkening of the skin is seen in patients on busulfan and is informally

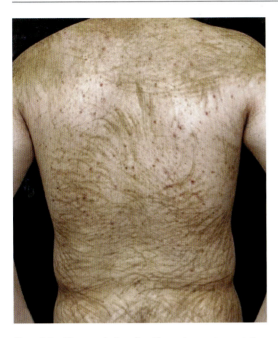

Fig. 8.2 Characteristic flagellate hyperpigmentation associated with bleomycin treatment (Reprinted from Chen YG, Huang CF, Dai MS. Young man with scratches on his back. Bleomycin-related flagellate hyperpigmentation. *Ann Emerg Med*. 2013;61:152–4. With permission from Elsevier)

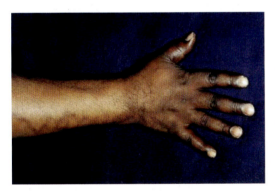

Fig. 8.3 Serpentine supervenous hyperpigmentation (Reprinted from Payne AS, James WD, Weiss RB. Dermatologic toxicity of chemotherapeutic agents. *Semin Oncol*. 2006;33:86–97. With permission from Elsevier)

referred to as the "busulfan tan." Serpentine supervenous hyperpigmentation or hyperpigmentation over the veins into which a chemotherapeutic agent is introduced is frequently reported after infusion of fluorouracil or docetaxel, shown in Fig. 8.3. Blue discoloration of the tongue and lunula has been reported after single-agent as well as combination chemotherapy and has been associated with several drugs including adriamycin, capecitabine, cyclophosphamide, doxorubicin, hydroxyurea, and tegafur. Increased pigment of the nail bed also commonly occurs during cancer treatment with chemotherapeutic agents.

While hyperpigmentation may be very distressing for some patients, it begins to fade slowly over several months after the drug is discontinued, and generally requires no additional intervention.

Acral Erythema

This well-known cutaneous complication of cancer chemotherapy treatment is known by many names, including Burgdorf's syndrome, palmar-plantar erythrodysesthesia syndrome, palmar-plantar erythema, hand-foot syndrome, and toxic erythema of the palms and soles. Despite its various designations, all of the aforementioned terms refer to the same distinct clinical entity: an intensely painful, symmetrical, well-demarcated, erythematous rash on the palms and soles that may occasionally involve the dorsum of the hands and feet, shown in Fig. 8.4a–c. A prodrome of burning and tingling in the extremities precedes the eruption of the tender erythema and is usually followed by edema and occasionally vesicle or frank bullae formation.

It is important to differentiate chemotherapy-associated acral erythema from the acral erythema of graft-versus-host disease (GVHD). Acral erythema of chemotherapy may be distinguished from GVHD by identifying the classic triad of systemic involvement that accompanies GVHD and includes cutaneous injury plus alterations in gastrointestinal and hepatic function. Chemotherapy-induced acral erythema is not associated with systemic manifestations.

Cytarabine is a commonly reported cause of acral erythema, causing cutaneous injury in a dose-dependent fashion. Additionally, acral erythema is the principal skin toxicity associated with fluorouracil use when administered as an infusion or orally, however, the incidence is greatly diminished when given as a bolus. Other agents that reportedly cause acral erythema

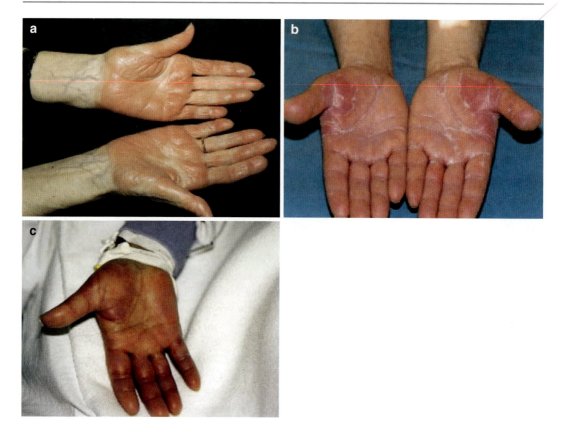

Fig. 8.4 (**a**) Palmar erythema and tenderness. (**b**) Palmar erythema with desquamation. (**c**) Palmar edema, ertheyma, and blistering (**a–c** Reprinted with kind permission from Springer Science + Business Media, BV. Nagore E, Insa A, Sanmartin O. Antineoplastic therapy-induced palmar plantar erythrodysesthesia ("hand-foot") syndrome. Incidence, recognition and management. *Am J Clin Dermatol*. 2000;1:225–34)

include hydroxyurea, methotrexate, paclitaxel, gemcitabine, etoposide, and cisplatin.

The primary goal of management is symptomatic relief, which is generally accomplished through the use of cool compresses and analgesics. Pyridoxine is occasionally given to help with any associated dysesthesia. Potent topical and systemic corticosteroids have also been reported to lessen the severity of the reaction and may be considered in some patients. If the symptoms prove to be intolerable, alteration or cessation of chemotherapy treatment may be indicated.

Neutrophilic Eccrine Hidradenitis (NEH)

Originally reported after cytarabine use in a patient with acute myeloid leukemia (AML), neutrophilic eccrine hidradenitis (NEH) has since been documented after administration of a variety of chemotherapeutic agents in patients with varying malignancies. NEH most often occurs after combination chemotherapy and is seen in both children and adults. Patients commonly present with nonspecific symptoms, including fever and a rash distributed over the head, neck, trunk, or extremities. The number and morphology of the lesions varies greatly, with single or multiple erythematous to violaceous lesions presenting as macules, papules, nodules, pustules, or plaques. While the majority of lesions are asymptomatic, some patients may report tenderness or pain. NEH has a very distinct histopathology, therefore skin biopsy plays a pivotal role in the diagnosis of NEH due to the non-specific nature of the clinical presentation. The pathophysiology is poorly understood, however excretion of the

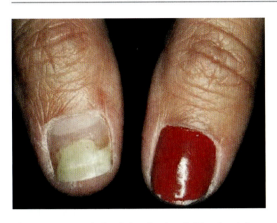

Fig. 8.5 Onycholysis of the distal nail (Reprinted from Payne AS, James WD, Weiss RB. Dermatologic toxicity of chemotherapeutic agents. *Semin Oncol.* 2006;33:86–97. With permission from Elsevier)

toxic agent via sweat ducts is thought to contribute.

Most cases do not require treatment, as spontaneous resolution generally occurs within 1–4 weeks after withdrawal of the offending agent. It is important to note that approximately 60 % of patients experience a recurrence of symptoms if chemotherapeutic treatment is re-initiated. Systemic corticosteroids and dapsone have been reported to be efficacious in non-resolving cases.

Onychodystrophy

Nail changes are often observed in association with the administration of numerous chemotherapeutic agents. Painful onycholysis or suppurative onycholysis has been reported with docetaxel and paclitaxel, as shown in Fig. 8.5. Other drugs known to induce various nail toxicities include estramustine, gefitinib, and the anthracyclines. Eliciting a history of chemotherapy administration usually yields the correct diagnosis, however, nail clippings for potassium-hydroxide and fungal culture help to rule out other common nail disorders considered in the differential diagnosis. Nail clippings can also be sent to the lab for PAS staining, which will show dermatophyte and yeast infections and has less false negatives that cultures.

Beau's lines are transverse ridges presenting in the nail that correspond to cycles of chemotherapy. The ridges move distally and disappear when treatment is discontinued. Transverse leukonychia presenting as multiple white lines may also appear in conjunction with chemotherapy cycles.

There is no consensus treatment for onychodystrophy due to chemotherapy; however, several modalities may be employed depending on the clinical situation. Antibiotics are administered when deemed appropriate by culture. Pain management is a major goal due the extremely painful nature of the majority of nail conditions. In the case of subungal abscess formation, nail plate avulsion may be necessary to relieve pressure and reduce pain.

Miscellaneous Drug Reactions

Several chemotherapeutic agents are known to produce miscellaneous cutaneous reactions. Long-term therapy with hydroxyurea is known to induce ulcerations of the malleoli of the lower extremities and mimic the cutaneous manifestations of dermatomyositis. Several drugs, bleomycin among them, produce a Raynaud phenomenon in some patients, which may or may not be accompanied by digital necrosis. Bleomycin is also noted to cause characteristic flagellate erythema. Acquired cutaneous adherence or "sticky skin" is characteristic of doxorubicin and ketoconazole. Granulocyte-macrophage colony stimulate factor is associated with a drug-induced Sweet's syndrome. Flushing is another reaction produced by several available chemotherapeutic agents.

Erythematous papules that evolve into pustules appearing on the face and trunk within 5 days of treatment initiation are commonly reported following the use of dactinomycin. Methotrexate and granulocyte colony stimulating factor have also been named as culprits in producing a similar acneiform reaction.

Additionally, some chemotherapy drugs exacerbate pre-existing skin disease, such as the inflammation of actinic keratoses observed after the use of fluorouracil and, to a lesser extent, dacarbazine, vincristine, dactinomycin, docorubicin, and cisplatin. Topical corticosteroids provide some relief, however the mechanism of this reaction remains unclear. The actinic keratosis may resolve after the reaction has occurred. In a similar fashion, paclitaxel and cytarabine are known to cause inflammation of seborrheic keratoses. Psoriasis patients who receive high-dose methotrexate have reported ulceration of pre-existing psoriatic plaques as well as the development of reversible cutaneous lymphoma, and interferon gamma and interleukin 2 also reportedly exacerbate psoriasis.

Mucocutaneous Effects of Tyrosine Kinase Inhibitors and Monoclonal Antibodies

As the molecular pathways that lead to unregulated cell proliferation and, ultimately, cancer are further elucidated, selective therapies that specifically target aberrant molecules in these pathways are being developed. Among these, tyrosine kinase inhibitors and monoclonal antibodies have quickly gained popularity and possess the potential to revolutionize modern cancer treatment. Despite their more selective mechanism of action, their use is still associated with adverse effects, the majority of which involve cutaneous injury.

Inhibitors of Epidermal Growth Factor Receptor (EGFR)

Overexpression of the epidermal growth factor receptor (EGFR) has been linked to the development of chemo-resistance and portends a poor prognosis in several cancers. The targeting of the EGFR is now a therapeutic intervention in many solid tumors with several classes of drugs currently under investigation.

The agents that target EGFR with the most well-characterized cutaneous side effects are the monoclonal antibody, cetuximab, and two small molecule inhibitors of the tyrosine kinase of EGFR, gefitinib and erlotinib. Cutaneous adverse effects are the most common side effect associated with the use of these agents and occur in

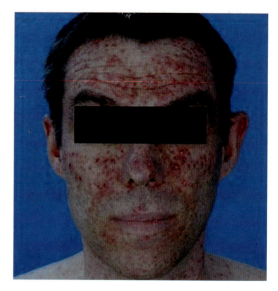

Fig. 8.6 Acneiform eruption from EGFR inhibitor. Facial folliculitis in a patient treated with cetuximab (Reprinted from Robert et al. (2005). With permission from Elsevier)

approximately 50 % of patients. Of the skin toxicities described, folliculitis is the most commonly encountered.

Clinically, the inflammatory papules and pustules arise in an acneiform distribution on the face, as seen in Fig. 8.6, but may also involve the chest and upper back. In some patients, diffuse involvement of the entire body has been reported. The severity of the eruption appears to be agent-specific, with cetuximab folliculitis being more extensive when compared to gefitinib and erlotinib.

Alterations in keratinocyte differentiation or chemokine expression have been proposed as the potential etiology of the rash but this has not yet been fully characterized. Interestingly, the severity of the folliculitis appears to be associated with improved treatment response and survival outcomes, however more investigation is needed to thoroughly understand the relationship as well as the mechanism.

If left untreated and the EGFR inhibitor continued, the rash will most likely wax and wane in severity, with the majority of lesions demonstrating improvement over time. While culture is often negative, antibiotics are useful in some patients, possibly due to their anti-inflammatory effects. If the folliculitis becomes intolerable,

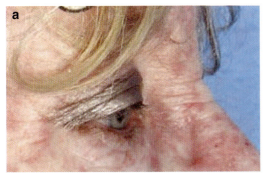

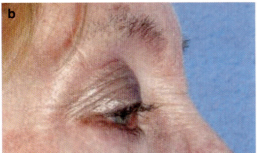

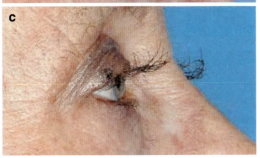

Fig. 8.7 (**a–c**) Progressive trichomegaly in a patient treated with erlotinib (Reprinted from Robert et al. (2005). With permission from Elsevier)

discontinuation of the EGFR inhibitor for approximately 1–2 weeks has been reported to improve lesions as well.

Other commonly reported mucocutaneous toxicities associated with EGFR inhibitor use include alterations in scalp hair texture and/or growth, progressive eyelash trichomegaly, shown in Fig. 8.7, paronychial inflammation and xerosis, or drying of the skin.

Tyrosine Kinase Inhibitors

Several other small molecule inhibitors of various kinases are currently being used for cancer treatment, and induce significant cutaneous

toxicity in patients. Imatinib, an inhibitor of the kinase BCR-ABL, is considered first-line for patients with chronic myelogenous leukemia and has been reported to produce a non-specific skin rash in 30–40 % of these patients. Other drug-induced cutaneous manifestations associated with imatinib use have also been reported, such as vasculitis, Stevens Johnson syndrome, acute generalized exanthematous pustulosis, oral lichenoid reaction, and toxic epidermal necrolysis.

Sorafenib and sunitinib are two additional targeted therapies that have shown great promise in the treatment of certain cancers. Acral erythema is a common adverse effect that occurs between 2 and 4 weeks after treatment initiation with either agent. The reaction appears to be dose-dependent and resolves upon discontinuation of the drug.

Painless subungal splinter hemorrhages and reversible alterations in hair and skin pigmentation have also been frequently reported side effects seen in patients undergoing therapy with sorafenib or sunitinib. Facial erythema often appears in patients 1–2 weeks after treatment initiation with sorafenib, and periocular edema has been known to occur commonly in patients treated with imatinib and occasionally in patients on sunitinib. Neither reaction requires treatment and generally resolves spontaneously over several weeks.

Cutaneous Side Effects of Radiation Therapy When Used in Conjunction with Systemic Chemotherapeutics

Radiation Recall

Radiation recall refers to the phenomenon where induction of chemotherapeutic treatment incites an inflammatory reaction in a previously irradiated site. The most common manifestation of radiation recall is a cutaneous response, however inflammation of other organ systems has also been reported. The classic culprits are doxorubicin and dactinomycin, however recall dermatitis has been documented after the use of several chemotherapeutic agents.

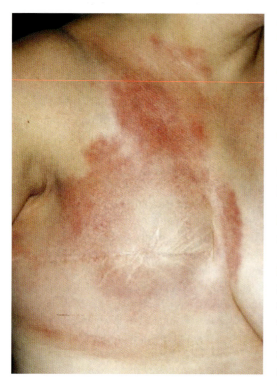

Fig. 8.8 Radiation recall dermatitis (Reprinted from Payne AS, James WD, Weiss RB. Dermatologic toxicity of chemotherapeutic agents. *Semin Oncol.* 2006;33:86–97. With permission from Elsevier)

Radiation recall dermatitis may occur anywhere from 8 days to 15 years after radiation therapy, and symptoms may manifest within hours to days after administration of the offending agent. Any previous irradiated area is susceptible to this cutaneous reaction, which is typically characterized by a painless or painful erythema, seen in Fig. 8.8. Vesiculation, desquamation, edema, and pruritus may or may not occur with necrosis and ulceration reported in severe cases.

The severity of the reaction is thought to be associated with the interval between radiation therapy and chemotherapy initiation, with shorter intervals resulting in more severe reactions. Higher doses of radiation given also appear to correlate with a greater severity of recall dermatitis Susser et al. (1999).

The mechanism of the reaction remains unknown but may be linked to a DNA repair defect. The dermatitis generally clears without treatment, and management is symptomatic. Systemic corticosteroids may significantly improve symptomatology, potentially allowing for continuation of the chemotherapy regimen.

Radiation Enhancement

Radiation enhancement is another potential complication when radiation therapy and chemotherapy are administered in the same patient. Radiation enhancement specifically refers to an increase in the toxicity of radiation therapy when administered concomitantly with chemotherapy. By definition, the two modalities must be administered together or within 7 days of each other, and result in greater toxicity when combined than either therapy administered alone. Similar to radiation recall, radiation enhancement has been reported to occur commonly in the skin, but has also been documented in virtually every other organ system.

The most commonly associated agents include bleomycin, dactinomycin, doxorubicin, fluorouracil, hydroxyurea, 6-mercaptopurine, and methotrexate.

The clinical presentation is reminiscent of radiation recall dermatitis with a natural course of self-limiting resolution over days to months. Treatment is supportive and long-term complications may include skin atrophy, fibrosis, and telangiectasia.

Conclusion

Patients undergoing cancer chemotherapy are particularly susceptible to complications from treatment. In addition to drug and hypersensitivity reactions that are inherent to most exogenous medications, cancer chemotherapy agents carry the unique potential for inducing cutaneous toxicity. Recognizing predictable patterns of cutaneous injury as well as the timeline in which they occur (Table 8.1), aids in the rapid diagnosis of these adverse effects, thereby reducing morbidity and mortality.

Table 8.1 Timeline for cutaneous reactions to chemotherapy drugs

Reaction		Presentation	Resolution
Chemotherapy-induced alopecia	Anagen effluvium	First noticed within 7–10 days after treatment initiation, most prominent at 1–2 months	Begins to regrow once chemotherapeutic agent is discontinued
	Telogen effluvium	Weeks to several months after a severe stressor	Regrows over time
Mucositis		Within 1–7 days	Heals spontaneously within 2–3 weeks
Extravasation	Irritant	Within 2–3 days	Disappears spontaneously over ensuing weeks
	Vesicant	Initial symptoms may appear immediately or develop days to weeks later	Ulcerations heal very slowly; may lead to permanent sequelae
		Ulceration occurs over several weeks	
Hyperpigmentation		Generally appears between the first and sixth month of therapy	Gradually fades over 6 months to a year after termination of chemotherapy treatment
Acral erythema		2–4 weeks	Will resolve upon discontinuation of offending agent but may recur with increased severity if treatment is resumed
Neutrophilic eccrine hidradenitis		2 days to 3 weeks	Clears spontaneously in 1–4 weeks after the offending agent is discontinued without scar formation
Radiation recall dermatitis		8 days to 15 years after radiation therapy and within hours to days after chemotherapy administration	Clears within hours to weeks after chemotherapy is discontinued
Acneiform eruption of EGFR inhibitors		May appear as early as 1 week after treatment initiation	Will persist but wax and wane in severity if drug is continued; will resolve if drug is discontinued

Suggested Reading

Alley E, Green R, Schuchter L. Cutaneous toxicities of cancer therapy. Curr Opin Oncol. 2002;14:212–6.

Bernstein EF, Spielvogel RL, Topolsky DL. Recurrent neutrophilic eccrine hidradenitis. Br J Dermatol. 1992;127:529–33.

Bronner AK, Hood AF. Cutaneous complications of chemotherapeutic agents. J Am Acad Dermatol. 1983;9:645–63.

Cox K, Stuart-Harris R, Abdini G, Grygiel J, Raghavan D. The management of cytotoxic-drug extravasation: guide-lines drawn up by a working party for the Clinical Oncological Society of Australia. Med J Aust. 1988;148:185–9.

DeSpain JD. Dermatologic toxicity of chemotherapy. Semin Oncol. 1992;19:501–7.

Duvic M, Lemak NA, Valero V, Hymes SR, Farmer KL, Hortobagyi GN, et al. A randomized trial of minoxidil in chemotherapy-induced alopecia. J Am Acad Dermatol. 1996;35:74–8.

Flynn TC, Harrist TJ, Murphy GF, Loss RW, Moschella SL. Neutrophilic eccrine hidradenitis: a distinctive rash associated with cytarabine therapy and acute leukemia. J Am Acad Dermatol. 1984;11:584–90.

Hood AF. Cutaneous side effects of cancer chemotherapy. Med Clin North Am. 1986;70:187–209.

Johnson TM, Rapini RP, Duvic M. Inflammation of actinic keratoses from systemic chemotherapy. J Am Acad Dermatol. 1987;17:192–7.

Koppel RA, Boh EE. Cutaneous reactions to chemotherapeutic agents. Am J Med Sci. 2001;321:327–35.

Laack E, Mende T, Knuffmann C, Hossfeld DK. Hand-foot syndrome associated with short infusions of combination chemotherapy with gemcitabine and vinorelbine. Ann Oncol. 2001;12:1761–3.

Larson DL. Treatment of tissue extravasation by antitumor agents. Cancer. 1982;49:1796–9.

Soto E, Fall-Dickson JM, Berger AM. Oral complications in cancer therapy. In: DeVita VT, Lawrence TS, Rosenberg SA, editors. Cancer: principles and practice of oncology. Philadelphia: Lippincott; 1993. p. 2385–94.

Pearce HP, Wilson BB. Erosion of psoriatic plaques: an early sign of methotrexate toxicity. J Am Acad Dermatol. 1996;35:835–8.

Robert C, Soria JC, Spatz A, Le Cesne A, Malka D, Pautier P, et al. Cutaneous side-effects of kinase inhibitors and blocking antibodies. Lancet Oncol. 2005;6:491–500.

Susser WS, Whitaker-Worth DL, Grant-Kels JM. Mucocutaneous reactions to chemotherapy. J Am Acad Dermatol. 1999;40:367–98; quiz 99–400.

Tosi A, Misciali C, Piraccini BM, Peluso AM, Bardazzi F. Drug-induced hair loss and hair growth. Incidence, management and avoidance. Drug Saf. 1994;10:310–7.

Wyatt AJ, Leonard GD, Sachs DL. Cutaneous reactions to chemotherapy and their management. Am J Clin Dermatol. 2006;7:45–63.

Cutaneous Reactions to Corticosteroids

9

Peniel Zelalem

Abstract

Corticosteroids, both topical and systemic, are common treatments for various skin diseases. Since the discovery of their antiinflammatory and immunosuppressive effects, they have been employed in treating various autoimmune and inflammatory skin conditions. Their common and ubiquitous use has brought several adverse effects both systemic and dermatologic. These adverse reactions include hypersensitivity reactions to the components of the drug, skin atrophy, steroid rosacea, and several bacterial, viral, and fungal infections secondary to immune compromise. Since steroids are used to treat various skin conditions, it is vital to recognize worsening of skin disease from underlying skin condition versus a complication of topical or systemic corticosteroid use.

Keywords

Corticosteroid • Skin atrophy–steroid induced • Steroid rosacea • Hypersensitivity reactions • Bacterial cutaneous infections • Viral cutaneous infections • Fungal cutaneous infections • Opportunistic infections • Cutaneous manifestation of disseminated infections

Introduction

Corticosteroids, both topical and systemic, are common treatments for various skin diseases. Since the discovery of their anti inflammatory and immunosuppressive effects, they have been employed in treating various autoimmune and inflammatory skin conditions. Their common and ubiquitous use has brought several adverse effects both systemic and dermatologic. This chapter will focus on the dermatologic effects of corticosteroids such as hypersensitivity or allergic reactions, direct drug effects, and diseases secondary to immunosuppression.

Hypersensitivity

Although corticosteroids are anti-inflammatory, allergic and hypersensitivity reactions do occur. When considering the wide use of corticosteroids

P. Zelalem, MD
Internal Medicine, University of Kansas Medical Center, 3901 Rainbow Boulevard, Kansas City, KS 66160, USA
e-mail: pzelalem@kumc.edu

J.C. Hall (ed.), *Skin Diseases in the Immunocompromised*,
DOI 10.1007/978-1-4471-6479-1_9, © Springer-Verlag London 2014

for variety of illnesses, the documented cases of hypersensitivity reactions can be considered rare. However, one must have heightened suspicion in order to differentiate worsening of underling disease condition that steroids are being used to treat from hypersensitivity reaction to the steroid agent. Hypersensitivity reactions can be classified as immediate or type 1 hypersensitivity and delayed or type 4 hypersensitivity. Immediate hypersensitivity includes urticaria, diffuse angioedema, brochospasm, and shock. Delayed hypersensitivity reactions can present as Stevens Johnson Syndrome, allergic contact dermatitis, systemic contact dermatitis, exanthematous pustulosis, maculopapular exanthematous, morbilliform eruption, or exfoliative dermatitis. Although rare, Stevens Johnson Syndrome characterized by bullous lesions and ulcerations can occur.

Allergic contact dermatitis can occur to topical, inhaled or intranasal corticosteroids. It can be erythematous vesicular, bullous, or eczematous. The face, nose, and eyelids can develop perioral dermatitis due to inhaled or intranasal corticosteroids. Sensitivity to one agent may not necessarily cause sensitivity to all.

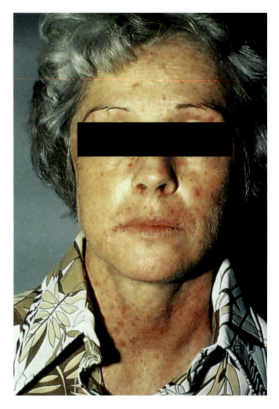

Fig. 9.1 Corticosteroid-induced rosacea in a patient who previously did not have rosacea. Shows inflammatory papules in a photo distribution on face and neck

Direct Drug Effects

Chronic use of both topical and systemic steroids can result in skin atrophy, which is one of the common side effects of steroids. It manifests as skin thinning and easy bruising. It may present as striae, telangiectasia, cigarette-paper atrophy, milia, subcutaneous fat atrophy, or poikiloderma. Skin thinning maybe reversible by discontinuing the steroid agent, however, striae and telangiectasia may remain permanent.

Steroid rosacea, as seen in Fig. 9.1, may occur with use of both systemic and topical corticosteroids. It presents as erythematous maculopapular rash that may or may not have pustules. It usually resolves with discontinuation of agents, however use of oral tetracycline or erythromycin may be necessary to reduce rebound rosacea. Steroid acne, shown in Fig. 9.2, can be seen with systemic or topical corticosteroids and consists

of monotonous symmetric red papules without cysts or comedones.

Along with the more superficial atrophy (called cigarette-paper wrinkling atrophy), mentioned earlier in the chapter and seen in Fig. 9.3, there is a unique syndrome of deep-skin, subcutaneous, and underlying muscular atrophy at the site of intramuscular steroid injection, usually with triamcinilone, as seen in Fig. 9.4. As deep as it may be, it usually resolves over several months to a year.

Secondary to Immunosuppression

Corticosteroids, with both acute and chronic use, result in varying degrees of immunosuppression. Immunocompromised individuals are susceptible to skin pathogens that affect immunocompetent individuals as well as wide variety of opportunistic infections. Corticosteroids are used to

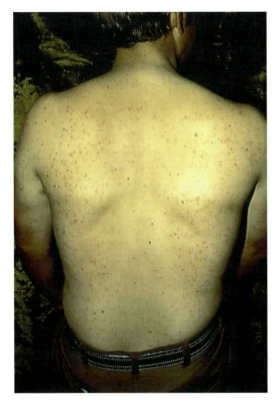

Fig. 9.2 Corticosteroid-induced acne with monotonous symmetric papules without comodones or cysts

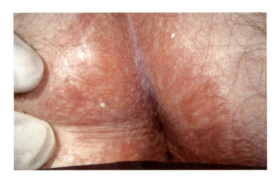

Fig. 9.3 Telangiectasias, milia, and atrophy from chronic clobetasol ointment use for lichen simplex chronicus in perirectal area

treat various skin conditions due to their anti-inflammatory and immunosuppressive properties. Due to these properties, they inhibit different paths of the immune system, making it more difficult to protect or fight against infections. They also affect collagen and fibrous tissue, causing the skin to lose its protective barrier function thus making it easier for pathogen invasion and spread.

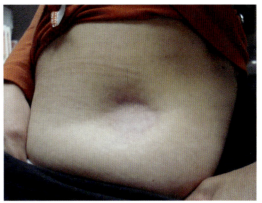

Fig. 9.4 Deep-skin, subcutaneous, and muscle atrophy from 80 mg of Kenalog given in buttocks for rheumatoid arthritis

Due to the anti-inflammatory effect of steroids, skin lesions may be different from their typical presentation. In this section, we will discuss bacterial, viral, and fungal infections in patients that are immunocompromised secondary to corticosteroid use. We will also discuss skin malignancies that have been reported in steroid induced immunocompromised patients.

Bacterial

In the immunocompromised, common pathogens can present in a typical manner, however, they may also have altered presentation due to immunosuppression. In addition, uncommon bacterial skin pathogens such as gram negative bacilli and mycobacterium species may more commonly be seen. Various skin lesions could be manifestations of systemic disease as well as cutaneous spread of systemic infections. In this chapter, we will briefly discuss common skin infections and emphasize infections more commonly seen in those with immune suppression secondary to chronic steroid use.

Common bacterial skin pathogens include *staphylococcus aureus*, *group A streptococcus*, and coryneform bacteria as well as less common but well described pathogens such as mycobacterial and actinomycele species. Common manifestations are cellulitis, erysipelas, staphylococcal scalded skin syndrome, impetigo, folliculitis, (seen in Fig. 9.5), boils, and trichomycosis. Eczematoid dermatitis can occur secondary to

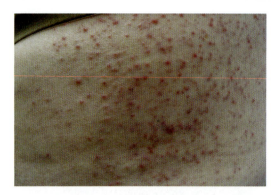

Fig. 9.5 Corticosteroid-induced folliculitis in a patient on 7 months of high-dose systemic corticosteroids for an autoimmune disease. It covers all of the patient's back in a symmetric pattern with perifollicular pustules and papules

staph aureus or coag negative staph colonization of underlying skin lesions. In addition, superinfection with staph or strep in conditions such as bullous pemphigoid treated with steroids can result in worsening of the lesion. Secondary infections such as intertrigo, which is overgrowth of normal flora, cause an inflammatory skin reaction.

In patients with chronic steroid use, typical and atypical presentations of mycobacteria have been identified. These can be caused by various mycobacterial species both slow growing and fast growing, such as *M. Marinum, M. Knasassii, MAI, M. Abscessus, M. Chelonei, M. Fortuitum, M. Ulcernans,* and even *M. Tuberculosis.* They can present as papules and nodules. *M. Heamophilum,* though rare, has been reported in immunocompromised patients. Actinomycetoma, caused most commonly by *actinomyces isrealii,* can manifest as hard, erythematus lesions which may transform into purulent discharges. *Nocardia asteroides,* although rare, does occur in the immunocompromised as a systemic infection with cutaneous manifestations as well as isolated skin lesions. It may present as nodules and ulcerations as well as abscesses. Bacillary angiomatosis secondary to *bartonella henselae* or Quintana is manifested by red vascular papules or nodules.

Viral

Individuals with chronic steroid use are also at higher risk for developing viral infections. They

are at increased risk to develop cutaneous or systemic infections with the common cutaneous viral pathogens as well as opportunistic infections. Localized skin diseases can be caused by HSV, varicella zoster, mulluscum contagiosum, and papillomavirus. Generalized skin diseases can be caused by measles, rubella, enteroviruses, parvovirus, HSV, togaviruses, flaviviruses, bunyaviruses, and arenaviruses. In this section, we will focus on viral cutaneous infections commonly seen in the immune-compromised secondary to corticosteroid use.

Herepes simplex virus and vericella zoster are commonly found in the immunocompetent and have higher incidences and severity of illnesses with increased risk for disseminated infections. Reactivation of latent viral infections occurs with immune suppression. Herpes simplex may present as localized lesions of herpes labialis and genitalis seen as chronic herpatic ulcers, verrucous tumors mimicking squamous cell carcinoma, and even skin infarction. Varicella zoseter lesions may present in milder forms as well as extensive zoster lesions with multi-dermatomal involvement depending on degree of immune suppression. Immunosuppression also puts one at higher risk for disseminated zoster infections as well as post herpatic neuralgia.

Molluscum contangiosum is sexually transmitted as well as via other means of skin contact. Lesions appear as skin-colored or erythematus umbilicated papules. It can have widespread disease that is resistant to treatment. This is commonly seen in HIV patients as well steroid dependent patients.

Cytomegalovirus (CMV) can cause diseases involving multiple organ systems. Various skin lesions have also been seen with CMV infection secondary to immune suppression. Cutaneous lesions can present as hyperpigmented nodules, plaques, ulcers, a maculopapular rash, or vesicles. It can involve skin mucosa of the oropharynx or anal mucosa.

Human papilloma virus (HPV) can cause warts on extremities and genitals. In the immunocompromised, warts may be multiple, and verrucous, either causing or mimicking a squamous cell carcinoma. Lesions can be reactivated with

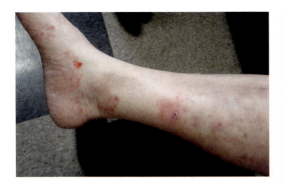

Fig. 9.6 Tinea in cognito treated with topical and intralesional corticosteroids for 6 months and now with extensive tinea and majocchi's granulomas of foot, ankle, and lower leg. KOH was positive and excellent response to 1 month of oral terbinafine

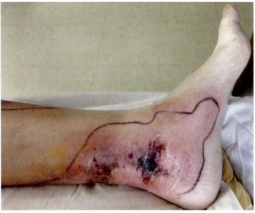

Fig. 9.7 This renal transplant patient had his systemic corticosteroids increased to treat what was thought to be a vasculitis over his medial maleolus. Erythema and pectechia are seen surrounding a gangrenous area covered by a hemorrhagic crust. Peripheral desquamation is also seen. The skin biopsy and culture showed Cryptococcus, and the systemic corticosteroids which appeared to worsen the condition were decreased

topical or systemic steroid use. Genital warts have been reported during topical steroid treatment for conditions such as genital lichen sclerosis et atrophicus.

Fungal

Incidences of cutaneous and systemic fungal infections have increased with increased use of immunosuppressive treatments. Corticosteroid use, whether by weakening skin integrity or by weakening T cell lymphocyte mediated immunity, predispose to fungal skin infections such as various opportunistic infections with candida, aspergillus, and cryptococcus, as well as primary pathogens such as histoplasma, coccidioides, and strangyloides.

Tinea incognito, seen in Fig. 9.6, is a dermatophytoses with different appearance from typical presentation due to use of systemic or topical corticosteroids. Dermatophytoses can be caused by fungi in the genera Microsporum, Epidermophyton, and Trichophyton. These organisms invade and colonize keratinized tissue of skin, nails, and hair. It usually presents as prurtic, erythematus inflammatory lesions in a ring-like format with inflammation worse at the outer ring. Due to the inflammation caused by these infections, lesions can be wrongly treated with topical steroids. The steroids initially may decrease the inflammation, however, with time they will cause extension of the infection. Deep Majocchi granulomas appear with time. It can mimic common skin conditions such as lupus erythematosus, rosacea, psoriasis, or eczema. It usually involves trunk and face, however it may occur in any area that topical corticosteroids are used.

Candidiasis is common. It can occur secondary to topical steroid application as well as inhaled and systemic corticosteroids. C. albicans is most commonly isolated, followed by C. neoformis. Infection can be localized to skin manifesting as an erythematous rash or can be a cutaneous spread of disseminated disease characterized by various morphology such as subcutaneous nodules, pustules, ulcerations, or intradermal bullae. Thrush secondary to inhaled steroids is commonly seen.

Cryptococcus, seen in Fig. 9.7, is another opportunistic infection commonly seen in various immunocompromised states. Skin lesions can present as subcutaneous nodules, ulcers, or pustules. Cutaneous lesions may be present isolated, however they can also be signs of disseminated disease. Biopsy and culture is usually required to make definitive diagnosis.

Aspregillus infection is usually systemic, involving multiple organ systems. A small percentage of immunocompromised people may

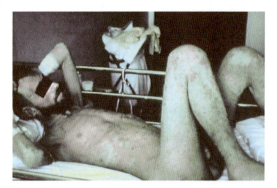

Fig. 9.8 This AIDS patient was treated for weeks with extensive topical corticosteroids, which seemed to only worsen his condition. He was being treated for psoriasis. He is covered in a thick adherent scale. A potassium hydroxide preparation of the scale revealed scabies and he slowly responded to anti-scabetic therapy

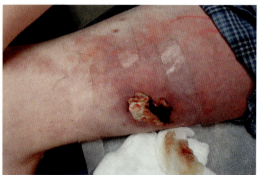

Fig. 9.9 Cutaneous histoplasmosis with extensive area of erythema becoming more violaceous as the area of necrosis and then full-thickness skin loss to muscle is approached. The patient had been on systemic corticosteroids for rehumatoid arthritis for over three decades. Initial biopsies were compatible with pyoderma gangrenosum and for over 6 months increasing predisone was given. The erythema improved but then worsened as full-thickness skin necrosis developed. Repeat biopsies with one for culture and one for histopathology were positive for cryptococcus neoformans. Urine and serum antigen were found to be positive for the same organism. Complete resolution with scar occurred with prolonged (1 year) systemic anti-fungal therapy

have cutaneous involvement. Cutaneous infections may present as nodules, papules, or plaques. It may also have ulcerations and abscesses and occasionally resemble bacterial cellulites.

Other conditions such as Scabies incognito, Pityrosporum folliculitis, and Coccidioides immitis have also been reported. There is report of scabies converting to Norwegian scabies, shown in Fig. 9.8, with the application of topical corticosteroids. Pityrosporum folliculitis can present with pruritic papules and pustules, which may be confused with steroid acne; however KOH reveals budding yeast cells with histology showing budding yeast in follicles. Coccidioides immitis may present as solitary verrucous plaque or nodules.

Cancer

Several skin malignancies such as Kaposi sarcoma, which are common in immunocompromised state secondary to HIV and chemotherapy, have been reported in patients with immunocompromise secondary to steroid use.

Conclusion

There are some general rules to be followed regarding use of topical steroids. Use the lowest potency that is effective. Use the topical steroid for shortest amount of time that is

necessary. Use the mildest potency possible on the face, genitalia, and intertriginous areas. Topical steroids are divided into seven groups depending on potency, with group 1 the most potent and group 7 the least potent. As a general rule, group 1 should be used for no longer than 2 weeks daily without a 1 week rest, or start it on a Monday–Wednesday–Friday schedule. Not only are there concerns about topical side effects detailed earlier in this chapter, but systemic side effects with suppression of the adrenal-pituitary axis, diabetes mellitus, and hypertension can occur among other side effects.

Clobetasol cream and ointment is the topical I use from the super-potent group. There is a midrange group of which triamcinilone cream and ointment are my choices. There is a mild-potency group which includes Cloderm, Locoid cream and lotion, and Desowen cream and ointment. Hydrocortisone is the mildest potency and is available over the counter in 1 and 2.5 % cream and ointment.

After prolonged use of the more potent groups, it may be necessary to titrate down to the lower groups to get control of the disease you want with the mildest therapeutic regimen possible.

The following Fig. 9.9 indicates some important points about corticosteroid patients. Remember that the disease may be rare since the immune status is so fundamentally altered. The disease is often extensive and sampling error when a biopsy is done is a common problem. When in doubt, repeat the biopsy. Finally, do not confuse a good response with diagnosis since the profound anti-inflammatory effect of corticosteroids can make virtually any disease look better at first. If the disease first improves and then worsens, the biopsy should be repeated—at multiple sites is always a good idea. Often the biopsy should be done at the active border and at the more involved interior of the area in question. Failure to get the correct diagnosis is always a hazard in this group of patients.

Suggested Reading

Ference JD, Last AR. Choosing topical corticosteroids. Am Fam Physician. 2009;79(2):135–40.

Fisher DA. Adverse effects of topical corticosteroid use. West J Med. 1995;162(2):123–6.

Hengge UR, Ruzicka T, Schwartz RA, Cork MJ. Adverse effects of topical glucocorticosteroids. J Am Acad Dermatol. 2006;54(1):1–15; quiz 16–8.

Morman MR. Possible side effects of topical steroids. Am Fam Physician. 1981;23(2):171–4.

Torres MJ, Canto G. Hypersensitivity reactions to corticosteroids. Curr Opin Allergy Clin Immunol. 2010;10(4):273–9.

Cutaneous Reactions to Tyrosine Kinase Inhibitors

10

Barbara Melosky

Abstract

Tyrosine kinase inhibitors (TKIs) are a new and unique class of orally administered, small- molecule therapeutics that have found their way into the standard of care treatment in almost all types of malignancy. The number of TKIs being developed and the number of indications for which they are being tested and approved is growing exponentially. As promising as TKIs are in helping patients avoid some of the side effects of traditional cytotoxic chemotherapy, they do come with a variety of cutaneous side effects. These are unique and variable and include skin rashes of many different types and severities, dry skin, hand–foot syndrome, pruritus, ocular, and hair and nail changes.

As patient survival is often directly correlated with successful therapeutic drug delivery, the management of TKI-induced skin diseases is critical. Making a correct clinical diagnosis of a TKI side effect ensures proper treatment and may avoid discontinuation or reduction of the medication.

TKIs can be grouped into three main classes based on the molecular pathway inhibited. These include (1) EGFR and the HER family inhibitors; (2) VEGF/PDGF/mixed inhibitors and (3) other inhibitors, including the BCR-ABL c-KIT and RET inhibitors. Characteristic skin conditions are associated with each of these classes of TKIs, which are described along with management strategies.

The key to successful management is clinician and patient education. Several general principals need to be emphasized: TKI-induced skin rashes are inflammatory in nature and not contagious; patients treated with TKIs should be instructed to use an alcohol-free emollient cream applied

B. Melosky, MD, FRCPC
Division of Medical Oncology, British Columbia
Cancer Agency Vancouver, 600 10th Ave W,
Vancouver, BC V5Z 4E6, Canada
e-mail: bmelosky@bccancer.bc.ca

J.C. Hall (ed.), *Skin Diseases in the Immunocompromised*,
DOI 10.1007/978-1-4471-6479-1_10, © Springer-Verlag London 2014

twice daily, preferably to their entire body; patients should avoid sun exposure and use protective clothing and broad spectrum UVA/UVB sunscreen. Care should be taken when treating cutaneous manifestations, as the wrong treatment can exacerbate the side effects.

Keywords

Tyrosine kinase inhibitor • TKI • Cutaneous manifestations • Skin rash • Epidermal growth factor receptor • Adverse event • Hand–foot syndrome • Vascular endothelial growth factor

Introduction

Tyrosine kinase inhibitors (TKIs) are targeted therapeutics used to treat a range of diseases and disorders, primarily cancers. This unique class of orally administered, small-molecule therapeutics has found their way into the standard of care treatment in almost all types of malignancy. TKIs may help patients avoid some of the side effects of traditional cytotoxic chemotherapy, where toxicities usually involve bone marrow stem cell involvement. However, as promising as the TKIs are, they do come with a variety of side effects which may sometimes be severe and life threatening.

TKI-related skin diseases, which usually manifest as rashes or dry skin, may seem minor in comparison to other TKI-related side effects. As with all cancer treatments, education for both the physician and patient is important, as often patient survival is directly correlated with successful therapeutic drug delivery. Although the exact pathophysiology of many of these skin manifestations remains vague or unknown, successful identification and management of these cutaneous side effects is important to ensure an adequate quality of life and treatment compliance for these patients. Making a correct clinical diagnosis of a TKI side effect ensures proper treatment, and may avoid discontinuation or reduction of the drug.

The number of TKIs being developed and the number of indications for which they are being tested and approved is growing exponentially. The purpose of this chapter is to describe the TKIs used in oncology with an emphasis on epidermal growth factor receptor (EGFR) family

and vascular endothelial growth factor (VEGFR) inhibition, to examine the cutaneous manifestations of TKIs, and discuss management strategies for patients experiencing TKI-related skin toxicities. This chapter does not attempt to review the efficacy of these different agents, which are discussed elsewhere.

Understanding Tyrosine Kinase Inhibitors (TKIS)

Kinases are intercellular enzymes that play important roles in cell development and have been implicated in cancer development and growth. Tyrosine kinases are an important kinase subgroup that specifically transfers a phosphate group from the coenzyme adenosine-5′-triphosphate (ATP) to tyrosine residues in cellular proteins.

The phosphorylation of cellular proteins by kinases is an important communication mechanism within a cell. Messages are conveyed via precise and sequential series of kinase reactions in a signal transduction cascade, and this can regulate cellular activities and functions including cell growth and mitosis. Tyrosine kinases can sometimes function as "on" or "off" switches; mutations can cause tyrosine kinases to become stuck in either the "on" or "off" position, which often causes upregulated cell signaling or activity leading to uncontrolled cell growth. This dysregulation of the cell communication machinery is often a necessary step in the development of cancer. Therefore, inhibiting this communication cascade with a TKI would be desirable as it may effectively inhibit certain types of cancers.

Tyrosine kinase inhibitors represent a relatively new therapeutic class. The concept of tyrosine kinase inhibition was first described in 1988, with the discovery of a small molecular weight molecule that could inhibit tyrosine phosphorylation. This first TKI specifically inhibited the epidermal growth factor receptor (EGFR) cascade. Following this, it was shown that it was possible to synthesize TKIs that could discriminate between closely related proteins such as EGFR and Human Epidermal Growth Factor Receptor 2 (HER2). This important discovery illustrates how the concept of targeted therapy emerged, and how TKIs can be grouped into classes based on their molecular targets. As one can imagine, small changes to the molecular structure of this class of molecule may change the target of the inhibitor as well as the side effect profile. For this reason, scientists are focusing on developing new and improved TKIs as therapies for a variety of malignancies.

TKIs may have a wide range of side effects which can include almost any organ system. Some of these side effects can be severe and life-threatening and may include hematologic toxicities such as venous thromboembolic events, anemia, infection and clotting issues, liver toxicity, cognitive effects, loss of fertility, gastric issues, kidney changes, cardiac problems, seizures, eyesight changes, muscle pain, and blood sugar issues. Different TKI's may differ in the types and the severity of these side effects.

Some tyrosine kinase inhibitors work on cell surface receptors while other tyrosine kinase inhibitors work on targeted pathways deep within a cell. Many TKIs inhibit multiple pathways through mixed inhibition, which can make it difficult to determine which specific pathway is associated with a certain toxicity. A successful treatment strategy is more likely to fail if the pathway responsible cannot be identified.

The cutaneous side effects of TKIs were first observed during the randomized clinical trials (RCT) that were conducted to test the efficacy of EGFR-inhibiting TKIs. As the purpose of these RCTs was to determine drug efficacy, the primary endpoint was patient survival and response. As a result, the cutaneous side effects observed were often poorly documented, and treatment was often vaguely described. In addition, there were difficulties in interpreting the cutaneous side effects observed in these trials because the rash was graded according to the National Cancer Institute Common Toxicity Criteria (NCI CTC) version 2.0 and Common Terminology Criteria for Adverse Events v3.0. The grading systems used were designed for medications and diseases before the time of targeted therapy, and may not have accurately reflected the clinical situation. As an example, a grading scale based on the percentage of body skin involvement could not accurately document the severity of a rash that manifests on the face of a patient. Although severe (grade III), the rash may be recorded by that system as grade I as only 10 % of the body skin surface is affected.

The Concept of Targeted Therapy: TKI Targets, Examples, and Indications

The TKI field is expanding exponentially, with a constant evolution in the numbers and types of pharmaceutical TKI's being developed and approved. Currently, hundreds of clinical trials featuring TKIs are being conducted. Many new TKIs will continue to emerge, and the number of TKIs in use and the numbers of diseases for which they are indicated will continue to expand. As the pathways of tumorigenesis are shared, a specific TKI may be used to treat more than one type of malignancy, which complicates the landscape still further.

For the purposes of exploring the cutaneous side effects, in this article TKIs are grouped into three main classes based on the molecular pathway inhibited. These include (1) EGFR and the HER family inhibitors; (2) VEGF/PDGF/mixed inhibitors and (3) other inhibitors, including the BCR-ABL, c-KIT and RET inhibitors. There are characteristic skin conditions associated with each of these classes, described in more detail in the following sections. The different TKIs described in this chapter are not meant to be a comprehensive list, but are examples to illustrate the range of skin conditions resulting from their use.

Table 10.1 Example of TKIs to be discussed and their current indications

Molecular pathway inhibited	Example of target: TKI	Current indication
EGFR/HER family	EGFR/HER 1: gefitinib, erlotinib	Non small cell lung cancer (NSCLC)
	EGFR/HER1, HER2, HER3. HER 4: afatinib	Non small cell lung cancer
	HER2: lapatinib	Breast cancer
VEGF/PDGF/Mixed inhibitors	Sunitunib, sorafinib, pazopanib, axitinib	Renal, hepatocellular, neuroendocrine carcinoma
	Regorafinib	Colorectal carcinoma
Other: BRAF, BCR-ABL, c-KIT, ALK, RET	BRAF: vemurafenib	Melanoma
	RET: vandetanib	Medullary thyroid carcinoma
	Others:	
	BCR-ABL: imatinib, nilotinib, dasatinib	Chronic myelocytic leukemia (CML)
	c-KIT: imatinib	Gastrointestinal stromal tumors (GISTs)
	Anaplastic lymphoma kinase: crizotinib	Non small cell lung cancer

Table 10.1 illustrates the three classes of TKIs discussed in this chapter. This table includes the cellular molecular pathways that are inhibited, specific molecular targets (if known), some examples of currently approved tyrosine kinase inhibitors, and current indications for which some of these inhibitors are used. This table is not intended to be conclusive, and is certain to change as more TKIs and indications are approved in the future.

Class 1: Epidermal Growth Factor Receptor and the HER Family Inhibitors

The HER (Human Epidermal Growth Factor) receptor family contains four members: EGFR (otherwise known as HER1), HER2, HER3, and HER4. The first-generation of EGFR inhibitor TKI's such as gefitinib and erlotinib, are very specific, blocking only HER1, whereas second-generation EGFR inhibitor TKI's such as afatinib, block several members of this family. The inhibitors in this class have shown efficacy against malignancies in tissues originating from the epidermis, lung, and breast as well as pancreatic malignancies. Future trials may show these inhibitors to be efficacious in other epidermal-derived malignancies as well.

EGFR is expressed in the basal layer of the epidermis, and its roles include stimulation of epidermal growth, inhibition of differentiation, and acceleration of wound healing. As the name of this receptor is "epidermal," it is no surprise that inhibitor toxicity may include the epidermis. Pathophysiological effects of EGFR inhibition include impaired growth and migration of keratinocytes, and the expression of inflammatory chemokines by these cells, which results in inflammatory cell recruitment. Not surprisingly, a histologic analysis demonstrates a mixed inflammatory infiltrate in the upper areas of the skin. This inflammation and subsequent cutaneous injury accounts for many of the symptoms observed in patients being treated with this class of TKI, including tenderness, papulopustules, and periungual inflammation.

Description of the Most Significant Dermatological Toxicities Observed

The most significant dermatological toxicities on epidermal-derived tissue observed with this class of TKIs are severe rashes, and can include a papulopustular eruption, dry skin, pruritus, and ocular and nail changes. The rash is very acne-like in appearance, and is accurately described as a papulopustular eruption. Other descriptions include the terms acneiform skin reaction, acneiform rash, acneiform follicular rash, acne-like

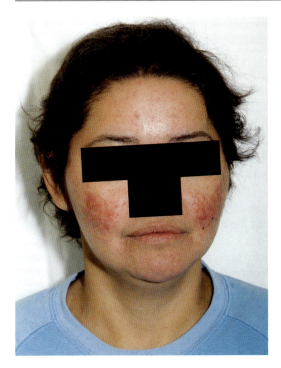

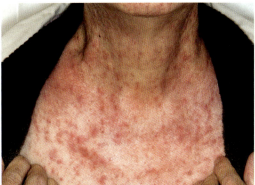

Fig. 10.2 A papulopustular eruption on the chest during treatment with erlotinib, an EGFR TKI, in addition to chemotherapy for a pancreatic malignancy. Because the recommended TKI dose in this setting is less than for NSCLC, the rash that is observed is usually milder in severity (Photo: ©BC Cancer Agency)

Fig. 10.1 A grade II papulopustular eruption on the face during treatment with erlotinib, an EGFR TKI, for stage IV non-small cell lung cancer. Note that the papulopustular eruption on her facial cheeks appears bilaterally. A differential diagnosis may include systemic lupus erythematosus (Photo: ©BC Cancer Agency)

rash, maculopapular skin rash, and amonomorphic pustular lesions. The rash may be triggered by sun exposure.

The EGFR-TKI-induced rash most often appears on the face and chest, but can be more widespread. Figures 10.1 and 10.2 show examples of how the rash manifests during the first few weeks of therapy. Figure 10.1 shows an example of a patient with a bilateral papulopustular eruption on her face. This patient with stage IV non-small cell lung cancer (NSCLC) was being treated with erlotinib third line therapy. The rash occurred after 14 days of treatment, at which time her chest X-ray showed an improvement, indicating that therapy was efficacious. Figure 10.2 shows a patient experiencing a papulopustular eruption on his chest. This patient was being treated with erlotinib in addition to chemotherapy for a pancreatic malignancy. Because the recommended TKI dose in this setting is less than

for NSCLC, the rash that is observed is usually milder in severity than in a lung cancer setting.

There are several phases to the cutaneous manifestations. In the first week of TKI treatment, patients often experience sensory disturbances, erythema, and edema. In the second week of TKI treatment, patients experience papulopustular eruptions, followed by crusting in week 4. In the 4–6 weeks following, a background of erythema and dry skin can be seen in areas previously affected by the papulopustular eruption.

In addition to the skin rash, other cutaneous manifestations may be observed. These include pruritus and paronychial inflammation associated with the lateral nail folds of the toes and fingers, and after a longer period of treatment, paronychia infections may become a concern.

Figures 10.3 and 10.4 show the finger and toes of a patient with stage IV NSCLC treated with afatinib. The finger (Fig. 10.3) shows a splinter hemorrhage which can be very annoying and painful for the patient. Although the toes in Fig. 10.4 look quite severely involved, this patient was relatively asymptomatic in terms of her feet; most patients have more severe manifestations.

Management Recommendations for Skin Rash

Patient education is a very important aspect of management, and several important points need to be communicated and emphasized. First of all,

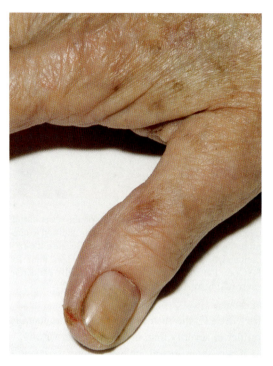

Fig. 10.3 A spinter hemorrhage on the hand of a patient treated with afatinib, a second-generation EGFR TKI, for stage IV non-small cell lung cancer. This would be classified as a potential side effect. These are treated with liquid bandage solution (Photo: ©BC Cancer Agency)

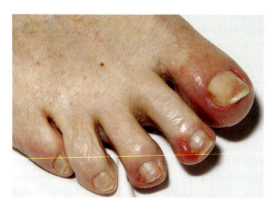

Fig. 10.4 Toes of the patient in Fig. 10.3 treated with afatinib, a second-generation EGFR TKI, for stage IV non-small cell lung cancer. Although the toes look quite severely involved, this patient was relatively asymptomatic in terms of the feet (Photo: ©BC Cancer Agency)

the rash is not contagious; the skin toxicity is not infectious, but inflammatory. Secondly, this skin rash is not acne, and so patients should be strongly discouraged from treating the rash with

over-the-counter acne medications, as acne medication is very drying and will exacerbate the pruritus. Third, as dry skin is almost universally experienced by patients taking this medication, they should be instructed to use an alcohol-free emollient cream applied twice daily, preferably to their entire body. Finally, since sun exposure may aggravate the pruritus, patients are advised to avoid sun exposure, and a broad spectrum sunscreen is strongly recommended.

The specific treatment algorithms for rashes caused by EGFR inhibitors vary widely throughout the different centers that use these agents in their clinics. Nonetheless, some basic principles may apply to all situations. Management guidelines utilized in the BC Cancer Agency Oncology Department (Table 10.2) are shown and discussed in further detail in the text below.

Mild reactions (NCI-CTC grade 1) are generally localized with no associated physical symptoms. Treatment options include topical low-medium potency corticosteroids. Other options include the addition of clindamycin 1 % gel to hydrocortisone 1 %, and the use of oral semisynthetic tetracyclines (i.e., doxycycline or minocycline). The EGFR inhibitor should be continued while the rash is being treated.

Moderate reactions (NCI-CTC grade 2) are more disseminated and can include symptoms such as tenderness or pruritus. The recommended treatment is hydrocortisone 1 % or 2.5 % cream ± clindamycin 1 % cream, as well as a 4-week course of an oral tetracycline antibiotic, such as doxycycline 100 mg or minocycline 100 mg twice daily. Minocycline can cause nausea in a small percentage of patients, and reduction to 100 mg daily may be better tolerated. As the rash from EGFR TKI may wax and wane, the treatment may need to be repeated at several intervals.

Severe reactions (NCI-CTC grade 3) are generalized, with major symptoms profoundly affecting activities of daily living. Though histological findings suggest that the papulopustular eruption has an inflammatory component, the use of topical oral corticosteroids is based on empirical data. A temporary 7- to 10-day discontinuation of the TKI involved is recommended, with subsequent reintroduction at a lower dose according to the

Table 10.2 BCCA guidelines for EGFR inhibitors rash

Grade	Toxicity	EGFR inhibitor
1	Macular or papular eruption or erythema with no associated symptoms	Maintain dose level of TKI Consider clindamycin 2 % and hydrocortisone 1 % in a lotion to be applied topically BID as needed
2	Macular or papulopustular eruption or erythema with pruritus or other symptoms that are tolerable or interfere with daily life	Maintain dose level of TKI Consider clindamycin 2 % and hydrocortisone 1 % in a lotion to be applied topically BID as needed + Minocycline 100 mg PO BID for 1–2 weeks or longer as needed
3	Severe, generalized erythroderma or macular, papular or vesicular eruption	Withhold EGFR TKI for 10–14 days When improvement to Grade 2 or less, continue at 50 % of original dose If toxicities do not worsen, escalate by 25 % increments of original dose until starting dose is reached If no improvement, discontinue Continue treatment with clindamycin 2 % and hydrocortisone 1 % in a lotion to be applied topically BID as needed + Minocycline 100 mg PO BID for 1–2 weeks or longer as needed
4	Generalized exfoliative, ulcerative or blistering skin toxicity	Discontinue treatment

Because early treatment of rash can prevent symptoms from becoming worse, clinicians are advised to assess patients weekly, and intervene when the first symptoms of rash appear

product monograph. Treatment with both a steroid cream and oral tetracycline as per moderate rash is encouraged during the interruption period. When treatment is reintroduced, dose escalation of the TKI being used is often possible.

Some guidelines, including the BCCA guidelines, include drug dose reduction to alleviate severe drug reactions. While side effects of the TKIs are often unpleasant, effort must be made to maintain patients on their cancer therapies. If a TKI is administered in only one dose, for example in the case of gefitinib, switching the patient to another TKI that has more flexible dosing is strongly recommended.

Management Recommendations for Rashes on the Scalp

A scalp rash may be successfully treated with the basic principles above, however a gel can be formulated because cream and lotion treatment can be unappealing in the hair or hairline area of the neck. As well, patients can often develop lesions and plaques on the scalp, which can be treated with topical clindamycin 2 % plus triamcinolone acetonide 0.1 % in equal parts of propylene glycol and water until resolution.

Management of Dermatological Toxicities Other Than Rash: Nail Changes, Dry Skin, Scaling and Hyperkeratosis, Eyelash Growth

Due to the lower frequency and visibility of additional toxicities when compared to rash, management recommendations are limited. Nail changes are usually mild, but like the rash, may be severe and symptomatic. Patients with splinter hemorrhages can be treated with liquid bandage. Oral doxycycline may be effective along with topical corticosteroids but in resistant cases, intralesional corticosteroid injections or removal of the nail plate may be beneficial.

As previously mentioned, dry skin in the trunk and extremities is very common in patients being treated with EGFR TKIs. Fragrance-free creams and ointments are recommended over lotions, which may contain alcohol. For scaling and hyperkeratosis, ammonium lactate and urea-containing preparations are also useful, but they should be used with care because of greater skin sensitivity in these patients.

Eyelash growth can be seen when epidermal growth factors are given for a prolonged period of time. Cutting the eyelashes intermittently to a shorter length can add to patient comfort. With prolonged use of EGFR TKIs, coarseness of the hair and central balding can also occur.

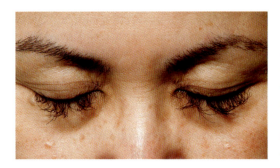

Fig. 10.5 TKI-induced eyelash growth in a patient treated with erlotinib, an EGFR TKI, for stage IV non-small cell lung cancer. This patient was treated with erlotinib for more than 3 years, followed with a prolonged course of afatinib, a second-generation EGFR TKI, with excellent response (Photo: ©BC Cancer Agency)

Figure 10.5 shows a patient with EGFR inhibitor-induced eyelash growth, treated with erlotinib for stage IV NSCLC adenocarcinoma. The patient was treated with erlotinib for over 3 years, and then was subsequently treated with a prolonged course of afatinib with an excellent response.

Relationship Between Toxicity of Rash and Efficacy in Patient Outcome

Interestingly, multiple trials of EGFR inhibitors have prospectively illustrated that toxicity may actually be related to the efficacy of the therapeutic. Patients who experienced the worse grade of rash had the greater response rates in their tumors and the longest survival while on therapy.

The foregoing finding is difficult to understand and explain. Is it just a correlative relationship indicating a good host immune system? Or is there a direct relationship between the EGFR receptor in the host's skin and the tumor? If the latter, then is prophylactic treatment, with rash incidence being delayed and decreased, safe? Is efficacy being sacrificed? The importance of this relationship is still evolving. This highlights the importance of correctly recognizing and treating the cutaneous side effects. By increasing patient tolerability the use of the TKI may be prolonged, leading to an improvement in patient outcomes such as survival.

Results are expected soon from the Pan-Canadian Trial NCT00473083: "*A Randomized Controlled Trial of Systemic and Topical*

Treatments for Rash Secondary to Erlotinib in Advanced Stage IIIB or IV Non-small cell lung cancer", in which patients starting an EGFR1 inhibitor were randomized to one of three arms for the management of their rash: (1) prophylactic minocycline for 4 weeks; (2) rash treatment according to grade; or (3) no treatment unless rash is severe. Primary outcomes include comparison of the groups for incidence of EGFR1 inhibitor-induced rash and to investigate if the rash caused by the EGFR1 inhibitor is self limiting. This ISO-patient trial is closed and outcomes are currently being analyzed.

In conclusion, tyrosine kinase inhibitors against the epidermal growth factor have become standard of care in cancers such as NSCLC. Skin toxicity is a major side effect to be expected and, indeed, may even be an indicator of therapeutic efficacy. Both physician and patient education are necessary to ensure compliance and proper drug delivery so that efficacy in terms of improvement in survival may be experienced.

Class 2: Vascular Endothelial Growth Factor Receptor/Platelet-Derived Growth Factor Receptor/Mixed Inhibitors

The vascular endothelial growth factor receptor (VEGFR) inhibitors, platelet-derived growth factor receptor (PDGFR) inhibitors and mixed inhibitors are classified in this second class of TKI inhibitors. These inhibitors are grouped in the same class together because most inhibit VEGFR and PDGRF in addition to other tyrosine kinases such as KIT, RET, etc. For this reason, these tyrosine kinases are known as "mixed", "dirty" or "multi-targeted." Examples of these inhibitors include the therapeutics sunitinib, sorafinib, pazopanib, and regorafinib.

For a more in-depth description of side effects and management strategies for VEGFRs, please refer to the excellent review by C. Kollmannsberger, et al. *Sunitinib therapy for metastatic renal cell carcinoma: recommendations for management of side effects*. The rest of this section addresses the cutaneous manifestations of these TKIs only.

The VEGFR pathway is a necessary pathway in normal physiology, regulating blood vessel formation and angiogenesis. During cancer development, tumors begin to express VEGFR when they reach a certain size, which then permits vessel growth into the tumor and the development of an independent blood supply. Thus, it is easy to conceptualize how anti-angiogenic strategies may be beneficial in many different tumors. TKIs that target the VEGFR are used to treat tumors such as renal, hepatocellular, neuroendocrine cancer and colorectal carcinoma. These cancers all share a similar characteristic: over-expression of the VEGF pathway.

As the name of this class of receptors includes "vascular," the side effect profile resulting from inhibition of this receptor can be predicted from the normal physiologic activity of this pathway. As VEGFRs are abundant in large blood vessels, the fact that inhibition of this pathway with a TKI leads to hypertension can be somewhat understood. It can also explain why many of this class can have severe side effects such as anemia, bruising, and immune deficiencies, as they involve central pathways necessary for cell survival and growth.

The mixed nature of these receptor inhibitors is reflected in a varied side effect profile. This makes it difficult to hypothesize the exact pathophysiology of the cutaneous effects and also makes it difficult to make accurate or effective treatment recommendations.

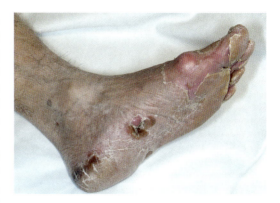

Fig. 10.6 Typical hand–foot syndrome resulting from sunitinib treatment. Feet are particularly affected as they are weight-bearing areas of the body; pathophysiology may involve capillary reconstruction in response to pressure (Photo: ©BC Cancer Agency)

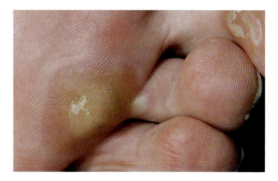

Fig. 10.7 Blister formation on the foot during therapy with sunitinib (Originally published as Fig. 2 in Kollmannsberger C, Soulieres D, Wong R, Scalera A, Gaspo R, Bjarnason G: Sunitinib therapy for metastatic renal cell carcinoma: recommendations for management of side effects. *Can Urol Assoc J*. 2007; 1(2 Suppl):S41–54. Photos courtesy of the Cleveland Clinic Taussig Cancer Institute)

Description of the Most Significant Dermatological Toxicities Observed

The most significant dermatological toxicities in patients taking TKls from this class include hand-foot syndrome (acral erythema), changes in hair color, skin rash, dry skin, skin discoloration, and subungual splinter hemorrhages. Skin toxicity typically occurs after 3–4 weeks of treatment.

Hand–Foot Syndrome

Hand–foot syndrome (also called acral erythema) is one of the more important toxicities that results from this TKI class, as it can be dose limiting, leading to a lower dose of the TKI administered

for treatment. The hand–foot syndrome presents as painful symmetric erythematous and edematous areas on the palms and soles. These effects are often preceded or accompanied by paresthesias, tingling, or numbness, and desquamation can also occur in severe cases. As well, painful hyperkeratotic areas on the pressure points surrounded by rings of erythematous and edematous lesions, and painful bullous lesions, blisters, or skin cracking can be observed. Figures 10.6, 10.7 and 10.8a, b illustrate some of the typical cutaneous toxicities on the feet of patients being treated with sunitinib. Figure 10.9 shows hand–foot syndrome in a patient treated with axitinib.

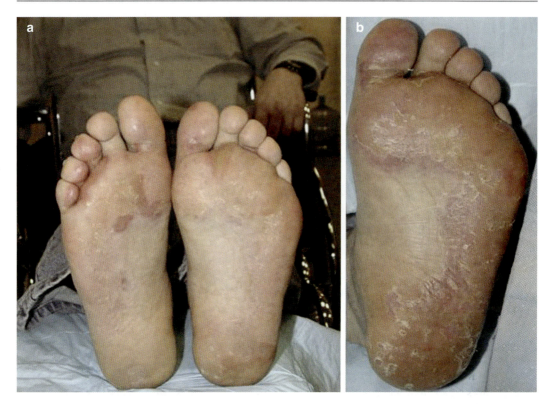

Figs. 10.8 (**a**, **b**) Hand–foot syndrome during sunitinib therapy. Image (**b**) shows the same left foot as in (**a**), but at a more advanced stage (Originally published as Fig. 1 in Kollmannsberger C, Soulieres D, Wong R, Scalera A, Gaspo R, Bjarnason G: Sunitinib therapy for metastatic renal cell carcinoma: recommendations for management of side effects. *Can Urol Assoc J*. 2007;1(2 Suppl):S41–54. Photos courtesy of the Cleveland Clinic Taussig Cancer Institute)

The hand-foot syndrome can resemble the more classic chemotherapy-induced hand–foot syndrome or palmar-plantar erythrodysesthesia that can arise with 5-fluorouracil, capecitabine, cytarabine, or doxorubicin. However, most patients with TKI-induced hand–foot syndrome have more localized and hyperkeratotic lesions that are distinct from classic chemotherapy-induced hand–foot syndrome.

Pre-existing hyperkeratosis on the sole of the feet seems to predispose patients treated with this second class of TKI, for painful soles, which have obvious negative impacts on mobility. In addition, patients may experience symptoms such as pain without any clinical findings.

The exact pathogenesis of TKI-induced hand–foot syndrome is still unknown. In mild grade 1 and 2 hand–foot syndromes, histologic

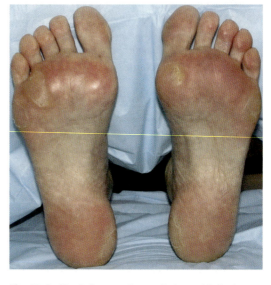

Fig. 10.9 Hand–foot syndrome during axitinib therapy (Photo courtesy of the Cleveland Clinic Taussig Cancer Institute)

changes to the endothelial cells in the dermis are observed. These changes are more pronounced in grade 3 hand-foot syndromes with peribullous lesions with vascular alteration, scattered keratinocyte necrosis, and intra-epidermal cleavage. One hypothesis for pathogenesis is that TKIs may damage the capillary endothelium, as both VEGFR and PDGFR are expressed in capillary vasculature. Frequent sites of impact (nails) or pressure (contact areas of the palms, soles) may possibly require continuous endothelial repair involving the VEGF receptor; VEGF pathway inhibition may cause abnormal small vessel repair in these areas, leading to the cutaneous manifestations of hand–foot syndrome.

Management Recommendations for Hand–Foot Syndrome

Management strategies for hand–foot syndrome include having a manicure and pedicure before treatment as a preventative measure. In more severe cases, TKI treatment interruptions or TKI dose reduction may be necessary, although this is discouraged from a therapeutic point of view. Patients should be advised to do the following:

- Use moisturizers, foot and hand-care products such as gel pad inserts and cotton gloves, and medication for pain management as required.
- Apply creams containing lanolin or urea to the hands and feet liberally and often, when therapy begins.
- Apply a sunscreen with a sun protection factor (SPF) of at least 30 to all exposed areas of the body.
- Decrease pressure on affected areas, staying off the feet when possible and avoiding friction or pressure to the hands.
- During treatment, shock absorbers may be used to relieve painful pressure points, and sandals seem to be helpful for some patients.
- Avoid tight-fitting shoes or rubbing pressure on the hands and feet, such as that caused by heavy activity, and avoid tight-fitting jewelry.

- Avoid shaving off blisters because this will cause the condition to worsen.
- Wear loose cotton clothes.
- Avoid using hot water to clean hands and feet. Instead use lukewarm water, and gently pat dry

Skin Rash

In patients taking VEGFR or PDGFR inhibitors, generalized erythema, maculopapular or seborrheic dermatitis-like rashes may appear. Although VEGFR/PDGFR TKI-induced rashes may be severe, they are much less severe or incidence than the previously discussed EGFR TKI-induced rashes. These rashes rarely require dose reduction and the symptoms tend to decrease over time.

Patients taking this second class should be advised to use moisturizing skin lotions or creams often, particularly after showers or before bedtime. If the skin is very dry, then urea-containing lotions and the use of colloidal oatmeal lotions may help to control TKI-associated skin rashes. In severe cases, steroid creams may be beneficial. In addition, patients should avoid hot showers, use sun protection, and wear loose-fitting cotton clothes.

Changes in Skin or Hair Color

Yellow discoloration of the skin or hair commonly occur in approximately 30 % of patients being treated with sunitinib and pazopanib. Yellow discoloration of the urine has been observed in conjunction with skin discoloration because of excretion of the drug and its metabolites. Although hair depigmentation occurs after 5–6 weeks of treatment, or as early as 2–3 weeks in facial hair, this effect is reversible as early as 2–3 weeks after treatment is discontinued. Figure 10.10 shows how successions of depigmented and normally pigmented bands of hair correlate with on and off periods of treatment.

Sunitinib-induced hair depigmentation is thought to be caused by blockade of c-KIT signalling and other receptors, which are thought to be involved in both melanocyte proliferation or differentiation, and proper pigment production.

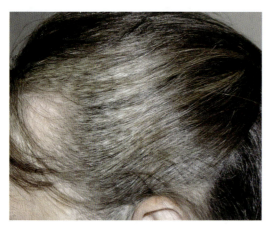

Fig. 10.10 Hair depigmentation during sunitinib therapy. This is reversible when treatment is discontinued (Originally published as Fig. 3 in Kollmannsberger C, Soulieres D, Wong R, Scalera A, Gaspo R, Bjarnason G: Sunitinib therapy for metastatic renal cell carcinoma: recommendations for management of side effects. *Can Urol Assoc J.* 2007; 1(2 Suppl):S41–54. Photos courtesy of Cleveland Clinic Taussig Cancer Institute)

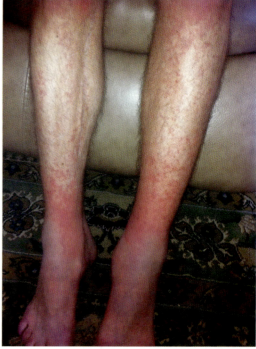

Fig. 10.11 Skin rash during BRAF inhibitor therapy (Photo courtesy of Alberta Health Services)

Class 3: Other Inhibitors: BRAF, BCR-ABL, C-KIT, ALK, RET

Other inhibitors include those that inhibit the BRAF, BCR-ABL, c-KIT, ALK, and RET pathways. These TKIs also have cutaneous manifestations, but are generally lower in incidence and severity than those targeting EGFR and VEGFR. Examples of this class of inhibitors include vemurafenib (BRAF), imatinib, nilotinib, dasatinib (BCR-ABL), imatinib (c-KIT), crizotinib (Anaplastic Lymphoma Kinase), and vandetanib (RET). These inhibitors will only be discussed briefly in this chapter.

BRAF: Class 1 RAF Inhibitors

BRAF TKI inhibition has become standard of care in cutaneous malignant melanoma. RAF inhibitors include the selective oral BRAF inhibitor vemurafenib, which was approved by the Food and Drug Administration (FDA) in August 2011 for the treatment of melanoma with a V600E BRAF mutation. BRAF-TKIs have some very interesting side effects, with cutaneous side effects being the most significant toxicity reported.

Mutations in BRAF (v-raf murine sarcoma viral oncogene homolog Bl) are thought to activate the mitogen activated signaling pathway (MAPK). This is recognized as another important signalling pathway that when activated results in cell growth and resistance to cell death. In this setting, BRAF inhibitors can be very efficacious.

The typical BRAF TKI-induced rash is described as a follicular hyperkeratotic rash over the ventral and dorsal midline and legs, as shown in Fig. 10.11. Verrucous hyperkeratotic lesions can be observed with keratosis pilaris at typical sites of the lateral aspects of the upper and lower limbs.

Other side effects of BRAF TKIs include cutaneous squamous cell carcinoma, which is reported in approximately 25 % of patients, and new primary melanomas reported in 2 % of patients. The majority of the excised lesions are classified as keratoacanthoma subtype or mixed keratoacanthoma subtype. Cases occur early in treatment, with a median time to first appearance of 7–8 weeks. Potential risk factors for squamous cell carcinoma include an age of over 65 years,

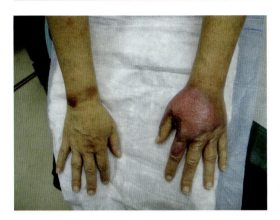

Fig. 10.12 Photosensitivity reaction during BRAF inhibitor therapy. Patient's left hand was exposed to sun while driving a car (Photo courtesy of Alberta Health Services)

prior skin cancer, mutations in the RAS gene, and chronic sun exposure. The pathogenesis of the squamous carcinoma is not fully understood but felt to be related to a paradoxical activation of the MAPK signaling pathway.

Management of BRAF Skin Rash

Dermatologic evaluations should be conducted prior to, and regularly during, treatment with vemurafenib. Monitoring for cutaneous squamous cell carcinoma and for new primary melanomas should continue for 6 months following discontinuation of the TKI. Patients presenting with cutaneous squamous cell carcinoma should have suspicious skin lesions excised, however TKI treatment interruption and/or dosage adjustment is not required in these cases.

Mild to severe photosensitivity has been reported in patients treated with RAF TKIs, including painful blistering in some cases. Photosensitivity is considered preventable in most patients by minimizing or avoiding sun exposure. Figure 10.12 shows an example of photosensitivity; this patient has blistering on the hand exposed to sunlight through the driver-side window. Dose modification is suggested for intolerable grade 2 or greater events.

RET Inhibitors

RET (rearranged during transfection) is a transmembrane tyrosine kinase expressed in the central and peripheral nervous system and in neural crest-derived cells. RET is involved in the development of enteric nervous system and renal organogenesis during embryonic life. Activating point mutations in the cysteine-rich area or the kinase domain of RET cause multiple endocrine neoplasia type 2 (MEN2), a group of familial cancer syndromes characterized by medullary thyroid carcinoma and pheochromocytoma. Rearranged forms of RET (termed RET/PTC) are detected in the majority of papillary thyroid carcinomas (PTC).

TKIs used to inhibit RET include vandetanib, a multitargeted inhibitor of several tyrosine kinases including RET, VEGFR and EGFR. In 28–71 % of patients treated with vandetanib, skin reactions with acneiform eruption, dry skin, pruritus, photosensitivity, or hand–foot skin reaction have been reported. Severe side effects are rare, affecting only 3–6 % of patients. In addition, paronychia, genital eruptions resembling intertrigo, photodistributed lichenoid drug eruption, and subacute cutaneous lupus erythematosus also have been reported. As with other TKIs, patients treated with vandetanib should be counseled to wear sunscreen and protective clothing when exposed to the sun.

Conclusion

The field of tyrosine kinase inhibitors is expanding and changing on a rapid basis. Currently many TKIs are approved to treat a multitude of cancers and that list will continue to grow as discovery continues. As more is understood about the molecular mechanics of tyrosine kinase inhibitors, they will be refined to become more efficacious and the associated toxicities will be reduced. Targeted therapy for cancer has arrived and is being applied as standard of care to most malignancies.

The skin manifestations of these TKIs are unique and variable. As research in this area continues, the pathophysiology of cutaneous manifestations continues to be examined and understood, and management strategies for these side-effects will evolve and improve.

The key to successful management of the cutaneous side effects from TKIs is clinician and patient education. Although this chapter recommends some specific strategies, several general principals need to be emphasized to patients. These general principals include the following:

- Patients being treated with TKIs should be instructed to use an alcohol-free emollient cream applied twice daily, preferably to their entire body.
- Patients need to avoid sun exposure as much as possible. When outdoors, patients should use protective clothing and broad spectrum UVA/UVB sunscreen.
- Care should be taken when treating cutaneous manifestations, as the wrong treatment (for example, acne medications) can exacerbate the side effects.

Maintaining patients on a therapeutic dose of the TKI results in improved survival in many instances, and thus must be encouraged. The effective management of side effects is an essential part of helping patients to stay on therapy at doses that impact their survival outcome.

Acknowledgements B. Melosky would like to thank the following individuals for providing photos: Cameron Heryet from the BC Cancer Agency, Vancouver BC; Michael Smylie from the Cross Cancer Institute, Edmonton, Alberta; and Laura Wood from the Cleveland Clinic Taussig Cancer Institute, Cleveland, Ohio.

Barb Melosky would also like to sincerely thank Dr. Christian Kollmannsberger for providing photos and for his expertise and advice on VEGF-Rs.

Suggested Reading

Dummer R, Rinderknecht J, Goldinger SM. Ultraviolet A and photosensitivity during vemurafenib therapy. N Engl J Med. 2012;366(5):480–1. doi:10.1056/NEJMc1113752.

Giacchero D, Ramacciotti C, Arnault JP, Brassard M, Baudin E, Maksimovic L, et al. A new spectrum of skin toxic effects associated with the multikinase inhibitor vandetanib. Arch Dermatol. 2012;148(12):1418–20.

Hartmann JT, Haap M, Kopp HG, Lipp HP. Tyrosine kinase inhibitors – a review on pharmacology, metabolism and side effects. Curr Drug Metab. 2009;10(5):470–81.

Lacouture ME. Mechanisms of cutaneous toxicities to EGFR inhibitors. Nat Rev Cancer. 2006;6(10):803–12.

Lacouture ME, Melosky BL. Cutaneous reactions to anticancer agents targeting the epidermal growth factor receptor: a dermatology-oncology perspective. Skin Therapy Lett. 2007;12(6):1–5.

Robert C, Soria JC, Spatz A, Le Cesne A, Malka D, Pautier P, et al. Cutaneous side-effects of kinase inhibitors and blocking antibodies. Lancet Oncol. 2005;6(7):491–500.

Cutaneous Manifestations of Aging and Immunodeficiency

11

Robert A. Norman and Zachary Henry

Abstract

Aging is defined as a time-sequential deterioration of living things that is prompted by increased susceptibility to disease and adverse events, leading to loss of viability and physiologic functions. In simpler terms, aging is characterized by the individual's inability to respond in a useful way to stress. Perhaps the most vital physiological component a person has for surviving aging is their body's immune system. Along with the ability to clear antigens from the body, the immune system is equally important in keeping the body's own physiology in check by monitoring for reactions that may go awry and unchecked, leading to malignancies, or helping the body rebuild and reshape itself in the face of any stress. Decreased ability to cope with stressors expected to be handled by the immune system could support the notion that aging may itself be considered a disease state. Although aging is accompanied by a decline in normal immune function of the B and T cells, aging is not reflected in profound changes in one of the many variables used to assess immune status with respect to a specific disease such as in HIV's viral load or T cell count. Without the benefit of specific laboratory-derived values to measure in discrete steps a shrinking of immune function, the concept of immunodeficiency being a disease state of the elderly might itself be arbitrary.

R.A. Norman, DO, MPH (✉)
Professor of Dermatology,
Nova Southeastern Medical School, Tampa, FL, USA

Private Practice,
8002 Gunn Highway, Tampa, FL 33626, USA
e-mail: skindrrob@aol.com

Z. Henry
Lake Erie College of Osteopathic Medicine, OMS IV,
Bradenton, FL, USA

J.C. Hall (ed.), *Skin Diseases in the Immunocompromised*,
DOI 10.1007/978-1-4471-6479-1_11, © Springer-Verlag London 2014

Keywords

Geriatrics • Elderly • Life expectancy • Life span • Immunodeficiency • Opportunistic infections • Aging • Herpes zoster • HIV • Seborrheic dermatitis • Angular cheilitis

Introduction

Aging is defined as a time-sequential deterioration of living things that is prompted by increased susceptibility to disease and adverse events, leading to loss of viability and physiologic functions. In simpler terms, aging is characterized by the individual's inability to respond in a useful way to stress. Perhaps the most vital physiological component a person has for surviving aging is their body's immune system. Along with the ability to clear antigens from the body, the immune system is equally important in keeping the body's own physiology in check by monitoring for reactions that may go awry and unchecked, leading to malignancies, or helping the body rebuild and reshape itself in the face of any stress. Decreased ability to cope with stressors expected to be handled by the immune system could support the notion that aging may itself be considered a disease state. Aging is not accompanied by a profound drop in one of the many variables used to assess immune status with respect to a specific disease such as viral load, T cell count, or gamma globulin, and this limits the ability to label an older person as immunodeficient. Without the benefit of specific laboratory-derived values to measure in discrete steps a shrinking of immune function, the concept of immunodeficiency being a disease state of the elderly might itself be arbitrary.

Aging Definitions

No internationally accepted standard to define someone as being "elderly" exists, nor has there ever really been any attempt to define characteristics that, once accumulated to a certain degree, officially shift a person's classification in their society from "adult" to "elder." The term "elderly" is an arbitrary term that, on a superficial basis, differs from culture to culture and region to region. Most people in developed countries would classify someone as being elderly when they approach the age they are capable of receiving pension benefits or reaching tax-exempt status; a generally agreeable age would be 65. While the United Nations has no official cutoff numerical criterion, it is known that they generally agree on the age of 60 as the point where any culture would agree that adult and elder reach an equilibrium. The difficulty in marking someone as elderly based on chronology comes as no surprise, seeing as how making a calendar age as the threshold of what is or isn't elderly would have to match up to a biological age, which definitely is not at all the same from person to person or culture to culture. So then there comes a point in medicine's attempt to define who is and isn't elderly and to try and make tangible the process of aging, the need to define a parameter that can be used universally and apply a definition does not change, something that in itself can convey more information than simply a number, although its application would have to still be relative to the reference group.

Life span suggests the average limit to which a member of a species will survive. Life expectancy is the proportion of that life span that a given member of the species will achieve. At some point, when a person's chronological and biological or functional age, or some blend of the two, reaches a certain percentage of life expectancy, one can be deemed elderly for the most part, from medicine's perspective. These quantities are constrained by their upper limit, which is set by the process of aging. Aging is defined as a time sequential deterioration of living things that is prompted by increased susceptibility to disease and adverse events, leading to loss of viability and physiologic functions. It is the degree to which physiologic functioning and adaptive responses are lost that paints a still somewhat unclear picture of what biologic age a person has attained. Aging is the process by which a living organism's disease state increases to the point that slightly less and less adverse situations are able to take a larger toll on it until it can no longer function.

Aging and Immunity

Perhaps the most vital component a person has for surviving the often harsh conditions and avoiding the friability of aging is their body's immune system. Aside from simply thinking of being necessary to clear antigens from the body, the immune system is equally important in keeping the body's own physiology in check by monitoring for reactions that may go awry and unchecked, leading to malignancies, or helping the body rebuild and reshape itself in the face of any stress. Decreased ability to cope with stressors would support the notion that aging, which by definition eventually brings about the onset of becoming "elderly," and is marked by an increase in disease states and inability to withstand stresses that would be expected to be handled by the immune system, is itself a disease state. That lack of strength in the face of physiologic adversity implies that this disease state is brought about by an ever decreasing efficiency of the human immune system.

Although it cannot be argued that people do become more prone to disease with age, there is varying validity to whether aging represents an actual state of immunodeficiency. Although aging is accompanied by a decline in normal immune function of the B and T cells, aging is not reflected in profound changes in one of the many variables used to assess immune status with respect to a specific disease such as in HIV's viral load or T cell count. Without the benefit of specific laboratory-derived values to measure in discrete steps a shrinking of immune function, the concept of immunodeficiency being a disease state of the elderly might itself be arbitrary.

Analysis of the aging body, albeit from a strictly physical standpoint without regard to being organic and arguably more complex, does point to some validity in the concept of a truly finite drop in immunity with age that can't be refuted. If you pour a glass of water out and allow it to form a puddle on a surface in your house, and just leave it alone for a day or two, when you come back to it would you expect it to still be there? The answer is no. At the same time, if you ask anyone with even a moderate degree of secondary education at what temperature water boils, they know it's 100° (in Celsius at atmospheric pressure). So, if it's not 100° Celsius in your house, and you aren't living at the top of Mount Everest, why did the water still dry up? The reason is that all systems will move into a state of maximum disorder if given the opportunity and not driven to do otherwise by outside forces. The water molecules in the puddle, being tightly bound to four others by hydrogen bonds in a neatly arranged network are much more ordered but energetically unfavorable compared to molecules in the vapor phase that move purposelessly through the air in the room freed from the restraints of their hydrogen bonds. This state of disorder minimizes the free energy of the system, and the energy lost in the process is known as entropy. When it breaks down, even the extremely complex and massive molecular structures that comprise a human cell are governed by the same laws of thermodynamics as the array of water molecules. Therefore, to allow genetically pre-programmed cell death, telomere depletion, or some other macromolecular structure or process to account entirely for the aging process alone would be insufficient. Under scrutiny, are the mechanisms that drive life simply large puddles of chemical potential that are ultimately subject to the same fate of thermodynamic instability as every other atomic particle? On a gross scale, manifestation of this instability would appear as a failure of the person to compete with stresses and maintain homeostasis—the overall purpose of a properly functioning immunity—and ultimately failure of every other organ system. This concept of ever-increasing entropy comprises the most basic component of what is known as the damage theory of aging.

Aging and Inflammation

While the damage theory of aging can propose that the root of decline in function and homeostasis is due to entropy on a global scale, this can be applied to the perspective of failing immunity specifically. It is strongly believed that as we age, over the course of decades of our bodies enduring pathology, be it trying to keep a latent infection of toxoplasmosis or herpes zoster under control, to every other stress and strain that requires some component of the immune system's action to guide us back into homeostasis, a degree of chronic inflammation begins. This chronic inflammation continues to grow and smolder in the internal environment until there comes a point where it continues even in the absence of an ongoing acute reaction to fuel it. Immunity's action to prevent damage in the acute phase comes with a long-term price. A major product of these excessive inflammatory responses includes the overproduction of reactive oxygen and nitrogen species that initiate redox reactions within the cellular environment. Left unchecked, these are thought to lead to a depletion of the cell's scavenging enzymes that are needed to inactivate the radicals when the oxidative stress is no longer necessary.

The inappropriately abundant radicals that result from an overworked and now slipshod inflammatory response directly facilitate the thermodynamic breakdown of the cells' molecular constituents, and extend to them their state of disorder. Their exothermic reactivity results in, for example, proteins losing their intricately arranged and structurally functional three-dimensional shapes and resorting to a more disordered yet energetically favorable string of purposeless amino acids. It is interesting that these same oxidative/reduction processes, when delicately orchestrated so that their free energy loss may be contained and coupled to a useful process as opposed to just dissipating as heat and promoting entropy, provides the electromotive force that indirectly drives all of life's vital workings by regenerating ATP via the mitochondrial transport chain. This is the major downside to chronic inflammation. These oxide and nitrogen radicals

are, however, absolutely necessary in the short term. They are one of the vital players in the immune system's destruction of foreign pathogens during the acute inflammatory response. The acute inflammatory process forms the basis of host defenses, tissue repair mechanisms, and a return to homeostasis when faced with stress. The heart of the problem, although seemingly paradoxical, behind the development of chronic inflammation leading to an unregulated immune system is that humans are living so much longer thanks to medical science. Human beings were meant to utilize the acute inflammatory response as a means of protection against their external environments so they may fulfill the same goal that Mother Nature intended for them, as is the case for every other living organism—to survive to reproductive age so that they may assist in the propagation of their species. This is the sole factor that determines an individual organism's "success" from an evolutionary standpoint.

We as a species have outpaced evolution's method of natural selection as the way to extend lifespan via advancements in medical treatment. As people are able to live longer, we are exhausting our immune responses far past what evolution has intended. The resulting excessive exposure to external and internal stresses and repeated cycling of activation and then (albeit progressively less and less successfully) deactivation of the acute immune response with continuous macrophage migration into tissues is what eventually tips the scale in favor of chronic inflammation, so that the damage due to the inflammatory response starts to outweigh the benefit of the acute response. This concept, called "inflammaging," is the result of the immunosenescence that inevitably must accompany the ever-increasing aging process/duration. Inflammation is the driving force behind the decrease in immune capacity, or relative immunodeficiency that allots the increase in likelihood and severity of disease process in the elderly.

In conjunction with using entropy and oxidative damage as a buttress for supporting the "inflammaging" process, there exists tangible evidence for a chronic inflammatory state that worsens with chronologic age. This evidence properly correlates with the notion that an overly activated but improperly regulated inflammatory process accompanies aging and, overall, decreases the efficiency of the immune system. This is made evident by an imbalance in the levels of inflammatory mediators that have been illustrated in laboratory research. Other in vitro and in vivo studies have provided plausible mechanisms to account for the manifestation of immunodeficiency with macromolecular and cellular dysfunctions. Given the fact that we are now living in a time of a worldwide "silver tsunami," when the aging population is growing at the fastest rate ever, perhaps we need to register a worldwide "silver alert" that reflects how our runaway immune systems must be primed to care for the current abundance of aging and stress.

These same inflammatory changes and similar correlations for immune dysfunction can be noted (to a much greater degree) in the already known chronic inflammatory state that develops with HIV infection. The chronic inflammatory state the body must assume to try and keep the virus contained and the way that it in itself contributes to immunodeficiency is in some ways exactly like, and in others at least analogous to, the inflammatory changes brought upon by an immune system simply worn out by age. It is feasible to compare HIV infection and the internal environment that it promotes to an acquired and heavily accentuated acceleration of the aging process from an immune perspective. Of all new HIV infections, 10 % occur in the elderly. Combined with the cumulative chronic inflammation of aging, the ability to fight off the HIV infection may be diminished.

Almost continuous lifelong exposure to antigens leading to chronic activation of macrophages and pro-inflammatory cells also results in an excessive production of inflammatory cytokines. The loss in functionality of the immune system with aging is demonstrated by increased tissue destruction and senescent cellular components that are less adequate with driving the internal environment back into homeostasis (in some instances actually pulling the body further out of balance) but still manage attempts to overexcite themselves in some cases with continuous production of stimulatory cytokines. One of the most notable examples is the gradual elevation of C-reactive protein. In acute illnesses, C-reactive protein can reach levels as high as 10,000 mg/dL. In terms of chronic inflammation, however, a low-grade but continuous level of 1–10 mg/dL has been correlated with many diseases deemed characteristic of aging, including dementia, cardiovascular disease, dementia, and metabolic syndrome. Even in older adults without overt disease or loss of physical and/or cognitive function, C-reactive protein rises at a slower rate. The upregulation of C-reactive protein is thought to be a response to other proinflammatory cytokines, namely tumor necrosis factor and interleukin 6. All of these work together in the activation of the complement cascade and progression of innate immune responses with tissue destruction, and organ dysfunction, all of which potentiate age-related diseases and immune-incompetency. HIV is associated with an even greater increase in these inflammatory changes, considering the fact that even if the peripheral blood is practically sterilized of virus, especially in cases of successful antiviral therapy, the virus continues to seed itself in the lymphoid organs where it replicates and destroys CD4+ T cells. While once assumed to be due to reactivation of or acute infection with EBV in the severely compromised host, it is now believed that the extreme levels of the B cell activating cytokine interleukin 6 associated with HIV are large contributors to the 120-fold increase in non-Hodgkin lymphomas seen in these patients (with an average age of onset in the general population being 66).

Another important factor contributing to inflammaging is nuclear factor kappa beta. This protein complex is bound to its inhibitory protein in the cytosol and is released in response to a multitude of stimuli, from viral or bacterial antigens, oxidized LDL, UV light, and free radicals. Once inside the nucleus, the nuclear factor activates transcription of genes encoding many cytokines used in the innate and adaptive immune responses (including interleukin 2). In T cells infected with HIV, the virus lays dormant until the T cell is activated either by antigens or cytokines. This activation triggers nuclear factor to enter the nucleus and connect to the long-terminal-repeat sequences that flank the HIV genome. This begins transcription of proviral DNA and ultimately leads to production of virons and lysis of the T cell. Tumor necrosis factor and other acute inflammatory cytokines produced by macrophages recruited to the site induce activation of more nuclear factor kappa beta. Under normal circumstances, this should activate a positive feedback loop to keep the immune system poised for defense, but in the case of HIV, allows the continued destruction of T cells and further viral replication.

Contrary to many of the inflammatory mediators and despite the enhancement of nuclear factor kappa beta, interleukin 2 actually shows diminished basal and stimulated production and responsiveness. This interleukin is responsible for promoting the growth and proliferation of T lymphocytes, further likening HIV to an exaggerated form of the chronic inflammation's immunosenescence. The lack of responsiveness is due in part to decreased rate of receptor production with respect to degradation. However, when administered in vitro, activators of protein kinase C and calcium ionophores brought about the proper response in T cells previously inert to the effect of interleukin. This shows that with age, disorder in the downstream signaling pathways that amplify the response to the ligand–receptor binding complex causes dampening of the physiologic effect. These molecular processes, which are linked to inflammaging, and can be explained by the damage theory of aging, are compounded by more profound and readily observable detrimental effects on the immune system with aging. Examples include a depletion of stem cells (believed to be a result of telomere depletion) and a lack of leukocyte progenitors, which leads to a decline in everything from phagocytes to antibody producing B cells. The cytotoxicity of natural killer cells declines, as well as the ability of dendritic cells to present antigens.

The inflammaging process could play a strong role in these defects for the same reason that many immune cells (including T lymphocytes) exhibit a lack of response to cytokines and macrophages lose their ability to control radical

release. Thymus involution, which results in a reduced capacity for the body to create naïve T cells, is a progressive process but is believed to eventually "catch up" to a person once they have aged past 55. This leaves them devoid of T cells that may be programmed to respond to antigens that are either brand new or infrequently encountered in that person's immune system. In this way, the elderly patient, even in a state of seemingly optimal health, naturally acquires a sort of functional deficiency in T cells. This demonstrates a more blatant manifestation of the detrimental effects that must constantly be taken into consideration as medical science attempts to circumvent evolution's plan. This lack of T lymphocyte stimulation and ultimate decline in maturation is probably a leading contributor to elderly susceptibility to foreign pathogens. Included would be acute infection with viruses like influenza, and their reactivation from latency, as is the case with herpes zoster.

Herpes Zoster

Herpes zoster is also common in HIV patients. For them, it is classified as being a category B diagnosis, meaning that it is not an AIDS defining illness, but it may be one of the first observations that immunity is waning, and its course and management could become complicated by opportunistic infections if the immune capacity decreases further. Despite being initiated by totally different mechanisms, their pathologies share a degree of overlap at the molecular and cellular levels, and so it makes sense that the conditions associated with the disease state of immunosenescence would also be noted (especially with increased severity) in the diseases attributed to the presence of HIV. These disorders, which are common in the elderly, are highlighted as being key milestones in the downward progression T cell deficiency in HIV patients. While a multitude of systems becomes affected by HIV, a great deal of observations to this depressed immunity become transparent via the integumentary system. Quite possibly the most obvious is the advent of herpes zoster, as seen

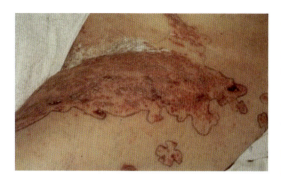

Fig. 11.1 An 81-year-old man with Alzheimer's disease with severe herpes zoster in the groin. In this age group severity of disease and postherpetic neuralgia are more common

in Fig. 11.1. This has a 20 % incidence during a person's lifetime and increases in incidence and risk of postherpetic neuralgia with age. All adults over 50 years of age should have a immunization for herpes zoster. The contraindications are severe immunosuppresion, but even that is a relative contraindication. Some experts recommend immunization before chemotherapy, transplantation, or beginning biologic therapy. Commonly referred to as shingles, this disorder can occur in anyone, but the odds increase with age or any scenario that involves immunosuppression as T cells lose their ability to combat the virus. Aside from the obvious cases, this can include people of any age on immunosuppressive drugs, radiation therapy, acquiring chickenpox at younger than 2 months of age, those affected by lymphoma, or in rare cases, even severe fatigue or emotional upset. Infection of a person who received the varicella vaccine as a child is possible but very unlikely.

Normally the varicella virus that caused the chicken pox is kept latent in dorsal root ganglia. Upon reactivation the virus travels up the sensory nerve root into the skin, bringing about the characteristic eruption of red swollen plaques. From these plaques, vesicles arise by about 3 days later. Like with herpes simplex infections, they will swell, rupture, bleed, and crust over within about 2 weeks. These are preceded by the prodrome of itching, burning, and pain (preherpetic neuralgia) 1 week before the eruptions. This may be accompanied by constitutional symptoms and regional lymphadenopathy. Two-thirds of herpes

zoster cases will appear in thoracic dermatomes, although any dermatome is possible, including trigeminal and sacral plexus. When affecting the ophthalmic division of the trigeminal nerve, it is referred to as ophthalmic zoster. The most serious ocular involvement includes activation in the nasociliary branch, leading to lesions on the tip and side of the nose with extensive ocular involvement. This is referred to as a positive Hutchinson sign and involves conjunctival, corneal, and scleral problems like anterior uveitis, neuropathic keratitis, perforation, glaucoma, optic neuritis, and retinal necrosis. The common prodrome in these cases would be headache, nausea, and vomiting.

When the rash involves the ear or inside the mouth, it is referred to as Ramsay Hunt syndrome and involves tinnitus, hearing loss, vertigo, nystagmus, and Bell's palsy due to infection of the geniculate ganglion. One of the most feared complications is immune-mediated encephalitis in these cases. If the inflammation of the dorsal nerve root is severe, atrophy and scarring of the dorsal root ganglion lead to post-herpetic neuralgia, described as the most feared complication and cause of morbidity. The hyperesthesia leaves the patient in a constant wearisome state of protection of the area of the neuralgia, as the slightest amount of pressure to the area initiates waves of sharp paroxysmal waves of excruciating pain that "leave most of its sufferers weary of existence."

First-line treatment of zoster involves vaccination for those 50 years and older without significant risks, and suppression of the active infection is achieved with 800 mg acyclovir five times a day for 1 week, valacyclovir 1,000 mg twice daily for 1 week, or famciclovir 500 mg twice daily for 1 week. In patients immunocompromised due to HIV infection, reconstitution of the immune system with HAART treatment in addition to the herpes specific antivirals is necessary to ensure successful treatment and ward off future attacks. The mainstay treatment option for post-herpetic neuralgia is nortriptyline, the tricyclic antidepressant with anticholinergic side effects. These drugs inhibit norepinephrine and serotonin reuptake in the central nervous system and increase nociceptive firing in the peripheral nervous system. Another less commonly used option is with pregabolin. Its side effects of weight gain, peripheral edema, dizziness and somnolence, as well as its classification as a schedule V controlled substance due to its ability to cause euphoria make it the second-line treatment.

Duration, severity, and odds of retaining the disease in the form of post-herpetic neuralgia all increase with the greater degree of immunosuppression the patient had prior to becoming symptomatic, i.e. someone who took a blow to their immune response due to reaching old age, being on prednisone therapy, or undergoing an extremely stressful emotional situation will have a less complicated course than someone who's HIV positive with a T cell count falling rapidly below 500 (the point at which category B infections become more expected, but still above the category C level of opportunistic infections who's threshold classically is said to sit around 200). Also, features that physicians, especially primary care, should be making note of are that shingles is generally limited to a single dermatome. Eruptions involving one or two adjacent dermatomes are much less likely, as are vesicles crossing the midline. Eruption that extends the full length of bilaterally symmetric dermatomes, or especially asymmetric dermatomes, is positively rare, and all should initiate further investigation into an underlying condition that could be facilitating the onset of shingles and not just write off the reactivation as being due to the immunosenescent state of old age.

Seborrheic Dermatitis

While much less severe, another common dermatologic condition that naturally increases in prevalence in the elderly but is severely exacerbated in states of extreme immune compromise is seborrheic dermatitis (SD), as seen in Fig. 11.2. It involves greasy, scaly, pruritic patches that are less demarcated than psoriasis and commonly involve areas spared by eczema (scalp, eyebrows, forehead, nasolabial fold, external meatus, chest, and axilla).

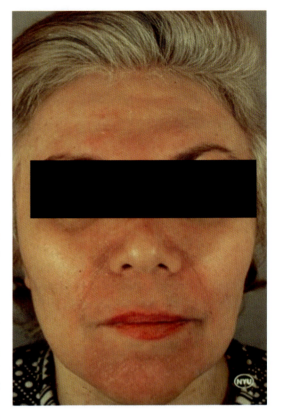

Fig. 11.2 Papulosquamous dermatitis with greasy scale accentuating the folds of skin. The scaling and erythema emphasizing the folds of the skin make the patient look older than she is. This pseudoaging is common on the eyelids

Seborrhea is believed to be due to an inflammatory response to the Malasezzia yeast, but other species of bacteria or fungi could be responsible. The pathogenesis of SD results from an overgrowth of Pityrosporum ovale (Malassezia furfur) in the sebum. Sebum is composed of triglycerides and esters, as well as fatty acids, cholesterol, and squalene. As the triglycerides and esters are broken down on secretion, individual free fatty acids accumulate. Recent research has shown Malasezzia to thrive in a free fatty acid medium. Malasezzia contain lipases that break down triglycerides and esters in a non-specific manner and create such an environment. They degrade sebum, free fatty acids from triglycerides, consume specific saturated fatty acids, and leave behind the unsaturates. Penetration of the modified sebaceous secretions results in inflammation, irritation, and scalp flaking. Skin cells die and are subsequently replaced by new skin cells in a never-ending cycle. In normal people this cycle takes about 1 month, and is usually not noticeable. On scalps where Malassezia thrives, the whole process can take less than half that time.

Seborrheic dermatitis typically affects areas of the skin where sebaceous glands appear in high frequency and are most active. The sebum secretion rate increases throughout the teens, remains steady through the 20s and 30s, then lessens with age. In males, the rate remains higher longer, into the 50s and 60s, but in females, the secretion rate drops quickly after menopause.

Human sebaceous glands (SG) are found over the entire skin surface (except the palms of the hands and soles of the feet), but sebum secretion is highest on the scalp, face, chest, and back. The distribution is classically symmetric, and common sites of involvement are the hairy areas of the head, including the scalp and scalp margin, eyebrows, eyelashes, mustache, and beard. Other common sites are the forehead, the nasolabial folds, the external ear canals, and the postauricular creases.

One of the characteristics of SD is dandruff; patients may complain of the scalp itching with dandruff, and because they think that the scale arises from dry skin, they decrease the frequency of shampooing, which allows further scale accumulation, resulting in greater inflammation and worsening symptoms. Treatment includes zinc soaps and selenium lotions to help suppress activity and maintain remissions of this chronic condition. Topical steroid creams illicit a quicker response. The most difficult and expansive cases are usually relieved by ketoconazole creams or ciclopirox olamine cream or gel. Metronidazole, tacrolimus, and elidel cream also have proven effective.

Seborrheic dermatitis is a common clinical finding in patients with neurological disease (an affliction of many elderly) and immunodeficiency. Immobility appears to play a significant component in generating conditions for disease pathogenesis. Neurological disease often results in a decrease in neuronal activity to areas where sebaceous glands exist in abundance, causing pooling of the sebum and thereby fostering conditions suitable for SD. Patients with immunodeficiency are also more prone to SD due to unopposed growth of Malasezzia. However, immobility may also be present in these patients due to a decrease in activity, further encouraging sebum collection and inflammation.

Over the last 21 years that our group and I have treated well over 200,000 patients in long-term care facilities, I (author RN) have noticed these consistent increases in SD in patients with neurologic or immunologic disease. Immobility plays a significant component in generating conditions for disease pathogenesis. Neurological disease often results in a decrease in neuronal activity to areas where sebaceous glands exist in abundance, causing pooling of the sebum and thereby fostering conditions suitable for SD. Patients with immunodeficiency are also more prone to SD due to unopposed growth of Malasezzia. However, immobility may also be present in these patients due to a decrease in activity, further encouraging sebum collection and inflammation.

The research and observations are consistent with an increased incidence of SD in patients with neurologic or immunologic disease. Dermatologists and other physicians should recognize the relationship between immobility caused by neurologic or immunologic disease to SD. Patients with histories of epilepsy, Down's syndrome, generalized neurological deficits, and immunodeficiency often demonstrate the role of immobility in facilitating the pathogenesis of SD. Seborrheic dermatitis is common in patients with Parkinson's disease; their decreased mobility may increase the pooling effect of sebum on the face and augment the growth of Malassezia yeasts.

Seborrhea and herpes zoster are both known to be category B infections in HIV-positive patients. Interestingly though, while the degree of seborrhea correlates directly with the rate of clinical deterioration, herpes zoster does not predict a faster progression to AIDS.

Angular Cheilitis

Another skin manifestation that may occur in aging is angular cheilitis. These erythematous

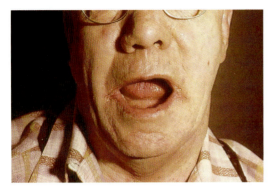

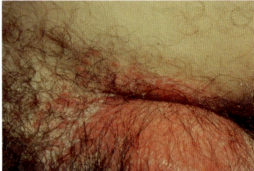

Fig. 11.3 Elderly male with malocclusion and crusted erythematous areas in the corner of the mouth, illustrating perleche caused by candida albicans

Fig. 11.4 Bright red erythematous dermatitis in the groin and scrotum with satellite lesions and an overhanging fringe of epidermal scale forming a cigarette-paper appearance. Commonly seen in elderly patients, especially when hospitalized or bed-ridden where fecal and urine soiling and a warm, wet environment from a constant reclining position all contribute to the problem

scaling crusty macules form bilaterally at the corners of the mouth, shown in Fig. 11.3. In some cases their severity becomes so advanced as to bleed and ulcerate. Beginning as a sore fissure, they worsen as patients lick and moisten the area in attempts to prevent further cracking. They can be caused by bacteria, but most commonly are fungal. The organisms pool in the intertriginous space of the corners of the mouth as they deepen with age. The increase in frequency in the elderly is especially notable when they have missing teeth or wear dentures, because both cause a loss of outer dimensions of the mouth. Angular cheilitis is one of the defining features of Plummer Vinson syndrome, may be induced by a multitude of vitamin/mineral deficiencies (B2, iron, or zinc) and also may be seen with medications that cause excessive drying of the skin, like isotretinoin. Typical treatment involves antifungal cream and a group V steroid. Mupirocin or bactroban applied two times a day is effective when the causative agent is yeast and bacteria.

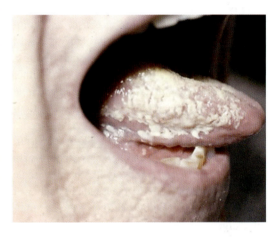

Fig. 11.5 Thick white coating of the tongue in an elderly male who turned out to have AIDS. This was related to a blood transfusion for heart bypass surgery before it was known that AIDS was viral and blood used for transfusion could be screened. It was the disease-presenting symptom

Candida albicans

Candida albicans is a yeast-like fungus of the normal oral, vaginal, and gut flora. Many factors including contraception, antibiotic therapy, diabetes, pregnancy, or anything that decreases cell-mediated immunity, can allow the yeast to become pathogenic. The primary lesion is a pustule, and the contents peel away to reveal a red,

denuded, glistening surface with a cigarette paper-like advancing border, seen in Fig. 11.4. Scale and inflammatory cells overflow in the mouth and/or vagina (wherever the primary infection is) and cause the characteristic cottage cheese-like material. The tongue is always involved, but it may spread to the trachea or esophagus. Diagnosis can be confirmed by observing pseudohyphae from the budding yeast. Concomitant HIV infection should be suspected in treatment-resistant cases. Chronic infection will involve firmly adherent, irregular, and velvety surfaces that coat the buccal mucosa and tongue, as seen in Fig. 11.5. The primary treatment is fluconazole (which may also be used prophylactically in chemo patients), but itraconazole, which is equally effective but less well tolerated, may need to be used in patients with chronic infection and/or HIV due to yeast's resistance to fluconazole is suspected. Ketoconazole and nystatin oral suspension are other options as well. Treatment of vaginal candidiasis is initiated with miconazole or clotrimazole creams.

Candidiasis is said to be recurrent when a patient has four occurrences in 1 year or three episodes in 1 year unrelated to antibiotic use. A commonly recurring infection in the elderly, Candidiasis' ability to affect the elderly does not lie primarily in their immunosenescence, as is the case of shingles, for example. While it can occur with no predisposing factor, the recurring theme of polypharmacy exhibited in the aging population is largely the inciting event in candida infection. Polypharmacy involves the unintentional overprescribing of medications, usually from multiple sources, to older people. These medications can have conflicting mechanisms of actions or compounding side effects. Complicated regimens requiring multiple dosings and time constraints can lead to some drugs being neglected, while other drugs may be accidentally taken in excess if previous dosings of that drug were simply forgotten or mistaken for a different medication taken around the same time that day. It's easy to see how this could arise, in the midst of taking ten different drugs from four different specialists, some three times a day, some on an empty stomach, some on a full stomach, some 12 h apart, etc. Medications such as steroids (oral or systemic) and antibiotics taken in the setting of polypharmacy leave the body susceptible to destruction of the normal protective flora, which allows candida to take the upper hand. Recurring candida, especially infections resistant to the first-line treatment in anyone (but unfortunately possibly overlooked in the elderly for various purposes) is a category B infection associated with HIV and should prompt further investigation, regardless of the rest of the symptomology, history of present illness, or known patient background.

Aging and Skin Cancers

The increased incidence of skin cancer in the elderly may occur from impaired immune responsiveness to light-induced malignant clones of epidermal cells. The decreased immune potential may come from the normal process of aging and the cumulative immunosuppressive effects of UV irradiation where the failure of the surveillance system allows the expression of cutaneous malignancy. Patients with one carcinoma have been shown to be at increased risk of developing additional skin tumors, and those with two or more basal cell carcinomas have a much greater chance to develop a new skin tumor within a year. Although this may represent a failure of the local immune system, it does not reflect a generalized immunoincompetence. Patients with early basal cell and squamous cell carcinoma generally have normal responses to skin testing and normal numbers of T- and B-lymphocytes. The continuing study of age-related changes that occur in the systemic immune system and cutaneous immune processes points to complex interactions of the two systems.

HIV and Aging

It is known that one million people in the United States are infected with HIV, but an estimated one-third of these do not know they are infected. With the production of highly active antiretroviral therapy, or HAART, in the mid 90s, the diagnosis has been downgraded from an absolute death sentence to a manageable chronic disease; living with HIV is now commonly likened to living with other chronic conditions such as diabetes. As people are living longer with the disease, the age of people infected with the disease is increasing with it. With the discovery of the disease in the early 1980s and throughout the early to mid-1990s and before it was heavily understood, the general public used stereotypes and prejudice to fuel a false image of HIV infection, and personal myths and beliefs to "fill in" missing information of the disease. While it is human nature to fear the unknown, the stigma of the disease that society created has unfortunately shifted HIV-positive individuals into a subset of the population—those false beliefs still exist today and have created an inaccurate sense of protection from them—those infected with the virus. By labeling us as "us" and HIV-positive individuals as "the other" it creates a separation and perhaps gives people a sense of comfort, a pseudo barrier that they can use to keep the malignancy at bay. It is with the help of this very barrier that the virus seems to be able to increase the rate at which it spreads, and go unnoticed throughout the population. The inaccuracy of this concept should easily be conceived by noting that the phenomenon of "normalcy" (with respect to any characteristic the majority group chooses to single out, not just sero-status) was an ideology constructed by Europeans only since the nineteenth century. Here, certain sets of personal ethics and beliefs of some persons were deemed superior to others', and these paved the way for characteristics to be designated as that of the group in power, or the "in-group" and who will be considered the other, or the "out group." This notion extends to all walks of life, maybe to a smaller degree, especially in developed countries, but is still utilized today. This makes for a deadly misconception in some cases, like when it is applied to a disease that can readily cross the borders of the "ins" and "outs" and have such devastating consequences as to be statistically deemed the second most common cause of death due to infection worldwide.

It should be noted that age is an independent risk factor for influencing clinical progression to AIDS; a retrospective case study conducted recently revealed diagnosis at age 60 accompanied a significantly shorter survival time. Before the development of HAART, survival if diagnosed HIV-positive before age 34 was 11 years, but that dropped to 6.6 and 4.4 years for diagnosis between ages 55 and 64 and after age 65, and for every 10-year increase in age at time of initial infection, there is a 43 % increase in mortality rate. In 2005, 15 % of newly diagnosed patients were over age 50 and 2 % were over 65! Studies have also shown that any person diagnosed with full-blown AIDS past the age of 35 has significantly low chances of surviving past 12 months,

let alone those diagnosed past age 60, at which case survival is deemed virtually impossible.

Heterosexual contact associated with transmission is on the rise, primarily among women and minorities of both genders, although the estimated annual percentage change of virus acquisition in males ages 50–59 rose 4.9 % from 1999 to 2004 and rose 6.8 % for females. Recent studies and surveys have shown that sexual activity is increasing in older adults. Theories for this increase include higher divorce rates, compounded by the increasing ease of acquisition of erectile dysfunction drugs, and wanting to live beyond the preconceived notions for what is or isn't characteristic behavior of an older person. People may have at one time lived consciously or even subconsciously according to these constraints, but as the popular trend (in developed countries at least) of "50 is the new 30" is allowed to become more and more mainstream, sexual activity among older adults becomes more prevalent.

When HIV first became an epidemic, the National AIDS Survey found that 85 % of respondents over age 50 reported inconsistent condom use, and more than 90 % of those over age 50 had never had an HIV test done, whereas 60 % of the subset of that population that was gay/ bisexual had, showing that a lack of awareness may very well have contributed to the growing trends displayed today in the older heterosexual population. What's even more disconcerting is that this applied only to the U.S.; in many developing countries such as Kenya, condom use is actually frowned upon because it is believed to promote promiscuity. People from many developing countries admit to never having seen one. Whether it is due to lack of concern about getting pregnant, or simply the perception that they are not at risk for sexually transmitted disease for reasons described above, condom use seems to decrease with aging past 50, especially with women, who seem to lack knowledge of personal risk and/or knowledge of methods for protection during risky behavior.

While it is primarily up to the individual to take responsibility for their own body, it seems even the healthcare field itself validates the misconception of who is or isn't more or less vulnerable to HIV; after all, despite the fact that 40 million people in the world are living with HIV, and approximately 2.8 million are over age 50 (including those due to new infections and those simply living longer with HAART), data from industrialized countries and the UNAIDS still primarily only reflects data on the epidemic up to age 49. It was only until just recently that the CDC officially implemented guidelines that voluntary HIV testing be done on all patients ages 13–64 regardless of risk, and those who admit to at least one risk factor should have repeat testing done at least annually. It also appears that the majority of newly reported infections in the older adult are not found during the acute stages, but many are stumbled upon incidentally through trial and error and while investigating other co-morbidities, and they are well into the chronic phases. This demonstrates failure of individual physicians to consider HIV infection in this particular population and also the possible underestimating of what could be opportunistic infections in these patients for simply severe exacerbations of disease that could be accounted for by the slightly suppressed immune system that comes with age regardless (shingles, for example). Older patients, while being more comfortable with themselves today as far as engaging in sexual activity, may still be very embarrassed to disclose this information to their physicians, and the physicians unfortunately may try and spare them this embarrassment by not asking, or simply would not even consider in their differential diagnosis that such activities and the repercussions they can have would apply to patients in this bracket.

Despite their knowledge of the disease, even healthcare providers allow preconceived notions to surmount what their clinical knowledge should tell them, and fail to consider HIV in this population. If this trend of new HIV incidence continues, knowledge of HIV infection and routine testing must become a more integral part of medicine in general, especially in primary care, as these physicians may be the ones initially approached with the chief complaint that will ultimately lead to diagnosis with the virus.

Furthermore, with respect to the already problematic issue of polypharm in the elderly population, knowledge of HAART will need to more heavily integrated into primary care medicine. The cholesterol-elevating effects of the protease inhibitors will require additional consideration when evaluating patients already prone to higher lipid profiles. Dosing regimens will need special care to account for the decreased metabolism of many drugs due to the cytochrome-inhibiting effects of drugs like ritonavir. While this effect is necessary to allot optimal therapy of the antivirals with regards to pharmacokinetics, the resulting increased blood levels of all the other patients' medications could be detrimental from their own individual side effects. On one hand, while not overtly harmful, the tendency of the nucleoside reverse transcriptase inhibitors (drugs which are absolutely paramount to antiretroviral treatment and make up the "backbone" of HAART therapy) to selectively promote apoptosis in facial and appendicular adipocytes via inhibition of the mitochondrial enzyme polymerase gamma would have severely harmful side effects to a patient's psyche when their manifestations of facial wasting is compounded by the already undesired destruction of skin elasticity through collagen depletion that comes with age. In the least, guidelines need to be updated for the twenty-first century to include more appropriate and thorough care of all patients. Co-morbid conditions associated with the immunocompromised and aging need to be better and more universally understood. The need for inclusion of HIV in the differential diagnosis of all patients, regardless of apparent risk factors, will enhance the physicians' ability to promote effective education, prevention, and treatment measures in not just the aging, but general population as well.

Seborrheic Keratose

There is a tumor of such dominant incidence in the aging population that it will be mentioned here. By far the most common benign tumors in the elderly are seborrheic keratoses. They can occur on any skin surface except the palms and

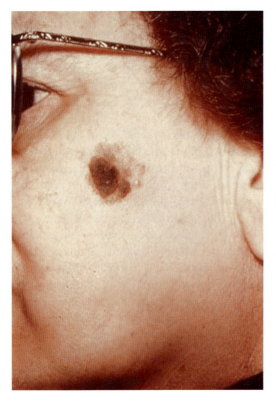

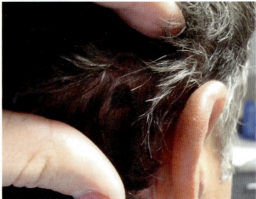

Fig. 11.7 Black tumor in the scalp that, although well demarcated, mimics a melanoma (more common in the immune-suppressed) with its dramatic black color. A biopsy is necessary to diagnose this benign seborrheic keratosis

Fig. 11.6 A typical seborrheic keratosis on the cheek of an elderly female. It is well demarcated with a superficial "stuck-on appearance." Increased markings of the lines on the skin give it a lichenified appearance and there are some white psuedohorned cysts

soles. They do not occur on mucous membranes. Although not caused by the sun, they can be seen in a photodistribution due to increased pigmentation by the sun and a tendancy to occur in sun-exposed areas in some patients. They tend to be inherited. Seborrheic refers to the sometimes greasy appearance and their appearance in areas of sebaceous gland prominence and keratosis means rough.

They can take many different forms, but a skin biopsy is usually definitive if the clinical diagnosis is in doubt. They are well-demarcated with a superficial "stuck-on" appearance. They have many colors but are most often various shades of brown, white, or black. They often have tiny white, brown, or black pin-head sized kereatotic circular papules within the tumor called pseudohorned cysts, as seen in Fig. 11.6. They may be asymptomatic or pruritic. In elderly patients

a thick keratotic type of seborrhea may be difficult to differentiate from a seborrheic kerotosis. Once a seborrheic keratosis is excoriated, it tends to take on the pink ill-defined characteristics of an actinic keratosis.

The argument that seborrheic keratosis and immune suppression be included in this text are multiple. Their frequency and variability are so overwhelming that they are in the differential diagnosis of many more obviously immune-related diseases most notably found in the elderly (see Figs. 11.7 and 11.8). There are molecular alterations in the seborrheic keratosis that have immune implications. Deoxyribonuclease(DNA) is decreased and ribonucleic acid and protein synthesis are decreased. There is some evidence of mutation of a gene coding for a growth factor receptor. Seborrheic keratosis can explode in numbers at the sight of skin inflammation. The sign of Lesar-Tr`elat is the dramatic increase in seborrheic keratosis sometimes are an erythematous base and is considered a paraneoplastic marker for underlying malignancy, especially gastrointestinal adenocarcinomas, breast, lung, and urinary tract.

Actinic keratosis, shown in Fig. 11.9, Actinic Keratotic tumor is the main differential diagnosis. They are caused by the sun and thus occur on sun-exposed areas. It is thought than sun exposure prior to 15 years of age is the most damag-

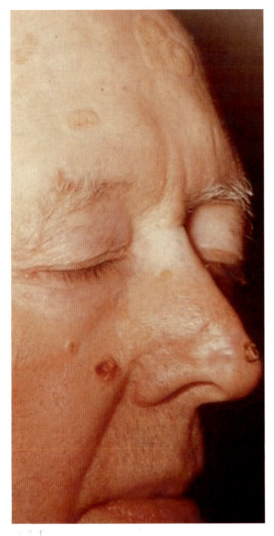

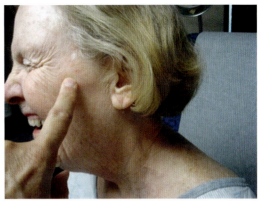

Fig. 11.9 Keratotic tumor arising on an ill-defined erythematous base. Rubbing the area is shown to cause the wince of the patient. Pain would be uncommon in a seborrheic keratosis, which would be more apt to itch if it caused any symptoms

cumulative and the more the exposure, the higher the risk, and damage is more common in the immunosuppressed population. The sun acts, as in all instances of ultraviolet-related disease, as a carcinogen and an immune suppressant.

Conclusion

We live in a time with a "silver tsunami" of aging. Investigating the concept of how and when we age, immunity, and dermatological manifestations in our elderly is a complex and challenging task.

Fig. 11.8 Forehead and most lateral tumor left malar area are typical seborrheic keratosis. They have a "stuck-on" appearance and brown pseudohorned cysts. The other two tumors on the medial cheek and nose are not as characteristic and the nasal lesion looks to have appeared near a scar site where a cancer may have been treated. Biopsy of these tumors showed basal cell cancers (more common in the immune-suppressed), thus illustrating the importance of a skin biopsy in more nondescript tumors

ing, but older patients still need to consider shade, outdoor activities before 10:00 AM and after 4:00 PM, sun-protective clothing (most notably broad-brimmed hats), and generous application of a broad-spectrum sunscreen preferably 30 min prior to sun exposure and repeated every hour if exposure to water or excessive sweating occurs. This is essential since ultraviolet light damage is

Suggested Reading

Abbas A, Aster J, Fausto N, Kumar V. Robins & Cotran pathologic basis of disease. Philadelphia: Elsevier Health Sciences; 2009.

Aspinall R, Andrew D. Thymic involution in aging. J Clin Immunol. 2000;20(4):250–6.

Bruunsgaard H, Pedersen AN, Schroll M, Skinhoj P, Pedersen BK. Decreased natural killer cell activity is associated with atherosclerosis in elderly humans. Exp Gerontol. 2001;37(1):127–36.

Cambier J. Immunosenescence: a problem of lymphopoiesis, homeostasis, microenvironment, and signaling. Immunol Rev. 2005;205:5–6.

Chung HY, Kim HJ, Kim JW, Yu BP. The inflammation hypothesis of aging: molecular modulation by calorie restriction. Ann N Y Acad Sci. 2001;928:327–35.

Cowley NC, Farr PM, Shuster S. The permissive effect of sebum in seborrhoeic dermatitis: an explanation of the rash in neurological disorders. Br J Dermatol. 1990;122(1):71–6.

Endo J, Norman R. Clinical cases in geriatric dermatology. London: Springer; 2013.

Endo J, Wong J, Norman R, Chang AL. Geriatric dermatology: part I. Geriatric pharmacology for the dermatologist. Am Acad Dermatol, Inc. 2013. http://www.jaad.org/article/S0190-9622(13)00063-7/abstract. Accessed 18 Apr 2013.

Franceschi C, Bonaf M, Valensin S. Human immunosenescence: the prevailing of innate immunity, the failing of clonotypic immunity, and the filling of immunological space. Vaccine. 2000;18(16):1717–20.

Fulop Jr T, Gagne D, Goulet AC, Desgeorges S, Lacombe G, et al. Age-related impairment of p56lck and ZAP-70 activities in human T lymphocytes activated through the TcR/CD3 complex. Exp Gerontol. 1999;34(2):197–216.

Gann, C. Sex life of older adults and rising STDs. ABC News Network, aired 3 Feb 2012. Available at: http://abcnews.go.com.

Habif T. Clinical dermatology—a color guide to diagnosis and therapy. 4th ed. New York: Mosby; 2004.

Hirschberg T, Hirschberg S. Everyday, everywhere. Global perspectives on popular culture. New York: McGraw Hill; 2002.

Howlader N, Noone AM, Krapcho M, Garshell J, Neyman N, Altekruse SF, et al. SEER cancer statistics review, 1975–2010. Bethesda: National Cancer Institute. http://seer.cancer.gov/csr/1975_2010/, based on November 2012 SEER data submission, posted to the SEER website, 2013. http://seer.cancer.gov/statfacts/html/nhl.html.

IRIN humanitarian news and analysis. [Internet] Global: HIV incidence rising in 50+ age group. Available at: http://www.irinnews.org/Report/83270/GLOBAL-HIV-incidence-rising-in-50-age-group. Accessed 12 Apr 2013.

IRIN humanitarian news and analysis. [Internet] Kenya: old but not cold: older people also at risk. Available from:http://www.irinnews.org/Report/75208/KENYA-Old-but-not-cold-older-people-also-at-risk. Accessed 12 Apr 2013.

Ito K, Hirao A, Arai F, Matsuoka S, Takubo K, Hamaguchi I, et al. Regulation of oxidative stress by ATM is required for self-renewal of haematopoietic stem cells. Nature. 2004;431(7011):997–1002.

Jenny NS. Inflammation in aging: cause, effect, or both? Discov Med. 2012;13(73):451–60.

Kane R, Ouslander J, Itamar Abrass I, Resnick B. Essentials of clinical geriatrics. 6th ed. New York: McGraw Hill Medical; 2009.

Koretsky M. Engineering and chemical thermodynamics. New York: John Wiley and Sons; 2003.

Maurer T, Berger T. Dermatologic manifestations of HIV. HIV InSite March 1998. University of California San Francisco. http://hivinsite.ucsf.edu/InSite?page=kb-04-01-01#S2.12.1X.

Min H, Montecino-Rodriguez E, Dorshkind K. Reduction in the developmental potential of intrathymic T cell progenitors with age. J Immunol. 2004;173(1):245–50.

Monaco C, Andreakos E, Kiriakidis S, et al. Canonical pathway of nuclear factor kappa B activation selectively regulates proinflammatory and prothrombotic responses in human atherosclerosis. Proc Natl Acad Sci U S A. 2004;101(15):5634–9. doi:10.1073/pnas.0401060101. PMC 397455. PMID 15064395.

Nguyen N, Holodniy M. HIV infection in the elderly. Clin Interv Aging. 2008;3(3):453–72.

Reiter GS. The HIV wasting syndrome. AIDS Clin Care. 1996;8(11):89–91, 93, 96.

Ro BI, Dawson TL. The role of sebaceous gland activity and scalp microfloral metabolism in the etiology of seborrheic dermatitis and dandruff. J Investig Dermatol Symp Proc. 2005;10(3):194–7.

Singh T, Newman AB. Inflammatory markers in population studies of aging. Ageing Res Rev. 2011;10(3):319–29.

Toy E, Briscoe D, Britton B, Reddy B. Case files: family practice. 2nd ed. New York: McGraw Hill Medical; 2010.

Wolf J, Weinberger B, Arnold CR, Maier AB, Westendorp RG, Grubeck-Loebenstein B. The effect of chronological age on the inflammatory response of human fibroblasts. Exp Gerontol. 2012;47(9):749–53.

UVA and UVB Therapy: Practical Applications and Implications for the Immunosuppressed Patient and Skin Disease

12

James R. Coster and Joseph A. Blackmon

Abstract

Phototherapy is an effective treatment option for a variety of skin disorders including psoriasis, photodermatoses, cutaneous T cell lymphoma, atopic dermatitis, vitiligo, and a number of sclerosing skin disorders. A variety of light sources can be used, either as a sole modality or in combination with sensitizing drugs, and treatments can be designed to address localized or diffuse skin conditions. Various types of light produce unique responses based on light energy/intensity and depth of penetration. The mechanisms by which various phototherapies impact target tissues are complex and it is clear that host immune responses play a key role in these processes.

Immunosuppressed patients present a number of unique challenges when phototherapies are employed. Given the fact that phototherapies mediate their effects via immune modulation, immunosuppression can alter both response and morbidity profiles. As such, treatment programs for immunosuppressed patients must be tailored and employed cautiously. Both acute and chronic morbidity profiles can vary considerably in immunosuppressed patients, and close clinical monitoring is essential during treatment. Long term follow up is often necessary. Most types of phototherapy are associated with a significant long-term risk of iatrogenic skin cancer in immunosuppressed patients. Absolute and relative contraindications must be carefully considered when immunosuppressed patients are being evaluated for phototherapy.

J.R. Coster, MD (✉)
Department of Radiation Oncology,
University of Kansas, School of Medicine,
3901 Rainbow Blvd., Kansas City, KS 66160, USA
e-mail: jcoster@kumc.edu

J.A. Blackmon, MD
Department of Dermatology, University of Kansas,
Kansas City, KS, USA

Keywords

Phototherapy • Photodynamic therapy • UVA • UVB • Narrow band UVB
• PUVA • Excimer laser • Psoriasis • Psoralen • Immunosuppression •
Organ transplant recipients • Non-melanoma skin cancer • Human immu-
nodeficiency virus

Introduction

Phototherapies of various types have been used
for centuries to treat a wide range of skin disorders. As our understanding of the pathophysiology of various skin disorders has evolved and
treatment technology has advanced, phototherapy has become an effective management option
for a variety of disorders including psoriasis,
other sclerosing skin disorders, cutaneous T cell
lymphoma, atopic dermatitis, photodermatoses
and vitiligo. Several types of phototherapy are
available to address specific skin conditions
including UVA, broad band UVB, narrow band
UVB, and both laser and non-laser excimer light.
UVA light can be combined with sensitizing psoralen drugs to enhance response.

Phototherapy utilizes non-ionizing ultraviolet
radiation which impacts both normal and diseased cells via a combination of complex mechanisms. The impact of phototherapy is mediated
by both DNA modulation and host immune reactions. Each type of light produces a unique
response based on depth of penetration and intensity. Light sources for various phototherapies can
deliver localized or full body exposure.

Phototherapy Treatment Options

Phototherapy, photochemotherapy, and excimer
laser therapy are established treatment options
for patients with psoriasis who do not respond
adequately to more conservative medical treatment. Psoralens are photosensitizing agents
which, when used in combination with UVA light
treatment, are highly effective in clearing psoriasis. Combined psoralen and UVA (PUVA) is very

effective in treating psoriasis and can produce
long periods of remission.

Narrowband UVB (nbUVB) is generally preferred in patients with psoriasis in its earlier stages.
Suberythemogenic doses of nbUVB will effectively
clear psoriasis in most patients over a period of
several weeks. NbUVB is more convenient than
PUVA and is associated with fewer long term
risks. In general, PUVA is used when appropriately administered UVB therapy proves ineffective or yields only temporary improvement.

PUVA is somewhat more challenging to
administer from a logistical standpoint, is more
costly than UVB therapy, and is associated with
side effects which require a higher level of clinical
attention and management. PUVA will induce a
clinically significant response in 80–90 % of psoriasis patients within 6–8 weeks of starting treatment. Clearing of psoriatic plaques is typically
complete within 10 weeks of starting PUVA.

In recent years biologic agents which directly
or indirectly modulate immune function have
become important tools for treating psoriasis.
PUVA and nbUVB are much more cost effective
than newer biologic agents and the role of each
must be considered in the context of each patient's
history and extent of disease. Additional variables which must be considered when a treatment
program is designed include skin type, the type
of light source to be used, dose per treatment and
treatment interval. Patients are monitored regularly to assess response and toxicity.

Challenges

Immunosuppressed patients present a number of
unique challenges when phototherapies are
employed. Given the fact that phototherapies

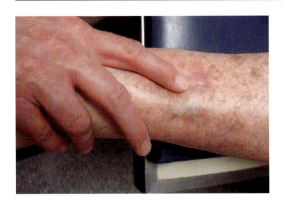

Fig. 12.1 Squamous cell carcinoma on the leg in a psoriasis patient. This is the main malignancy that is increased with phototherapies and can be easily missed as simply another area of psoriasis in psoriasis patients. Induration around an area of adherent hyperkeratosis, sometimes with pain, are important clinic signs

utilize immune modulation to produce host responses to disease, immunosuppression can alter response as well as acute and chronic morbidity profiles. As such, treatment programs for these patients must be designed with care and caution, and patients must be monitored vigilantly both during and after treatment. Immunosuppressed patients, therefore, are not typically good candidates for home-based UV treatment.

Long-term use of PUVA therapy can produce negative cosmetic effects such as photoaging, wrinkling, freckling, mottling, atrophy, elastosis, xerosis, and telangiectasia induction. Cataract formation can be induced by PUVA treatment as well\ and appropriate eye protection should be used. Skin cancers, particularly squamous cell carcinomas as shown in Fig. 12.1, are much more common in patients who receive PUVA treatment. UVB therapy is much less carcinogenic than UVA therapy. The risk of iatrogenic skin cancers is markedly higher in immunosuppressed patients who receive most types of phototherapy.

Absolute contraindications to PUVA include lupus erythematosus, xeroderma pigmentosum, porphyrias, Darier's disease, and trichothiodystrophy. A number of relative contraindications exist as well.

Biologic agents such as interleukin modulators, tumor necrosis factor modulators, and T cell blockers, may increase the risk of skin cancer with prolonged follow up. When these agents are used in sequential combination with phototherapy, even narrow band UVB, there is an increased incidence of carcinogenesis. Carcinogenic potential is heightened in all patients with chronic immunosuppression.

HIV photodermatitis and autoimmune depigmentation occur in a minority of HIV-seropositive patients and can be treated with phototherapy. UV therapies must be employed cautiously in these patients given the potential for heightened treatment sensitivity, variable response, and potential long term morbidities.

History

Modern phototherapy dates back to the late nineteenth century. In 1895 Niels Finsen first used a carbon arc lamp to treat lupus vulgaris. In 1923 Goeckerman used broadband UVB light and coal tar to treat psoriasis. Photosensitizing psoralen compounds were first identified in 1948 and the first synthetic psoralens were produced in 1964 to treat vitiligo. The value and efficacy of photochemotherapy was firmly established in 1974 when Parish published data confirming that combining 8-methoxypsoralen with UVA light was effective in clearing psoriasis in 21 patients.

An array of therapies utilizing ultraviolet light have been developed over the last several decades, including UVA, broad and narrow band UVB, and excimer laser treatment. Phototherapy incorporates the use of non-ionizing ultraviolet radiation. The mechanisms by which UVA and UVB treatment impact both normal and diseased cells are complex, involving both DNA modulation and host immune response. Each type of light produces a unique response of variable depth and intensity depending on wavelength and penetrance. UVA wavelengths are between 320–400 nm and the UVB range is 280–320 nm. UVA is subdivided into UVA1 (340–400 nm) and UVA2 (320–340 nm). UVB is subdivided into broadband UVB (280–320 nm) and narrowband UVB (311–312 nm).

Phototherapy and Photochemotherapy

While all light-based treatment is technically phototherapy, many clinicians refer to UVB treatment specifically as phototherapy. This treatment is used in patients with extensive disease, alone or in combination with topical tar. UVB injury produces a combination of immunomodulatory effects.

Narrow-band UVB (311 nm) is an alternative to standard (broadband—290–320 nm) UVB in the treatment of psoriasis. Suberythemogenic doses of narrow band UVB are more effective than broadband UVB in clearing plaque psoriasis. Apoptosis of T cells is also more common with 311 nm than with broadband UVB. However, the higher cost of narrow band UVB bulbs compared with broadband bulbs currently limits its availability. Patients receive near-erythema-inducing doses of UVB at least three times weekly until remission is achieved, after which a maintenance regimen is usually recommended to prolong the remission.

Photochemotherapy incorporates light therapy combined with sensitizing chemicals applied topically or administered systemically. PUVA incorporates the use of a light-activated chemical, psoralen, followed by exposure to UVA light. Psoralens are photosensitizing agents found in plants. They have been available in synthetic form since the 1970s. Psoralens are not active without UV light. When they are combined with exposure to UVA in PUVA, they are highly effective at clearing psoriasis.

UVA penetrates deeper into the dermis compared to UVB, targeting subepidermal components including blood vessels. A number of possible mechanisms have been postulated to explain PUVA's effects. With oral PUVA, patients ingest the photosensitizing drug, 8-methoxypsoralen, followed within 2 h by exposure to UVA. This regimen is undertaken two to three times weekly in increasing doses until the desired effect is achieved, after which the frequency of the sessions is decreased to a once or twice per week maintenance program. With bath PUVA, the psoralen capsules are dissolved in water, and affected skin (hands, feet, or total body) is soaked for 15–30 min prior to UVA exposure.

Some patients take psoralen prior to coming into the office/clinic for PUVA and increased photosensitivity is typically present starting 1 h after an oral dose and resolves after 8 h. There is an inverse relationship between wavelength and energy and as such longer wavelength UVA1 light produces less skin effect than broadband UVB.

Psoriasis

Psoriasis is one of the most common autoimmune diseases in the United States. It affects approximately 2 % of the world's population. Psoriasis typically manifests as red, lichenified plaques with silvery scale. It is a chronic, recurring, lifelong disease process thought to be due to hyperproliferation of skin cells induced by a poorly defined process of immune stimulation. Psoriasis has a variety of presentations. Most patients exhibit chronic or intermittent stationary plaques (psoriasis vulgaris).

Other manifestations include non-infectious pustules (pustular psoriasis), numerous small, scaly, red or pink, teardrop-shaped papules or plaques (guttate psoriasis), and widespread inflammation and/or exfoliation of the skin (psoriatic erythroderma). Involvement is occasionally limited to the hands and feet (palmoplantar disease). Psoriasis is generally classified as being mild (affecting <3 % of the body surface area), moderate (3–10 %), or severe (>10 % of body surface area). Severity of disease is also based on intensity of psoriatic changes in affected areas, response to treatment, and overall impact on patient quality of life. Less than 40 % of patients with psoriasis have moderate or severe disease.

The Psoriasis Area and Severity Index (PASI) is a commonly used tool to objectively grade the extent and severity of the disease. The percentage of skin involved by disease and severity of involvement within each area is scored and summed to arrive at a total ranging from 0 to 72. The body is divided into four sections: head

(H; 10 % of skin surface area); arms (A; 20 %); trunk (T; 30 %), and legs (L; 40 %). Each area is scored as follows:

- 0 % of involved area, grade: 0
- <10 % of involved area, grade: 1
- 10–29 % of involved area, grade: 2
- 30–49 % of involved area, grade: 3
- 50–69 % of involved area, grade: 4
- 70–89 % of involved area, grade: 5
- 90–100 % of involved area, grade: 6

The severity of involvement in each area is estimated by three clinical signs: erythema, induration, and desquamation, rated on a scale of 0–4. The sum of the severity parameters for each area is multiplied by the area score for that area. Each area score is then multiplied by its respective surface area (0.1 for head, 0.2 for arms, 0.3 for body, and 0.4 for legs). The sum of all four products is the PASI score.

Medical management of psoriasis may include bath solutions, moisturizers, topical corticosteroid ointments and creams, vitamin D ointment, retinoids, coal tar (Goeckerman treatment), anthralin, and immunosuppressive drugs such as methotrexate. Phototherapy, photochemotherapy and excimer laser therapy are established treatment options for patients with psoriasis who do not respond to more conservative medical treatment. For patients with resistant psoriasis biologic agents such as interleukin modulators (ustekinumab), and tumor necrosis factor inhibitors (adalimumab, etanercept, infliximab) may also be administered.

PUVA and UVB Therapies

PUVA, UVB, and excimer laser therapy are all appropriate treatment options for psoriasis. Each is safe and effective when used properly in appropriately selected patients. Narrowband UVB (nbUVB) is generally preferred in patients with earlier stage disease. Suberythemogenic doses of nbUVB will effectively clear psoriasis in most patients. For patients with Fitzpatrick skin types I through III, a three times per week schedule is typically preferred. A median of 20–25 exposures will typically yield excellent results.

PUVA is very effective in treating psoriasis of various stages and can produce long periods of remission. PUVA is somewhat more challenging from a logistical standpoint, is more costly than UVB therapy, and is associated with a higher rate of iatrogenic skin cancers than UVB treatment.

The number of treatment sessions required to achieve optimal results varies by UV modality, dosing regimen, skin type, and extent of disease. For nbUVB, 15–20 treatments are typically sufficient; for bbUVB, 20–25 treatments. Favorable responses are typically evident within 2–4 weeks of initiation of UV therapy.

Excimer laser treatment employs a specific energy of UVB light and is best used for relatively localized disease, involving less than 10 % of body surface area. One advantage of excimer laser treatment over other UV therapies is that treatment can be targeted more precisely, restricting dose to diseased skin and sparing unaffected areas. Much like PUVA and traditional UVB therapy, treatments are given two to three times per week for a period of 1–3 months. Remission times typically range between 3 and 6 months.

Indications for more aggressive and/or comprehensive therapy, include involvement of more than 10 % of body surface; involvement of vulnerable areas such as the face, hands, feet, and genitalia; poor response to localized therapy; and when variants such as pustular, guttate, and erythrodermic psoriasis are present. In these circumstances treatment options include phototherapy (broad and narrowband), photochemotherapy (PUVA), systemic agents such as methotrexate and retinoids, and biologic therapies. Patients who require chronic intermittent treatment are often managed with a strategy in which one of several treatments is employed in a rotating sequence which can be repeated. This strategy can reduce the risk for long term morbidities and may delay the emergence of refractory disease states.

PUVA has been proven to be more effective than some, but not all, of the biologic therapies for psoriasis that have been developed in recent years. Drugs such as infliximab, adalimumab, and etanercept, have shown great promise as targeted drug alternatives to more traditional options.

Patient convenience is another consideration when evaluating psoriasis treatments. Since phototherapy is time-consuming and is not always geographically available, drug therapies can be logistically appealing, though costly, alternatives to phototherapy.

While a host of new and intriguing biologic therapies have become available in recent years, phototherapy remains a key treatment strategy in the armamentarium of options available to treat a variety of skin conditions. Management options must be carefully selected and employed in immunosuppressed patients. Among patients who are already immunosuppressed, psoriasis does not typically respond well to topical steroids unless high concentration formulations are prescribed. Using higher potency topical steroids to treat large areas of skin leads to systemic absorption which can cause adrenal suppression and exacerbate systemic immunosuppressive processes.

Tar plus UVB (Goeckermann therapy) has been employed with marginal success by some clinicians, though an increased incidence of Kaposi's sarcoma has been reported in some patients during or soon after such treatment. Since Kaposi's sarcoma is known to arise more frequently in traumatized or inflamed skin (Koebner phenomenon) it is hypothesized that photochemotherapy may facilitate the induction process.

PUVA reduces T cell numbers in atypical infiltrates in the skin and may even eliminate circulating atypical T lymphocytes.

PUVA can be used to treat a variety of conditions in addition to psoriasis, including eczema, skin conditions associated with graft-versus-host disease, vitiligo, mycosis fungoides, large-plaque parapsoriasis, and cutaneous T-cell lymphoma.

Psoralens

Psoralens are a family of chemicals that absorb light in the UVA spectrum (320–400 nm). Light absorption causes these chemicals to become biologically activated. As noted previously, psoralens are not biologically active without proper light exposure. Activated psoralens

trigger heightened sensitivity to ultraviolet light and manifest as erythema. It is hypothesized that PUVA produces its skin effects via a number of mechanisms, including damage to epidermal cell receptors, modulation of T lymphocyte activity, and possibly direct DNA damage.

Two forms of the psoralen are available, 8-methoxypsoralen (8-MOP) and 5-methoxypsoralen. 8-MOP (methoxsalen) is the only psoralen available in the United States by prescription. 8-MOP can be given orally or applied topically. Topical 8-MOP is rarely used given its tendency to induce severe acute skin effects over a rather narrow usage spectrum. Methoxsalen has a relatively short half-life of up to 2 h, and 80 % is eliminated within 6–8 h. Peak serum and skin levels are seen 1–6 h after ingestion with a mean of 2 h.

UVA exposure typically begins 2–3 h after ingestion. Since 8-MOP causes nausea in some patients, it is best taken on an empty stomach. Patients who do not tolerate 8-MOP can be given a trial of 5-MOP, which is typically well tolerated but more costly. Psoralen is usually given orally but can also be used topically as a cream or water bath. PUVA bath treatment is somewhat cumbersome but offers an effective alternative to oral psoralen for patients who do not tolerate the latter.

An additional advantage of topical psoralen regimens is that is that higher skin concentrations of the drug are achieved, which shortens UVA treatment sessions. Such patients must be monitored closely as acute morbidities appear more quickly when topical psoralens are used. Careful pretreatment estimates of skin sensitivity should be used (minimal phototoxic dose estimate).

PUVA is typically administered two to three times per week. A once-per-week regimen is occasionally used for patients who face travel and have logistical problems attending more frequent sessions. The latent interval prior to manifestation of treatment benefit is prolonged when this regimen is used. Patients must take precautions to limit their environmental exposure to sunlight for 24 h after taking psoralens. In addition to the use of proper skin coverings and sunscreens, proper eye protection incorporating UVA-absorbing lenses must be used.

One to two hours after ingesting psoralen, patients are exposed to a fluorescent UVA light source. Light exposure is prescribed by the treating physician in units of energy. Total energy is dependent on type/quality of light source, bulb age, and duration of exposure. There are two methods by which initial UVA dose is calculated, one based on assessment of skin type and the other based on a trial dose of PUVA designed to assess individual response and tolerance. The clinical method is based on assessment of the patient's Fitzpatrick skin type, which is based upon how a patient's skin responds to sun exposure. The trial method (PUVA test) seeks to determine the minimal phototoxic dose (MPD), that is, the lowest UVA dose which will produce erythema 72 h after psoralen administration and UVA exposure. There is no consistent evidence that either approach yields better outcomes.

Light sources are available in a variety of housing devices depending on the surface area of the body being treated. Full-body exposure can be accomplished with the use of circular or hexagonal cabins equipped with longitudinally arranged fluorescent tubes. A combination of broadband and/or narrowband UVB tubes can be arranged between the UVA tubes to provide a wider range of energies. Such mixed UVA-UVB cabins typically incorporate 21 UVA tubes and 21 UVB tubes and can be programmed to emit one or a combination of energies of light. Cabins must be equipped with a ventilation system. Smaller, specially configured light boxes can be used to treat only the hands, feet, forearms, legs, face, or scalp.

The dose received by the skin is defined by multiplying light intensity by time of exposure. The dose is typically recorded in joules per cm^2, a descriptive value used for its convenience. Currently, treatment units are equipped with photometers with a maximum sensitivity of 360 nm, which enables the intensity of the UVA or UVB light in the booth to be checked instantaneously; as a precaution, each booth comprises two independent sensors. The cabins are also equipped with electronic dose programmers linked to the sensors so that exposure time may be adapted instantaneously to the UV light intensity and voltage parameters.

Modern PUVA boxes usually contain a device which monitors the amount of light energy to which the patient is exposed and will automatically end the treatment when the desired dose has been delivered. Initial exposures are relatively brief, generally about 30 s, but later can increase to 20 min or more depending on the UVA device and bulb type, patient skin type, skin tolerance, and pigmentation profile. Exposures should be separated by a minimum of 48 h in order to minimize the risk for burning. The duration of the treatments sessions is steadily increased over 20–30 sessions. The total number of treatment exposures is determined on a case-by-case basis depending on patient tolerance and response.

PUVA is more effective than broadband UVB, but is no more efficacious than narrowband UVB. Narrowband UVB is more convenient than PUVA and is associated with fewer long term risks. As such, PUVA is used only when appropriately administered UVB therapy proves ineffective and yields only temporary improvement. UVB is preferred in younger patients given the risk of skin cancer associated with large cumulative exposures to PUVA. Phototherapy for psoriasis is not curative. Remissions typically last approximately 6 months.

UVB treatment is preferred in patients with extensive limb and trunk disease which makes ongoing topical therapy challenging. UVB will effectively clear psoriasis vulgaris in more than 50 % of patients who receive at least 30 treatments.

PUVA is selected when UVB therapy proves ineffective. PUVA is typically more effective for patients who exhibit short remissions with UVB Therapy. PUVA is typically more effective than UVB in treating palmoplantar pustular psoriasis. PUVA will induce a clinically significant response in 80–90 % of psoriasis patients within 6–8 weeks of starting treatment. Treatments are somewhat time consuming in that they are administered three times per week. Clearing of psoriatic plaques is typically complete within 10 weeks of starting treatment. The impact of UVB treatment is seen more quickly, usually within 2–4 weeks.

Optimizing the process of selecting a starting dose for PUVA in immunosuppressed patients can be accomplished by testing a sample skin patch. After psoralen is ingested, a small area of skin is exposed to UVA. The minimum photo-toxic dose is that which produces uniform ery-thema 72 h post treatment. This becomes the starting dose for therapy.

Among other issues which must be considered when selecting treatment strategies for patients deemed candidates for phototherapy are cost and convenience. Psoralen costs approximately $50 to $75 per dose. Treatments are administered two to three times per week for more than 6 weeks in most cases. For patients who require ongoing therapy, PUVA has an annual cost of $3,500 to $4,500. Biologic agents such as infliximab cost $22,500 to $25,500 (2012 data). The durability of treatment effect in patients receiving PUVA is typically longer than that seen with biologic agents, though randomized data are lacking.

UVB Phototherapy Regimen

There is no standardized optimum treatment regi-men for conditions amenable to UVB therapy. Treatment must be tailored to suit the conditions of each patient. Variables which must be consid-ered when a treatment program is designed include skin type, the type of light source to be used, dose per treatment, and treatment interval. Patients are monitored regularly to assess response and toxicity. Treatment regimens should be as efficient as possible in order to limit poten-tial for acute and chronic toxicity.

Acute morbidities are typically limited to ery-thema and xerosis. Erythema evolves in 15–40 % of patients and when evident appears within 8–24 h of exposure.

In some cases UVB phototherapy can be undertaken in the patient's home. Treatment must be transitioned from the medical clinic under the close supervision of a physician, particularly in patients who have extensive disease (e.g., psoria-sis) which will require long-term treatment. Patients who are candidates for home-based UVB treatment must demonstrate good response to UVB in the clinic, must be motivated, reliable,

able to keep accurate records of exposure, willing to adhere to physician instructions regarding treatment, and agreeable to return to the clinic for routine follow-up. Most home devices employ narrowband UVB phototherapy and most patients who use home therapy are treating psoriasis. Home UVB treatment units are available for hand/foot treatment, and half body and full body therapy. Immunosuppressed patients are more prone to acute and chronic morbidities associated with UVB therapy and are generally best man-aged in the medical clinic. Immunosuppressed patients are not typically good candidates for home-based UV treatment.

Other Diseases Amenable to Phototherapy Treatments

Connective Tissue Disease, Including Cutaneous Graft Versus Host Disease (GVHD)

Connective tissue disease, also referred to as sclerosing skin disease, includes numerous condi-tions that affect the connective tissue in various parts of the body. Sclerosing skin diseases include necrobiosis lipoidica; systemic sclerosis; local-ized scleroderma, also known as morphea; sclero-dermoid GVHD; extragenital lichen sclerosus et atrophicus; lupus erythematosus; POEMS syn-drome; and rare sclerodermoid diseases such as eosinophilic fasciitis and pansclerotic morphea. Symptoms and treatment options vary according to each condition. In some diseases, topical ste-roids are effective and in others, phototherapy and photochemotherapy are indicated. Management strategies must be designed to suit each patient's disease status, presentation, and goals. The mech-anism by which phototherapies impact connective tissue disease processes is multifactorial and appears to involve suppression of inflammatory mediators, collagen promotors, and dermal fibro-blasts. Data from numerous systematic reviews, randomized controlled trials, and case series support the efficacy of UVA and PUVA for the treatment of most sclerosing skin diseases.

Cutaneous T-Cell Lymphoma, Including Mycosis Fungoides

Cutaneous T-cell lymphoma (CTCL) is a slowly evolving form of non-Hodgkin lymphoma of the T-cell. Early stages of the disease may present as distinctive lymphoid dermatoses, such as parapsoriasis, poikiloderma atrophicans vasculare, and follicular mucinosis (alopecia mucinosa). Two-thirds of CTCL cases are mycosis fungoides, a form of CTCL that evolves from scaly skin patches and plaques. Sezary syndrome is an aggressive form of mycosis fungoides. CTCL may initially be treated with topical chemotherapy agents. When topical treatments prove to be ineffective PUVA can be employed and is often quite useful in treating early stage CTCL in the patch and plaque phase.

The 2012 National Comprehensive Cancer Network guidelines list phototherapy as a treatment option for mycosis fungoides and Sezary syndrome. Specifically, recommendations are for nbUVB for patch and thin plaque stage disease and PUVA for the treatment of thicker plaques. The European Organization for Research and Treatment for Cancer (EORTC) consensus guidelines recommend PUVA as an option for the treatment of stages IA through III mycosis fungoides and Sezary syndrome.

PUVA's impact is typically limited to superficial foci of disease directly penetrated by UVA energy. There is no consistent evidence that PUVA induces an abscopal effect, whereby immune and other humoral factors activated by superficial treatment disseminate into sanctuary areas, resulting in an indirect treatment effect. Phototherapies are administered as palliative interventions but do not impact the overall survival rate in patients with CTCL.

Lichen Planus

Lichen planus is an inflammatory disease that usually affects the skin and/or the mouth and is characterized most often as planar, polygonal, pruritic, violaceous-colored papules sometimes coalescing into plaques. Since there is no cure for lichen planus, treatment is aimed at relieving symptoms. Milder cases may be treated with corticosteroid creams and ointments, anti-inflammatory drugs, and antihistamines. More severe cases may require oral or injectable corticosteroids, phototherapy, and photochemotherapy.

While published data are limited to retrospective case series analysis and anecdotal reports, PUVA and nbUVB phototherapy have proven to be effective interventions for most patients with lichen planus. Up to 75 % of patients will exhibit a complete response to treatment within 2 months and remissions prove to be quite durable in a substantial minority of patients. There is inconsistency across various reports, however, likely due to the heterogeneity of the extent and nature of the disease within patient populations as well as across the treatment regimens that have been employed. Some studies suggest that bath PUVA could be more effective than oral PUVA, though long-term outcomes have been variable.

Atopic Dermatitis/Eczema

UVB and PUVA are effective treatments for atopic dermatitis/eczema. The general principles that guide treatment of psoriasis can be applied to treatment of atopic dermatitis, though less intensive treatment is often sufficient. Phototherapy is particularly useful in patients with extensive truncal and limb eczema which has proven to be refractory to standard topical treatments and in patients who are poor candidates for protracted steroid therapy. The benefits of phototherapy for atopicdermatitis/eczema are not typically evident until at least 15–20 treatments have been given.

Photodermatoses

Photodermatoses are skin conditions that are aggravated by sunlight. The common photodermatoses include polymorphic light eruption, actinic prurigo, and chronic actinic dermatitis, also known as photosensitivity dermatitis. Solar urticaria is a rare photodermatosis characterized by pruritis, erythema, pain and wheal formation.

While avoidance of sun exposure, use of sunscreens, and topical and/or oral steroids are effective in controlling these processes in most patients, severe cases can be effectively treated with phototherapy. UVA, narrowband UVB, broad band UVB, UVA, and PUVA are all effective. Specific treatment modality must be tailored to the extent, severity, and skin type of each patient.

Vitiligo

Phototherapy can effectively treat vitiligo. It is hypothesized that PUVA stimulates melanocytes via activation of the c-AMP pathway. Vitiligo is best managed with narrowband UVB (as opposed to PUVA) when feasible. Treatments are administered two to three times weekly and can be carried out in the clinic or, in many cases, in the patient's home.

Side Effects of UVA and UVB Therapies

The acute skin effects of phototherapies are dose-mediated and as such, treatments can be titrated to response and tolerance. If topical corticosteroids are being used to control skin symptoms at the outset of PUVA therapy this regimen is typically continued until PUVA therapy has had a chance to begin to impact the disease process. Discontinuing topical steroids immediately prior to PUVA will often precipitate a rebound exacerbation.

Patients must be closely monitored during the early phase of treatment. Significant erythema/burning is uncommon but a minority of patients prove to be particularly sensitive to appropriately administered phototherapy. Symptomatic erythema appears in approximately 10 % of patients during a full course of treatment. Other acute morbidities include central nervous system symptoms such as nausea, headache, dizziness, and insomnia. CNS symptoms typically diminish or resolve with appropriate reduction in dosing.

Long-term use of PUVA therapy can produce negative cosmetic effects and is associated with higher rates of skin cancer. Cosmetic effects include photoaging effects such as wrinkling, freckling (ephelides), mottling (poikiloderma), atrophy, elastosis, xerosis, and telangiectasia formation. A higher incidence of cataract formation is seen as well. PUVA is mutagenic, carcinogenic, and immunosuppressive. As such, the most significant complication of PUVA therapy is skin cancer, particularly squamous cell carcinoma.

PUVA is associated with a significant increase in the incidence of squamous cell carcinoma, but only a modest increase in basal cell carcinoma. Large retrospective studies indicate that more than 25 % of patients followed for long periods of time following PUVA therapy go on to develop skin cancer. The risk of skin cancer increases measurably once patients receive at least 100–150 treatments and patients receiving at least 250 treatments exhibit a greater than ten-fold increase in squamous cell carcinoma. The incidence is higher still in patients with Fitzpatrick type I–II skin.

While the incidence of melanoma does not appear to increase significantly during the first 10 years after UV therapies, a small increase in incidence has been reported beyond 15 years of follow-up. Genital skin is remarkably susceptible to the carcinogenic effects of PUVA. The cumulative cancer incidence following significant exposure is increased more than 250-fold. As such, careful shielding of genitalia is particularly important when patients are undergoing PUVA treatment. Shielding the face, when feasible, will also diminish the long-term risk of iatrogenic cancer induction. The incidence of keratoacanthoma (Fig. 12.2) is also increased following PUVA therapy. There is no evidence that PUVA therapy raises risk for internal malignancy.

Human papilloma virus (HPV), including a cross section of numerous subtypes of the virus, appears to be a cofactor in the carcinogenic process by which PUVA impacts treated skin. HPV has been detected in up to 75 % of non-melanoma skin cancers in patients treated with PUVA. The ratio of squamous cell carcinoma to basal cell carcinoma is opposite that seen in the general population, and is similar to that seen in patients who have undergone organ transplantation,

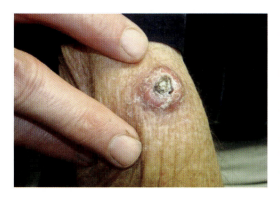

Fig. 12.2 A keratoacanthoma on the arm with symmetry, rapid growth, and a keratotic center. It is considered by many as a form of squamous cell cancer and is increases with phototherapy. Metastasis is very rare

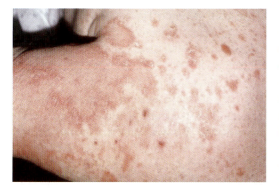

Fig. 12.3 Subacute cataneous lupus erththematosus has a variant that mimics psoriasis with a papulosquamous look. Phototherapy will make this worse instead of better. Telangiectasia and atrophy are signs seen in this example of subacute cataneous lupus on the back of the shoulder that help with the diagnosis. There is a rare variant of psoriasis that also may worsen with phototherapy

suggesting that immunomodulation may well play a significant role in the carcinogenic effect of PUVA.

There are a number of circumstances in which PUVA and UVB are contraindicated. Absolute contraindications include lupus eryhthematosus (Fig. 12.3) and presence of photodermatoses such as xeroderma pigmentosum, porphyrias, Darier's disease, and trichothiodystrophy. Patients who are medically unfit, such that their tolerance for potential dermatitis would be quite

limited, should not receive phototherapy. Pregnancy is a contraindication to PUVA (though UVB therapy can be considered during pregnancy). Relative contraindications to PUVA and UVB include a personal history of skin cancer, young age (due to the long-term risk of skin cancers), patients with certain types of epilepsy who are prone to seizure induction by exposure to fluorescent lamps, patients taking certain medications that can potentiate the effect of psoralen or induce heightened photosensitivity, history of significant burns or high-dose radiation therapy to targeted skin, atypical nevus syndrome, history of photosensitivity disorder (including lupus erythematosus and porphyria), and significant family history of skin cancers (especially when such cancers appeared at younger ages).

Patients with significant immunosuppression, whether genetic, acquired, or iatrogenic, constitute a high-risk group poorly suited to most forms of UV therapy. Depending upon the nature and extent of the skin condition to be addressed and the severity of immunocompromise, a favorable therapeutic ratio will exist for select patients. Immunosuppressed patients require particularly vigilant monitoring as they are prone to develop more severe treatment related morbidities and such side effects tend to evolve more rapidly and earlier in the treatment course compared with immunocompetent patients. Protective measures must be employed as rigorously as possible. UVB therapies pose fewer challenges than PUVA in this regard.

Evolving data suggest that biologic agents (such as T cell blockers, interleukin and tumor necrosis factor modulators) in and of themselves may increase the risk for skin cancer with prolonged follow-up. Used in sequential combination with phototherapy, even narrowband UVB, an increased incidence of carcinogenesis is seen. While there are limited data regarding acute and chronic morbidities associated with the use of biologic agents in immunosuppressed patients, such individuals are presumed to be at greater risk for treatment related carcinogenesis compared with immunocompetent patients. UVB therapy is much less carcinogenic than UVA.

Special Considerations in Immunocompromised Patients

Human immunodeficiency virus (HIV) has been linked to myriad cutaneous manifestations, some of which can be directly or indirectly caused by or treated with UV radiation therapy. HIV not only causes immunodeficiency but can also induce autoimmune disorders. HIV photodermatitis has been reported in up to 5 % of HIV-seropositive patients, encompassing a variety of clinical manifestations. African American patients exhibit much higher rates of photodermatitis than other races. A number of case reports have been published detailing outcomes among HIV-positive patients who present with or later develop vitiligo, which is a manifestation of autoimmune depigmentation. Standard treatment options for patients with vitiligo include, but are not limited to, ultraviolet radiation. Outcomes across various case reports suggest that UVB and PUVA treatment may be less effective in immunocompromised patients, and that repigmentation occurs in a minority of patients who respond well to highly active antiretroviral therapy (HAART).

Chronic actinic dermatitis, a condition belonging to the immunologically mediated photodermatoses, has also been linked to HIV infection. It typically presents as an eczematous eruption in sun-exposed areas. The age of onset is younger in the affected population versus the immunocompetent, and the prevalence of photosensitivity in the HIV population has been estimated at 5.4 %. Furthermore, worsening of immunodeficiency (a drop in CD4 count) typically shows a worsening of CAD. Eosinophilic pustular folliculitis (EPF), also known as Ofuji's disease, is an inflammatory dermatosis more commonly found in the Asian population. It typically presents as annular or isolated papules or plaques on the face or scalp usually with an associated systemic eosinophilia. There is an immunosuppression-associated variant that has been linked with HIV or an immunocompromised state. A case report did indicate that one patient benefited from UVB therapy, although the duration and frequency was not specified.

UV therapies must be used with caution in HIV-seropositive patients. UV therapy has been reported to worsen or even induce HIV-related skin disease in a minority of such patients. Kaposi's sarcoma, the first malignant tumor associated with HIV-infection, is a proliferative tumor of endothelial cells induced by the human herpes-virus 8 (HHV-8). PUVA therapy has been implicated as a possible inductive agent in the development of Kaposi's sarcoma in at least one patient not known to be HIV positive who was being treated for alopecia areata.

Patients who have undergone organ transplantation are at a significantly increased risk of developing precancerous actinic keratoses (AKs) and non-melanoma skin cancers as a direct result of the immunosuppressive medications required to maintain the graft. The incidence of squamous cell skin cancer is increased 65–250-fold and a ten-fold increase in basal cell carcinoma is seen compared with immunocompetent patients. The ratio of squamous to basal cell carcinoma is opposite of that seen in immunocompetent patients. The incidence of squamous cell carcinoma is <10 % 1 year post-transplantation, but increases to 82 % after 20 years. The incidence of malignant melanoma (3.4-fold) and Kaposi sarcoma (84-fold) is also increased in transplant patients, and risk increases continuously over time. Several factors contribute to the overall risk of developing skin cancer in this patient population, including exposure to ultraviolet radiation, especially UVB, co-infection with the human papilloma virus, duration of the graft, and immunosuppressant drug therapy.

Immunosuppressant drugs such as cyclosporine, azathioprine, and the calcineurin are all associated with an increased incidence of skin cancer. Early evidence suggests that drugs such as sirolimus and everolimus, which inhibit mTOR protein kinase, may actually reduce the risk of skin cancers in transplant patients compared with more traditional immunosuppressive drugs.

Transplant patients must be educated and cautioned regarding skin cancer risks and behavioral modification strategies that can reduce these risks. Minimizing UV light exposure and close follow-up in the medical clinic are critically important.

Aggressive management of precancerous and cancerous lesions helps optimize both quality of life and overall survival in this high-risk population. A number of treatment strategies can be useful, including topical 5-fluorouracil, cryotherapy, photodynamic therapy, imiquimod, and retinoids. Imiquimod and retinoids have demonstrated efficacy as prophylactic interventions as well.

Photodynamic Therapy

Photodynamic therapy (PDT) is the unique process that utilizes a photosensitizing substance, such as aminolevulinic acid (ALA) or its methyl ester methyl aminolevulinate (MAL). Both are precursors to protoporphyrin IX and when exposed to appropriate wavelengths of light and oxygen, produce reactive oxygen species that cause cell death specifically in rapidly dividing cells (i.e. precancerous actinic keratoses on the scalp). MAL offers advantages over ALA in terms of skin penetration, secondary to its improved lipophilicity, and greater specificity for neoplastic cells. The treatment is convenient, can target a large affected surface area of skin, and can be performed in the outpatient clinical setting. First, a keratolytic agent (salicylic acid 5–20 %, propylene glycol 20–50 %, carbamide 10–20 % or acetone) is applied to the treatment site. The photosensitizer is then applied topically, followed by a specific incubation period that is product specific. The patient then is exposed to a specific wavelength of light for a product-specific period of time. The FDA-approved Blu-U device uses ALA and is activated by blue light near the Soret band (~410 nm). Since there are other peaks in the excitation spectrum of porphyrins, other devices use MAL in conjunction with red light at approximately 635 nm to achieve similar results.

The efficacy of PDT in preventing the occurrence of new actinic keratoses (AKs) and non-melanoma skin cancer (NMSC) in organ transplant recipients (OTR) has been well documented. A 2010 study observed the use of cyclic blue-light source PDT every 4–8 weeks for 2 years in OTRs at high risk for squamous cell carcinomas (SCCs). The authors found a 95 % reduction in SCCs compared to baseline after the 24-month period. Wulf et al. investigated the use of a single session of MAL PDT in 27 renal transplant patients as primary prevention of new actinic keratoses, basal cell carcinomas, squamous cell carcinomas, keratoacanthomas, or warts. The results indicated a statistically significant longer mean time to occurrence of a new lesion in the PDT group (9.8 months versus 6.8 months in the control).

Pain during and after illumination is a common side effect experienced by patients undergoing PDT. There is also the inherent risk of further immunosuppression created by PDT intrinsic to its mechanism of recruiting inflammatory and pro-inflammatory cytokines. However, in an analysis of over 200 OTRs undergoing PDT with ALA/MAL, no study indicated damage to the transplanted organ.

Conclusion

Phototherapy is a comparatively safe and effective treatment strategy for appropriately selected patients with a variety of skin conditions, including psoriasis, cutaneous T cell lymphoma, various photodermatoses, vitiligo and atopic dermatitis. Several types of light therapy may be employed, with or without sensitizing psoralens, depending on the type and severity of the condition being addressed.

Phototherapy, photochemotherapy, and excimer laser therapy are established treatment options for patients with psoriasis who do not respond adequately to more conservative medical treatment. Combined psoralen and UVA (PUVA) is highly effective in treating psoriasis and can produce long periods of remission. Narrowband UVB (nbUVB) is generally preferred in patients with psoriasis in its earlier stages. Suberythemogenic doses of nbUVB will effectively clear psoriasis in most patients over a period of several weeks. NbUVB is more convenient than PUVA and is associated with fewer long term risks.

PUVA is somewhat more challenging to administer from a logistical standpoint, is more costly than UVB therapy, and is associated with side effects which require a higher level of clinical attention and management.

Immunosuppressed patients present a number of unique challenges when phototherapies are employed. Given the fact that phototherapies utilize immune modulation to produce host responses to disease, immunosuppression can alter response as well as acute and chronic morbidity profiles. As such, treatment programs for these patients must be designed with care and caution, and patients must be monitored vigilantly both during and after treatment. Immunosuppressed patients, therefore, are not typically good candidates for home-based UV treatment. Both acute and chronic morbidities can be greatly exacerbated in immunosuppressed patients. The risk of iatrogenic skin cancers, in particular, is markedly higher in immunosuppressed patients who receive most types of phototherapy. Absolute contraindications to PUVA include extant lupus eryhthematosus, xeroderma pigmentosum, porphyrias, Darier's disease, and trichothiodystrophy. A number of relative contraindications exist as well. HIV-seropositive patients and can be treated with phototherapy, but UV therapies must be employed cautiously in these patients given the potential for heightened treatment sensitivity, variable response, and potential long term morbidities.

Suggested Reading

Alldredge BK, Corelli RL, Ernst ME, Guglielmo Jr J, Koda-Kimble MA, Youngs LY. Applied therapeutics: the clinical use of drugs. Philadelphia: Lippincott Williams & Wilkins; 2013.

Antony FC, Marsden RA. Vitiligo in association with human immunodeficiency virus infection. J Eur Acad Dermatol Venereol. 2003;17(4):456–8.

Bangash HK, Colegio OR. Management of non-melanoma skin cancer in immunocompromised solid organ transplant recipients. Curr Treat Options Oncol. 2012;13(3):354–76.

Basset-Seguin N, Baumann Conzett K, Gerritsen MJ, Gonzalez H, Haedersdal M, Hofbauer GF, et al. Photodynamic therapy for actinic keratosis in organ transplant patients. J Eur Acad Dermatol Venereol. 2013;27(1):57–66.

Bilu D, Mamelak AJ, Nguyen RH, Queiroz PC, Kowalski J, Morison WL, et al. Clinical and epidemiologic characterization of photosensitivity in HIV-positive individuals. Photodermatol Photoimmunol Photomed. 2004;20(4):175–83.

Breuckmann F, Gambichler T, Altmeyer P, Kreuter A. UVA/UVA1 phototherapy and PUVA photochemotherapy in connective tissue diseases and related disorders: a research based review. BMC Dermatol. 2004;4(1):11.

Cribier B, Frances C, Chosidow O. Treatment of lichen planus. An evidence-based medicine analysis of efficacy. Arch Dermatol. 1998;134(12):1521–30.

Jemec GBE, Miech D, Kemény L. Non-surgical treatment of keratinocyte skin cancer. Berlin/Heidelberg: Springer; 2010.

Jensen P, Hansen S, Moller B, Leivestad T, Pfeffer P, Geiran O, et al. Skin cancer in kidney and heart transplant recipients and different long-term immunosuppressive therapy regimens. J Am Acad Dermatol. 1999;40(2 Pt 1):177–86.

Katoh M, Nomura T, Miyachi Y, Kabashima K. Eosinophilic pustular folliculitis: a review of the Japanese published works. J Dermatol. 2013;40(1):15–20.

Lehmann P, Schwarz T. Photodermatoses: diagnosis and treatment. Dtsch Arztebl Int. 2011;108(9):135–41.

Pariser DM, Bagel J, Gelfand JM, Korman NJ, Ritchlin CT, Strober BE, et al. National Psoriasis Foundation clinical consensus on disease severity. Arch Dermatol. 2007;143(2):239–42.

Philips R. HIV photodermatitis presenting with widespread vitiligo-like depigmentation. Dermatol Online J. 2012;18(1):6.

Picardo M, Taich A. Vitiligo. Berlin/Heidelberg: Springer; 2010. p. 91–4.

Popivanova NI, Chudomirova KN, Baltadzhiev IG, Abadjieva TI. HIV/AIDS-associated Kaposi's sarcoma with multiple skin-mucosal disseminations following ultraviolet (puva) photochemotherapy. Folia Med (Plovdiv). 2010;52(3):56–61.

Rival-Tringali AL, Euvrard S, Decullier E, Claudy A, Faure M, Kanitakis J. Conversion from calcineurin inhibitors to sirolimus reduces vascularization and thickness of post-transplant cutaneous squamous cell carcinomas. Anticancer Res. 2009;29(6):1927–32.

Tan AW, Lim KS, Theng C, Chong WS. Chronic actinic dermatitis in Asian skin: a Singaporean experience. Photodermatol Photoimmunol Photomed. 2011;27(4):172–5.

Ulrich C, Kanitakis J, Stockfleth E, Euvrard S. Skin cancer in organ transplant recipients—where do we stand today? Am J Transplant. 2008;8(11):2192–8.

Willey A, Mehta S, Lee PK. Reduction in the incidence of squamous cell carcinoma in solid organ transplant recipients treated with cyclic photodynamic therapy. Dermatol Surg. 2010;36(5):652–8.

Wulf HC, Pavel S, Stender I, Bakker-Wensveen CA. Topical photodynamic therapy for prevention of new skin lesions in renal transplant recipients. Acta Derm Venereol. 2006;86(1):25–8.

Skin Cancer in the Immunocompromised

13

Ting Wang, Daniel J. Aires, and Deede Liu

Abstract

Skin cancer in organ transplant recipients (OTRs) and other immunosuppressed populations is a significant health care concern. The more than two million American OTRs have a dramatically increased risk for developing squamous cell cancer, as well as a variety of other skin cancers, including basal cell cancer, melanoma, Merkel cell carcinoma, and Kaposi sarcoma. Skin cancer risk is also increased among patients receiving immunosuppressive treatment for various autoimmune diseases such as rheumatoid arthritis, inflammatory bowel disease, and psoriasis, and also patients infected with the human immunodeficiency virus. Management of cutaneous neoplasia in these at-risk populations includes topical therapies, photodynamic therapy, systemic retinoids, surgical excision, as well as multidisciplinary care involving patient education and frequent dermatological examinations. In OTRs and autoimmune patients the revision of immunosuppression is also a key treatment consideration for aggressive skin cancers.

Keywords

Immunosuppression • Organ transplantation • Inflammatory disease • HIV • Non-melanoma skin cancer • Melanoma • Merkel cell carcinoma • Kaposi sarcoma

T. Wang, MD, PhD • D.J. Aires, MD, JD
D. Liu, MD (✉)
Division of Dermatology, Department of Internal
Medicine, University of Kansas Medical Center,
3901 Rainbow Boulevard, Kansas City,
KS 66160, USA
e-mail: dliu@kumc.edu

J.C. Hall (ed.), *Skin Diseases in the Immunocompromised*,
DOI 10.1007/978-1-4471-6479-1_13, © Springer-Verlag London 2014

us< /br>

Introduction

Iatrogenic immunosuppression, primarily in organ transplant recipients (OTR), is increasingly common. Cutaneous cancers and precancerous lesions present unique challenges in these patient populations. Along with standard treatment, modification of immunosuppression is a key consideration. Patients with human immunodeficiency virus (HIV) or those receiving immunomodulatory medications are also at elevated risk for skin cancer; special considerations in these populations are also addressed below. Although much remains to be learned, consensus protocols and approaches can be helpful in treating.

Organ Transplantation

More than two million Americans are organ transplant recipients (OTRs). Compared to the general population, OTRs have a dramatically increased risk for developing a variety of skin cancers, including squamous cell cancer (SCC), basal cell cancer (BCC), melanoma, Merkel cell carcinoma, and Kaposi's sarcoma. Overall, nearly 50 % of OTRs develop skin cancer. In addition, skin cancers in OTRs tend to run a more aggressive course with increased morbidity and mortality compared to those in immunocompetent patients. Among the OTRs, non-melanoma skin cancers (NMSC), especially SCC, are the most common malignancies, accounting for more than 90 % of all skin cancers. In contrast to the general population where the ratio of BCC to SCC is 4:1, in OTRs the ratio is inverted and SCC is more common than BCC.

Although all OTRs are at elevated risk for skin cancers, a number of specific factors have been identified that increase risk even further. These risk factors are summarized in the list below. These include older age, male gender, increased UV exposure and duration of immunosuppression. Increased duration of immunosuppression is particularly associated with SCC. The risk appears to vary by skin type as well, with pale Fitzpatrick skin type I carrying the greatest risk.

Risk factors for skin cancer in OTRs
Fair skin
Increased sunlight exposure
Personal history of NMSC
Male sex
Types of organ transplant (heart > lung > kidney > liver)
Longer duration of immunosuppression
Longer post-transplant time
Level and types of immunosuppression[a]
History of lymphoma and CD4 lymphocytopenia
Autoimmune disorders (Rheumatoid arthritis, systemic lupus erythematosus, autoimmune hepatitis)
History of HPV infection
Dysplastic nevus[b]
History of melanoma in organ donor[b]

[a]Use of Azathioprine and calcineurin inhibitors associate with higher risk of skin cancers
[b]Higher risk factor for development of melanoma

The type of immunosuppression also appears to play a role. In transplantation, there are generally considered to be two phases of immunosuppression. The first phase, induction therapy, occurs preoperatively and immediately post-transplantation, and the second phase, maintenance therapy, commences after the immediate post-transplantation period and is continued over the long-term. Different immunosuppressive regimens are generally used for these two phases. Muromonab-CD3 (OKT3) and anti-thymocyte globulin (ATG) are often used in the induction phase. OKT3 is a murine monoclonal IgG2a antibody that binds to the T cell receptor-CD3 complex on the surface of circulating T cells, initially leading to activation, but subsequently inducing blockage and apoptosis of the T cells. The T-cell depletion effect by ATG is thought to occur through complement-dependent lysis, T-cell activation and apoptosis, modulation of leukocyte/endothelium interactions, induction of B-cell apoptosis, blockage of dendritic cell function, and induction of regulatory T and natural killer T cells.

A much broader range of immunosuppressants is used in the maintenance phase. These include corticosteroids, azathioprine, mycophenolate mofetil (MMF), calcineurin inhibitors (cyclosporine and tacrolimus), and rapamycin inhibitors (sirolumus and everolimus).

Corticosteroids exert their immunosuppressive effects via multiple mechanisms, including NFkB and AP-1 inhibition, lymphocyte apoptosis, decreased immunoglobulin and IL-2 production, and decreased NK cell activity. Mycophenolate mofetil inhibits inosine monophosphate dehydrogenase needed for de novo purine synthesis; this in turn prevents proliferation of T and B lymphocytes. Cyclosporine reduces IL-2 production and helper T-cell and cytotoxic T-cell proliferation by inhibiting calcineurin, the enzyme that activates transcription factor NFAT-1. Tacrolimus binds to FK506-binding protein, which inhibits calcineurin and NFAT-1 via a different pathway. Thiopurines, which include azathioprine, 6thioguanine and 6-mercaptopurine, exert their immunosuppressive effects by interfering with key processes in T cell activation. Sirolimus and everolimus both inhibit activation of T and B cells by IL-2 by binding to FKBP-12, which blocks the mammalian target of rapamycin (mTOR).

During maintenance, azathioprine is associated with greater incidence of SCC versus MMF, MMF combined with cyclosporine A, or MMF combined with tacrolimus. In contrast to azathioprine, sirolimus has demonstrated a protective effect against skin cancers, particularly SCC and Kaposi's sarcoma. Nonetheless sirolimus tends not be a first line agent as it is associated with doubled risk of other serious adverse events, including proteinuria, edema, diarrhea, hyperlipidemia, myelosuppression, impaired wound healing and thrombotic microangiopathy. While skin cancers generally manifest during the maintenance phase of treatment, some studies have revealed increased SCC and BCC risk during induction therapy using OKT3 or ATG.

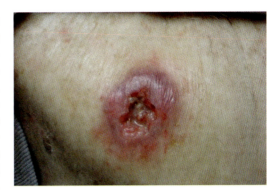

Fig. 13.1 Large squamous cell cancer on the back that was treated by MOHS surgery. These tumors are particulary worrisome in immune-suppressed patients where metastasis is more common. Erythema, induration, ulceration, and exophytic fleshy tumor are all indicative of a squamous cell cancer

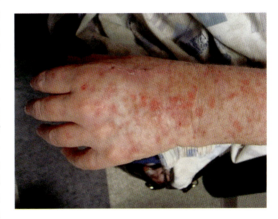

Fig. 13.2 Extensive actinic keratosis over the back of hand and extensor forearm with keratotic tumors arising on ill-defined erytheamatous base. These are often painful to the touch and feel very rough. Risk of malignant transformation to a squamous cell cancer is probably more common in an immune-compromised state

population. The mean time to diagnosis of first non-melanoma skin cancer has been reported to be 4–9 years after kidney transplantation.

Squamous Cell Carcinoma

Squamous cell carcinoma (SCC), shown in Fig. 13.1, is the most common skin cancer in OTRs, occurring 65–250 times more frequently than in general population. Moreover, SCC in OTRs carries a higher metastatic risk of around 8 %, in contrast to the 0.5–5 % risk in the general

Pathogenesis

The development of SCC is thought to be multifactorial, with etiological factors including UV radiation, immunosuppressed status, and presence of HPV infection. Multiple steps are likely to be involved in carcinogenesis, with the first step probably being the development of actinic keratosis (AK), shown in Fig. 13.2. Although each individual AK lesion is estimated to have a 0.6 % per year risk of progression to SCC, in one study approximately two-thirds of SCCs originated from AKs, which emphasizes the importance of treating AKs early. Because in most studies to date on invasive SCC, there is limited data on squamous cell carcinoma in situ (SCCIS) in OTRs. The risk of progression of SCCIS to invasive SCC has been estimated to be 3–5 %.

It is well known that in SCC and AK, UV radiation results in both immunologic tumor tolerance and DNA damage, such as mutations in the tumor suppressor gene p53. It can also activate several oncogenic pathways, including RAS and cMYC in SCCs, and NF-κB and TNF in AKs, respectively. Interestingly, all these genes are downstream of epidermal growth factor receptor (EGFR), whose overexpression has been noted in SCC with worse clinical outcome. Several hyperproliferation-related genes and stress markers, such as keratin 6 (KRT6) and KRT16, are upregulated by UV as well. Of note, high-risk strains of human papillomavirus (HPV) may also play a role in the pathogenesis of SCC in OTRs via actions of two oncoproteins, E6 and E7, both of which ultimately inhibit the p53 pathway. Aberrations in these pathways ultimately lead to apoptosis inhibition and uncontrolled proliferation by tumor cells.

Clinical Features

Clinically, AKs usually present as erythematous scaly papules on sun-exposed areas. They tend to be chronic and progressive. AKs are generally diagnosed clinically without histologic evaluation. However, in an OTR the clinician should have a low threshold to biopsy an AK-like lesion that is persistent or demonstrates atypical clinical features to rule out SCC, particularly in OTRs.

SCCs usually present as rapidly growing erythematous hyperkeratotic or ulcerated pap-

ules or plaques. They can also present as verrucous papules, mimicking warts. Accurate diagnosis of SCC relies on histopathologic examination.

Management—General Considerations

All OTRs will benefit from skin cancer-oriented screening and education before transplantation, and also from regular examination afterward. Although all OTRs are considered to have higher risk for skin cancers, clinicians need to be aware of the key factors that predispose certain sub-populations of OTRs to even higher risks, as detailed in the bulleted list discussed early in "Organ Transplantation." These include prior history of skin cancer, multiple AKs, fair complexion, older age, history of HPV infection, and longer duration and intensity of immunosuppression. Patients should be educated to avoid unprotected sun exposure, especially during peak UV hours of 10 a.m. to 2 p.m, to practice sun protection with sun-protective clothing and application of broad-spectrum sunscreen with SPF > 30 to exposed areas, and to cease tanning bed use. Patients should be taught to perform skin self-examinations, and recognize common pre-malignant and malignant skin lesions. Based on the individual's risk for developing skin cancers, OTRs need to return to the office for follow-up at appropriate time intervals.

Actinic Keratosis and Warts

Early treatment of AKs and warts is critical to prevent progression to SCC. Standard therapies include cryotherapy, curettage with electrodessication, topical 5-fluorouracil, and photodynamic therapy. Treatment-resistant warts and AKs, or those with atypical clinical features, should be examined histologically to rule out SCC. Alarming features include bleeding, ulceration, pigmentation, large surface area or edema, rapid growth, or location on high-risk areas such as lips or ears.

Less Aggressive SCC

Treatment decisions for SCC should be guided by aggressiveness based on the risk factors outlined below. These include lesion history, size, location, and histopathology.

Risk factors suggesting aggressiveness of SCC
Clinical features
Size>0.6 cm on H zone of face (central face, eyebrows, eyelids, periorbital, nose, lips, chin, pre- and post-auricular, temple and ears), hands, feet and genitalia
Size>1.0 cm on forehead, cheeks, neck and scalp
Size>2.0 cm on trunk and extremities
Location of scalp, central face, ear, lip, genitalia, nail unit
Recurrent nature
Occurrence in a scar, or in the field of prior radiation
Rapid growth
Ulceration
Satellite metastasis
Histologic features
Poor differentiation
Perineural involvement
Invasion of subcutaneous fat

Furthermore, full-body skin exam and palpation of draining lymph nodes should be performed if they have not been done recently. Less aggressive SCC can be treated with destructive techniques such as electrodessication and curettage (ED&C), cryosurgery, or surgical excision with postoperative margin assessment. Obtaining a margin of 4–6 mm beyond surrounding erythema is recommended.

Aggressive SCC Without Metastasis

For aggressive SCC, surgical excision with complete removal is recommended. The highest cure rate with the best conservation of normal tissue can be achieved with Mohs micrographic surgery. High cure rates can also be achieved by excision with intraoperative frozen section but this requires expertise of both the surgeon and the pathologist. Conventional excision with postoperative margin evaluation is also valuable, but this has a lower cure rate compared to Mohs. However, conventional surgery is valuable when Mohs is unavailable, or when the lesion is too large to achieve complete clear margin. Guidelines by Stasko et al. recommend a margin of 6–10 mm of clinically normal skin beyond surrounding erythema and into the subcutaneous fat tissue.

For high-risk SCC, adjuvant radiation therapy is indicated in the following scenarios: inability to achieve clear margin, re-excision not feasible, perineural disease, multiple metastases to lymph nodes, and extranodal spread. For inoperable tumors or in poor surgical candidates due to other comorbidities, radiation therapy can be considered as the primary therapy.

Sentinel lymph node biopsy (SLNB) is not routinely recommended for high-risk SCC. A recent study of 20 patients suggested that SLNB may offer prognostic information, but at this time it has not been established which patients stand to benefit, and what the ultimate role of SLNB will be in treating SCC in OTRs.

Aggressive SCC with In-transit Cutaneous Metastasis

It is well defined that cutaneous SCC metastasis usually occurs in sequential steps, first spreading along lymphatics to adjacent areas, next arriving in draining lymphatic basins, and ultimately metastasizing to distant locations. In-transit cutaneous metastasis is defined as a cutaneous metastatic focus located between the primary tumor and the closest lymph nodes. Clinically, in-transit metastasis can appear as subtle gray-white to skin-colored papules that are not contiguous with the primary tumor. Patients with such lesions should be referred for full oncological assessment of lymphatic involvement and distant metastasis. Imaging studies such as computed tomographic (CT) and/or magnetic resonance imaging (MRI) can help evaluate tumor spread. If no other metastasis is identified, then primary and satellite lesions should be removed via Mohs or conventional surgery. These patients also need to be evaluated for possible postoperative radiation. If further metastases are found, the treatment regimen will depend on the nature of the metastases, as detailed in the next sections.

Aggressive SCC with Palpable Lymphadenopathy or Further Metastasis

Patients with palpable lymphadenopathy should be referred to oncology and/or surgical oncology for tissue sampling via fine-needle aspiration or open node biopsy. A complete oncological evaluation is warranted. The following options could be considered: therapeutic lymphadenectomy or parotidectomy for tumors involving the parotid, adjuvant radiation therapy, initiation of chemoprevention, and revision of immunosuppression regimen. Optimal approaches often involve multidisciplinary consultation with relevant experts from dermatology, pathology, the transplant team, and medical, surgical, and radiation oncology. Adjustment of immunosuppression regimen may range from simple dose reduction, discontinuation of one or more of several immunosuppressive agents, and substitution of alternate therapies. The risks of tumor progression need to be weighed against the possibility of allograft rejection.

At present, the efficacy of systemic chemotherapy for metastatic SCC has not been well established. However, recent studies suggest potential roles for two newer agents, cetuximab and capecitabine. Cetuximab is a monoclonal antibody directed toward the epidermal growth factor receptor (EGFR). It inactivates EGFR via direct binding, which subsequently inhibits cell proliferation and promotes apoptosis. Cetuximab has been approved for treatment of advanced or metastatic head and neck SCC. Some studies suggest efficacy of cetuximab against cutaneous SCC, including a phase II clinical trial. However, it should be noted that there is an issue of emerging resistance, which may limit the utility of this treatment. Furthermore, there are two reports of fatalities due to diffuse alveolar damage after use of cetuximab for SCC in single-lung transplant recipients. Thus, the utility of cetuximab for treating SCC in OTRs needs further investigation. Common adverse effects of cetuximab include acneiform eruption, skin desquamation, cardiotoxicity, pulmonary toxicity, diarrhea, and hypersensitivity reactions.

Capecitabine is a 5-fluorouracil (5FU) prodrug. After enzymatic conversion to 5FU, it inhibits DNA and RNA synthesis. Capecitabine is approved as therapy for metastatic breast and colon cancer. A number of studies showed subtle improvement of SCC and AKs but also decreased incidence of new SCC, BCC, and AKs in OTRs. Adverse reactions include fatigue, hand–foot syndrome, neutropenic fever, and diarrhea. Overall, although cetuximab and capecitabine are potentially promising treatment modalities, more investigations are warranted to fully establish their efficacy and safety for SCC in OTRs.

Chemoprevention

Chemoprevention or chemoprophylaxis refers to suppressing or reversing carcinogenesis via topical or systemic agents. Chemoprevention is often considered for OTRs and other patients at risk of developing multiple, invasive, or metastatic SCC, as outlined below.

Indications to consider chemoprevention
>5–10 NMSCs per year[a]
NMSC developing at accerlerating rate[a]
Several NMSCs in high risk locations particularly head and neck[a]
High risk NMSC with >20 % risk of metastasis[a]
Metastatic NMSC[a]
Eruptive keratoacanthoma
Numerous AKs

[a]Risk factors for development of numerous or high-risk NMSC includes immunosuppression (OTRs, hematologic malignancies, chronic immunosuppressive therapy, human immunodeficiency virus infection), chronic radiation or UV radiation exposure, chronic arsenic exposure, genetic syndromes such as Nevoid BCC syndrome, xeroderma pigmentosum, epidermodysplasia verruciformis

It is important to note that the goal of chemoprevention is to reduce the number of new NMSCs to a manageable level rather than completely eradicate new NMSCs. Several chmopreventive agents have been studied for effectiveness and safety in the OTR population, which are explained below.

Retinoids

Retinoids are vitamin A derivatives with antiproliferative properties that regulate differentiation, apoptosis, and cell cycle arrest. Acitretin, isotretinoin, and etretinate have been shown to reduce the incidence of SCC, BCC, and AK; acitretin and isotretinoin are available in the United States. Most retinoid studies have demonstrated efficacy in decreasing new skin cancers and suppressing recurrence or progression of high-risk SCC. Oral retinoids are thus often recommended for OTRs at risk for multiple, invasive, or metastatic SCCs. On the contrary, the use of oral retinoids in prevention of BCC is controversial and not routinely recommended. One should also be aware of the existence of a rebound effect with emergence of difficult-to-control new SCCs upon discontinuation of oral retinoids.

Systemic Retinoids

Systemic retinoids are highly teratogenic and thus absolutely contraindicated during pregnancy, lactation, or at any time in women of childbearing potential who cannot achieve effective contraception. Other major potential adverse events and risks include mucocutaneous dryness, liver injury, hypertriglyceridemia, increased intracranial pressure, myalgia, and bone pain. Thus, additional contraindications include moderate to severe liver dysfunction, concomitant hepatotoxic medication, alcohol abuse, kidney dysfunction, and uncontrolled hyperlipidemia. Both acitretin and isotretinoin should be started at lower doses, with the goal of reaching a target dose of 15–25 mg per day and 0.5 mg/kg per day, respectively, based on the patient's clinical response, side effects, and laboratory values. Acitretin is usually considered the first choice as it has more longterm data. However, in women of childbearing age, isotretinoin is often preferred due to its shorter half-life. Women are also advised to use two forms of contraception for 3 years after discontinuing acitretin and 1 month after discontinuing isotretinoin.

Patients receiving systemic retinoids should have a complete history and physical exam, complete blood count, glucose, creatinine, liver function tests, fasting lipid panel, and hepatitis screen at baseline, and repeat history and physical exam, creatinine, liver function tests, and lipid panel every month for the first 3 months then every 3 months.

Topical Retinoids

Topical retinoids have been used to treat BCC and SCC in situ with an approximately 50 % resolution rate. They have also been evaluated as possible chemoprevention agents. The largest randomized double-blind study of a topical retinoid vs. vehicle control involved more than 1,100 patients who were followed for 1.5–5.5 years. There was no difference between topical tretinoin 0.1 % cream and vehicle in reducing NMSC or AK counts. Thus, routine use of topical retinoids for chemoprevention cannot be supported at this time.

Adjustment of Immunosuppression Regimen

With the increasing understanding of the many potential adverse effects of immunosuppression regimens on infection risk, general immune function, bone density, metabolism and mental health, many transplantation programs now reduce immunosuppressant medications to the lowest possible level consistent with proper graft function. It is also well accepted that a more aggressive approach toward reduction of immunosuppression can be taken with kidney or liver versus heart allograft recipients. This is partly due to the fact that kidney transplant recipients may return to dialysis in the setting of allograft failure, and liver allografts display lower intrinsic immunogenicity and tend to recover better from rejection.

Several studies have demonstrated that dose reduction of immunosuppression results in improved outcomes for patients with aggressive SCC, multiple new SCCs, or metastatic SCC. Regimen adjustment can involve different approaches including (1) reduction of current immunosuppression to the lowest level maintaining good graft function; (2) discontinuation of one or more if patient is on multiple medications; and (3) conversion from a regimen based on calcineurin inhibition to one based on mTOR inhibition via sirolimus or everolimus.

One study reported that although both sirolimus and calcineurin-inhibitor based groups demonstrated stable allograft function, sirolimus was associated with a doubled incidence of serious adverse events such as proteinuria, edema, diarrhea, hyperlipidemia, myelosuppression, impaired wound healing, and thrombotic microangiopathy. It is typically considered only after the organ graft function stabilizes and surgical wounds heal.

In practice, adjusting the immunosuppression regimen is often difficult due to the increased risks of acute or accelerated chronic rejection. While immunosuppression should be managed by the transplant team, the dermatologist can play a critical role by quantifying skin cancer risks and ideally controlling them to allow optimal graft support. Table 13.1 provides a guidance for reduction of immunosuppression based from an expert consensus issued by the International Transplant Skin Cancer Collaborative (ITSCC) and the Skin Care in Organ transplant Patient Europe (SCOPE).

Photodynamic Therapy

Photodynamic therapy (PDT) refers to field therapy with red or violet light after topical incubation with a protoporphyrin sensitizer. The most common sensitizers are 5-aminolevulinic acid (ALA) or methyl-esterified ALA (mALA). When photoactivated by the light source, protoporphyrins generate reactive oxygen species that preferentially destroy dysplastic and cancerous cells. Red light has a longer wavelength than violet, so red may be more effective for treatment of deeper lesions. However, side effects of red light include more prolonged erythema and pain.

Although PDT has been commonly utilized to treat AKs, warts, and superficial NMSCs, its role in chemoprevention of NMSC is more controversial. Experimental studies in hairless mice have demonstrated that PDT can delay the development of UV-induced skin carcinomas. However, given its effectiveness in treating precancerous skin lesions, ready availability, and good safety profile, PDT can be considered as an option for areas with field cancerization, especially in patients who are not candidates for systemic retinoids or immunosuppression regimen adjustment.

Topical 5-Fluorouracil

5-Fluorouracil (5FU), a pyrimidine analog, interferes with DNA synthesis and ultimately induces cell cycle arrest and apoptosis. Topical 5FU is approved for treatment of AK and superficial BCC. Topical 5FU under occlusion has been reported to successfully treat SCCIS as well as BCC. 5FU field treatment can decrease the numbers of Aks, thus theoretically reducing the risk of SCC, however, the role of 5FU in chemoprevention in OTRs will benefit from further study.

Topical Imiquimod

Imiquimod activates innate and adaptive immunity via binding to toll-like receptors 7 and 8 (TLR7 and TLR8). Binding triggers secretion of a variety of pro-inflammatory cytokines including interferon-α, tumor necrosis factor-$\pm$, and interleukin-6. Imiquimod is approved by the FDA to treat AKs, superficial BCC and genital warts. In OTRs there is a theoretical concern that imiquimod, as an immune response enhancer, might interfere with the patient's systemic immunosuppression. There is a single report of post-imiquimod renal graft rejection in a patient; of note this patient had previously rejected two prior kidneys in the absence of imiquimod. Against this, there have numerous case reports on safe use of imiquimod in individual OTRs, and, more importantly, three larger imiquimod studies showing no graft-related complications in a total of 81 OTR patients. In a randomized, blinded, placebo-controlled study of 14 renal transplant patients using imiquimod on areas up to 60 cm^2, seven had less skin atypia, viral warts, and squamous skin tumors on treated skin at 1-year follow-up. Renal function was not adversely affected.

Table 13.1 Expert consensus on reduction of immunosuppression for skin cancers

Numbers of NMSC per year	Level of reduction to consider		
	Kidney transplant	**Heart transplant**	**Liver transplant**
≤1 (negligible risk of mortality over 3 years)	Mild	None	Mild
2–25 (0.5–2 % risk of mortality over 3 years)	Mild	Mild	Mild
>25 (5 % risk of mortality over 3 years)	Moderate	Mild	Moderate
SCC	**Level of reduction to consider**		
	Kidney transplant	**Heart transplant**	**Liver transplant**
Average risk (1–5 % risk of mortality over 3 years)	Mild	None	Mild
Moderate risk (5 % risk of mortality over 3 years)	Mild	Mild	Mild
High risk (10 % risk of mortality over 3 years)	Moderate	Mild	Moderate
Very high risk (25 % risk of mortality over 3 years)	Moderate	Mild	Moderate
Metastatic (50 % risk of mortality over 3 years)	Severe	Moderate	Moderate
Untreatable (90 % risk of mortality over 3 years)	Severe	Severe	Severe
Melanoma	**Level of reduction to consider**		
	Kidney transplant	**Heart transplant**	**Liver transplant**
Stage IA (1–5 % risk of mortality over 3 years)	Mild	None	Mild
Stage IB (5 % risk of mortality over 3 years)	Mild	Mild	Mild
Stage IIA (10 % risk of mortality over 3 years)	Moderate	Mild	Moderate
Stage IIB (25 % risk of mortality over 3 years)	Moderate	Mild	Moderate
Stage IIC/III (50 % risk of mortality over 3 years)	Severe	Moderate	Moderate
Stage IV (90 % risk of mortality over 3 years)	Severe	Severe	Severe
Merkle cell carcinoma	**Level of reduction to consider**		
	Kidney transplant	**Heart transplant**	**Liver transplant**
Early (10 % risk of mortality over 3 years)	Moderate	Mild	Moderate
Aggressive (50 % risk of mortality over 3 years)	Severe	Moderate	Moderate
Metastatic (90 % risk of mortality over 3 years)	Severe	Severe	Severe
Kaposi's sarcoma	**Level of reduction to consider**		
	Kidney transplant	**Heart transplant**	**Liver transplant**
Cutaneous and oral (1 % risk of mortality over 3 years)	Mild	None	Mild
Visceral (50 % risk of mortality over 3 years)	Severe	Moderate	Moderate

Adapted from Otely et al. Reduction of immunosuppression for tansplant-associated skin cancer: expert consensus survey. Br J Dermatol. 2006;154(3)395–400

Key: *Mild*–Poses mild risk to allograft that is often reversible but need medical attention

 Moderate–Poses moderate risk to allograft that is partially permanent

 Severe–Poses severe risk to allograft that could result in need to resume idalysis in kidney allograpt, or re-transplantation or death in heart and liver allografts

In a retrospective study of 24 OTRs (18 kidney, 4 kidney-pancreas, and 2 heart), imiquimod applied three times a week for 9 weeks showed partial responses in 50 % of the AK-treated patients and 42 % of wart-treated patients without graft function compromise. In a prospective, multicenter, randomized, placebo-controlled safety and efficacy study of imiquimod for the treatment of AK in 43 kidney, heart, and liver transplant patients over a 16-week period, no signs of graft rejection were detected and the complete histologic clearance rate was 62.1 % vs 0 % for vehicle patients. Efficacy was within the range previously observed in non-transplanted populations. Thus, it appears that imiquimod may be safe and effective in reducing cutaneous dysplasia and development of squamous tumors in OTRs. That said, larger and lengthier studies would help confirm these results, and at this time many dermatologists still prefer other topical agents such as 5FU over imiquimod.

Topical Diclofenac Sodium

Topical diclofenac sodium is thought to induce apoptosis and inhibit angiogenesis via its activity as an inhibitor of cyclo-oxygenase (COX-2). Diclofenac 3 % gel is approved to treat AKs, and has shown efficacy in immunosuppressed patients. In a study of 32 OTRs, diclofenac 3 % gel safely and effectively treated AKs and reduced invasive SCC 2 years post-treatment. Further investigations could help confirm its role in chemoprevention.

Other Reagents and Issues

A recent double-blind placebo-controlled randomized trial of the COX2 inhibitor celecoxib for chemoprevention of skin cancer showed reduced numbers of SCCs and BCCs in the celecoxib arm but no alteration in AK incidence. Although the mechanism is not well understood, elevated prostaglandin may be important in generating SCC, and COX2 inhibition may prevent this. Results of epidemiologic studies on NSAIDS and SCC have been conflicting. The role of NSAIDS in SCC chemoprevention needs further clarification.

Ingenol mebutate is an active agent in the sap of the plant Euphorbia peplus that induces cell death and immune response. It has been approved for topical treatment of AKs, but its role in SCC has not been studied.

In a recent phase III study, oral difluoromethylornithine (DFMO) has been shown to be effective and safe for reduction of new SCCs. It inhibits ornithine decarboxylase, which may play an important role in promoting SCC development. Further studies are ongoing to define its utility in chemoprevention.

Multiple nutritional approaches have been associated with decreased risk of SCCs, including reduction of dietary fat, consumption of perillyl alcohols found in cherries and spearmint, and caffeine intake. It should be noted that the above associations are based on very limited data. Vitamin D has been a popular topic in recent years although recent studies support only a role in skeletal health. In this spirit, a meta-analysis failed to demonstrate any association between SCC and vitamin D intake.

Basal Cell Carcinoma

Basal cell carcinoma (BCC), shown in Fig. 13.3, is the most common skin cancer in the general population and the second most common cancer in OTRs. There is an approximately 10–16-fold increased risk of BCC in OTRs versus immuno-

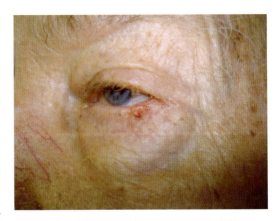

Fig. 13.3 Translucent pink fleshy tumor on the edge of the lower eyelid with a central dell with evidence of recent bleeding. MOHS surgery is the treatment of choice to avoid eye damage and minimal eyelid scarring

competent individuals. BCC appears about 7 years post-transplantation. Like all other skin cancers, it occurs earlier in heart transplantation patients than in kidney transplantation patients.

Pathogenesis

Numerous studies have demonstrated the role of Hedgehog (Hh) signaling pathway in the development of BCC. The Hh pathway is a key regulator in embryogenesis and cell differentiation. Hh is a soluble protein that binds its cell surface receptor, Patched (PTCH1). In the absence of Hh, PTCH1 inhibits the activity of another cell surface molecule called Smoothened (SMO). When Hh binds to PTCH1 it no longer inhibits SMO, thus activating the pathway. Ninety percent of BCCs possess PTCH1-inactivating mutations, and 10 % possess SMO-activating mutations. Both mutations lead to activation of the Hh signaling cascade even in the absence of Hh. This, in turn, leads to cell cycle progression and ultimately carcinogenesis.

Clinical Features

The clinical presentation, histologic features, and treatment modalities of BCC in OTRs do not differ significantly from those in the general population. Most present as pearly papules with telangiectasia. In a study of over 2,000 transplant recipients, approximately 7 % developed BCC; nodular BCC predominated on the head and neck area while superficial BCC was the most common subtype in extracephalic sites.

Management

Prognosis and treatment of BCC in OTRs do not differ greatly from those in the general population. Superficial BCC can be treated with cryosurgery, ED&C, topical 5FU, topical imiquimod, or conventional surgical excision with histological margin assessment. Invasive BCC can be treated with surgical excision as first-line therapy. Mohs is indicated for aggressive types (Fig. 13.4) like

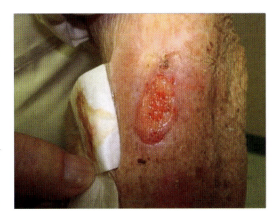

Fig. 13.4 Exophytic bleeding tumor on the upper outer arm. Tumors this large are not uncommon in the immune compromised

morpheaform, infiltrating, or perineural involvement, or recurrent BCC. Mohs is also indicated in areas where tissue sparing is important such as face, or areas where closure is challenging, such as fingers or shins. Metastatic BCC is exceedingly rare. In patients with metastatic BCC or locally invasive BCC that is not amenable to surgery or radiation, vismodegib is a promising new therapy approved in 2012. Vismodegib inactivates the Hh pathway by inactivating SMO. Vismidegib does carry a substantial adverse events profile including muscle cramps (72 %), alopecia (64 %), and dysgeusia (55 %). In life-threatening BCC or metastatic BCC, adjustment of the immunosuppression regimen should be discussed with the transplant team. As of now, there is limited data demonstrating the chemoprotective effect of mTOR inhibitors in BCC.

Melanoma

The incidence of cutaneous melanoma in OTRs is about four times higher than that of the general population, ranging from 0- to 17-fold in various studies. Melanoma, shown in Fig. 13.5, accounts for approximately 6 % of skin cancers in OTRs but is associated with outsized mortality risk. Melanomas make up an even higher proportion of the skin cancers in pediatric OTRs, with one study reporting 12 % of all pediatric OTR cancers. The mean time to diagnosis of melanoma

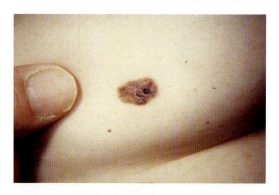

Fig. 13.5 Multicolored, roughly surfaced malignant melanoma on the breast. It is larger than 6 mm and the edge is not smooth. This is slightly more common in the immune suppressed, and metatstatic potential is significant

after transplantation ranges from 4 to 11 years. Risk factors include ultraviolet exposure, multiple and dysplastic nevi, and a family history of melanoma.

There are three main categories of melanoma in OTRs: (1) pre-existing melanoma before transplantation; (2) de novo melanoma developing post-transplantation; and (3) melanoma derived from the organ donor.

Pre-existing Melanoma Before Transplantation

Although several studies found no increased recurrence or other worse outcomes for OTRs with a history of melanoma prior to transplantation, Penn et al. reported a nearly 20 % recurrence rate in 31 OTRs with history of melanoma. Thus, many experts now recommend a waiting period before transplantation based on the nature of a prior cutaneous melanoma. It has been proposed that no waiting time is needed for patients with melanoma in situ, a 2-year waiting time for melanoma with Breslow thickness < 1 mm or negative SLNB, and 5-year wait time if thickness is > 2 mm. History of positive SLNB or metastatic melanoma is often considered to be a contraindication for organ transplantation. Depth-based waiting periods generally apply only to kidney transplantation where patients can receive dialysis treatment while they wait, but recent melanoma may be taken into account when assessing the suitability of other organ transplants.

De Novo Melanoma Developing Post-transplantation

The incidence of post-transplant primary melanoma is two- to four-fold higher than that in the general population. Importantly, the survival rate is markedly poorer in OTRs versus the general population, especially if Breslow thickness is more than 1.5–2 mm.

Although donor-derived melanoma is rare, melanoma is nonetheless one of the most often reported and deadly donor-derived malignancies. Multiple case reports and case series have reported instances of melanoma transmission from organ donor to recipient. The donor transmission has been proposed to be a result of undiagnosed melanoma, melanoma dormancy, latent recurrence, micrometastasis, and/or circulating tumor cells. It is possible that melanoma cells can remain dormant in an immunocompetent donor for years only to be reactivated in the context of the immunosuppressed organ recipient. In renal transplant patients, removal of the allograft and treatment of associated metastases should be performed. However, in heart, lung, or liver transplant, reduction of immunosuppression with treatment of metastases and/or urgent re-transplantation may be the only salvage options. Melanoma is thus one of only a small number of malignancies for which a recent policy paper of the ad hoc Disease Transmission Advisory Committee (DTAC) of the Organ Procurement and Transplantation Network/United Network for Organ Sharing (OPTN/UNOS) recommends that any prior history makes an individual ineligible to serve as an organ donor. A comprehensive history and examination of skin looking even for the presence of scars that might indicate prior melanoma excision is recommended to exclude prior melanoma history in potential organ donors.

Merkel Cell Carcinoma

Merkel cell carcinoma (MCC) is a rare yet highly aggressive neuroendocrine tumor that originates from Merkel cells located in the basal layer of epidermis. MCC accounts for approximately 7–8 % of skin cancers in OTRs, which is approximately five to ten-fold higher than in the general population. Mean time to diagnosis of MCC in OTRs ranges from 3.8 to 11 years post-transplantation. Mortality of post-transplantation MCC is high, with a 5-year survival rate of less than 50 %. Risk factors include UV exposure, age, and degree of immunosuppression. MCC predominantly affects Caucasian men over 50 years old and typically arises on sun-exposed areas, particularly the head and neck.

The etiology of MCC is unclear, although numerous studies have suggested that Merkel cell polyomavirus (MCPyV) may contribute to tumor development. Usually MCC presents as a solitary, rapidly growing, asymptomatic, reddish to bluish dome-shaped nodule, often ulcerating. The diagnosis of MCC relies on histopathologic examination.

Treatment of MCC depends on the extent of disease. Radiation therapy may confer survival benefits for all stages of MCC. Sentinel lymph node biopsy is recommended. For local disease, local wide excision or Mohs micrographic surgery is recommended. For metastatic disease, complete dissection of involved lymph nodes, and multi-agent chemotherapy in addition to radiotherapy may be indicated. Similar to melanoma and high-risk SCC, revision of immunosuppression should be considered if feasible. Table 13.1 presents an overview of expert consensus on reduction of immunosuppression for various skin cancers.

Kaposi's Sarcoma

Kaposi's sarcoma (KS), seen in Fig. 13.6, is a rare vascular tumor that can affect skin, mucosal surfaces, and visceral organs. It is 84–500-fold more common in OTRs than in the general population and accounts for approximately 5 % of skin cancers in OTRs. KS often develops slightly

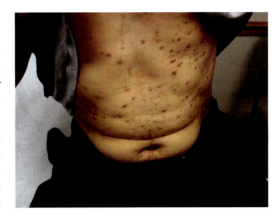

Fig. 13.6 Purple tumors scattered over the abdomen in a pityriasis rosea-like distribution. This is in an HIV-positive patient. Kaposi's sarcoma can also be induced by iatrogenic immunosuppression and will dissipate when the incriminating chemotherapy is reduced or eliminated

sooner post-transplantation than SCC, with mean onset at 13 months after transplant. Mucocutaneous lesions compose 75 % of KS cases, and tend to be diagnosed much earlier than visceral KS (2.6 vs 9.1 years). Classic KS has a male predominance with male to female ratio of 17:1. However, in immunocompromised patients, KS occurs slightly more frequently in females, with one-half to two-thirds of cases occurring in females. In OTRs KS tends to have a more aggressive course, with a 69 % 5-year survival rate. Risk factors include older age, male gender, Hispanic or Middle Eastern ethnicity, and greater immunosuppression—particularly with systemic steroids, azathioprine, and cyclosporine.

Pathogenesis

Although human herpes virus 8 (HHV-8) is known to play an essential role in development of KS, the route of progression from HHV-8 to KS is not fully understood. One of the HHV-genes encodes a viral G-protein coupled receptor (GPCR) that can activate the Akt/mTOR pathway, which ultimately results in dysregulation of the cell cycle and inhibition of apoptosis. In immunosuppressed mice these then induce angioproliferative tumors that are histologically identical to KS. Interestingly, mTOR inhibitors, such as sirolimus and everolimus, both prevent KS development and induce KS remission in transplant recipients; in contrast calcineurin inhibitor immunosuppression promotes KS development. Much data indicates that KS requires not only HHV-8 infection, but also other cofactors such as immunosuppression.

Clinical Features

Similar to KS in the general population, KS in OTRs has three clinical and histological stages: patch, plaque, and tumor. Cutaneous KS often presents as an enlarging, irregularly bordered, bluish to violaceous patch on a distal lower leg, which may then evolve into plaques or tumors. KS diagnosis depends on histologic examination, including immunohistochemical staining for HHV-8.

Management

Currently the first-line therapy for KS in OTRs is to switch from calcineurin inhibitors to sirolimus. In one case series, all 15 kidney transplant patients with KS went into remission months after switching from cyclosporine to sirolimus. However, subsequent studies reported only transient benefit and even refractory response in some patients. Local lesions can be treated with surgical excision, intralesional doxorubicin, and/or radiotherapy. Very early and superficial lesions may be treated with lasers, such as the pulsed dye laser and carbon-dioxide laser, but caution is advised due to the risk of incomplete treatment and recurrence. Electrochemotherapy, an emerging treatment for cutaneous lesions, is an option as well. For rapidly progressive disease with visceral involvement, oncology consultation should be obtained for consideration of systemic chemotherapy.

Immune-Mediated Inflammatory Diseases

Immune-mediated inflammatory diseases (IMIDs) are characterized by unmitigated inflammation that results from, or is triggered by, dysregulation of the normal immune response. IMIDs include autoimmune conditions, such as rheumatoid arthritis (RA) and inflammatory bowel disease (IBD), as well as non-autoimmune inflammatory diseases such as psoriasis. Treatment of inflammatory diseases focuses on inhibition of inflammation and usually involves modulators of immune responses, such as corticosteroids and "biologics" such as tumor necrosis factor (TNF) inhibitors. Inflammatory diseases generally are associated with an increased cancer risk both from the effect of the inflammatory disease itself as well as the consequences of the therapies being used.

Inflammatory Diseases and Skin Cancer Risks

Patients with RA have a 70 % increased risk of NMSC. This is elevated further in RA patients who receive prednisone, TNF inhibitors, and/or methotrexate. Risks of developing melanoma and Merkel cell carcinoma are also increased in patients with RA. In psoriasis, a recent meta-analysis also showed an increased risk of skin cancer. However, melanoma risk was not increased. Patients with ulcerative colitis were similarly shown to have increased risk of Kaposi's sarcoma.

Inflammatory Disease Treatments and Skin Cancer Risks

Several common anti-inflammatory drugs have been shown to increase the risk of skin cancer. Accumulating evidence has demonstrated increased risks of NMSC in patients taking thiopurines, which include azathioprine, 6-thioguanine and 6-mercaptopurine, particularly those with IBD. Cyclosporine significantly increases the risk of NMSC in RA and all types of skin cancers in psoriasis. Methotrexate is a folic acid analog that inhibits DNA synthesis and cell proliferation. The risk of NMSC is increased in psoriasis patients treated with methotrexate. In patients with RA, methotrexate doubles the risk of NMSC when combined with anti-TNF agents and also increases the risk of melanoma.

The newer anti-TNF agents are strong modulators of both innate and adaptive immune responses that inhibit multiple signaling pathways such MAP kinases and NF-κB. Anti-TNFs have been approved for treatment of RA, psoriasis, psoriatic arthritis, IBD, ankylosing spondylitis, and juvenile idiopathic arthritis. Of the many studies investigating the effect of anti-TNFs and malignancy risks, most of the randomized studies have been either too small or of inadequate duration to demonstrate statistically significant effects. Several meta-analyses have also yielded conflicting associations between the use of anti-TNFs and skin cancers. Further studies are needed to elucidate the malignancy risk of chronic anti-TNF use.

Several other immune-modulating medications that have recently come into use for IMIDs may also carry increased risks for skin cancers, and will require long-term studies. Rituximab is a CD20 monoclonal antibody that induces apoptosis of B cells and down-regulates the B-cell receptor. It has been approved for the treatment of RA and granulomatosis with polyangiitis (formerly called Wegener's granulomatosis). There is sparse data on the risk of skin cancer with rituximab; however, a recent report did not observe an increased risk in RA patients.

Ustekinumab, an IL-12/23 blocking antibody that inhibits Th1 and Th17 pathways, is approved for treatment of psoriasis and psoriatic arthritis. To date, no increased risk in skin cancers has been reported. Observational data for anakinra, an interleukin-1 (IL-1) receptor antagonist approved for treatment of RA, has not demonstrated an increased incidence of skin cancer in RA patients. Tocilizumab is a monoclonal antibody to the IL-6 receptor and is approved for RA and juvenile idiopathic arthritis. A recent meta-analysis found no increased rate of malignancies in RA patients receiving tocilizumab. These newer agents have not yet been shown to increase the risk for skin cancers.

Treatments for skin cancers in patients with IMIDs are the same as that for the general population. There are no formal recommendations for enhanced surveillance in this group although it seems reasonable that patients who have been treated with thiopurines, cyclosporine, and methotrexate would benefit from regular dermatologic examinations.

Human Immunodeficiency Virus and Acquired Immunodeficiency Syndrome (HIV and AIDS)

There has long been recognition of increased cancers in the HIV/AIDS population.

Kaposi's sarcoma (KS), for example, was one of the original AIDS-defining diagnoses. Before the introduction of antiretroviral therapy (ART), the incidence of KS was 1:3 in HIV-infected homosexual men. The incidence of KS has declined to around 1:20 with the wide use of ART; however this is still significantly increased compared to incidence of 1:100,000 in the general population. ART either alone or in combination with systemic and local therapy has a crucial role in treating KS.

Patients with HIV infection also have a higher incidence rate of NMSC. A recent study reported a 2.6-fold increased incidence of SCC in HIV-positive patients compared to HIV-negative patients. This is significantly lower than the >65-fold higher rates of SCC among the organ transplant population. The incidence of BCC is about two-fold higher in HIV patients and interestingly this appears to be limited to men, suggesting the contribution of other confounding factors such as income, sex, and sexual orientation. CD4 counts less than 500 among HIV-positive patients associated with an increased risk of SCC but not of BCC. While the course of NMSC in OTRs tends to be more aggressive, the course of NMSC in HIV patients was found to be similar to that in general population. Treatments for the NMSC in HIV patients are similar to those modalities utilized in the general population.

Melanoma was reported to have a 2.6-fold increased risk in HIV-positive subjects. One study noted a shorter disease-free duration and poorer survival rate for HIV-positive melanoma group. Given the limited data, the relationship between HIV infection, ART, CD4 count, and melanoma incidence/course remains unclear. Treatment options for melanoma in HIV/AIDS patients are similar to those in the general population except for the addition of ART.

Conclusion

Skin cancer is a common problem in immunosuppressed patients, regardless of the basis for immune impairment. Optimal patient outcomes depend on awareness and vigilance on the part of the dermatologist and the general health care team. Skin cancer tends to be especially important in OTRs who suffer from both greatly elevated incidence and significantly higher mortality.

Although many different types of skin cancer are more frequent in this population, SCC and melanoma stand out. Patients who take immunosuppressive medications for other reasons or have immunodeficiency syndromes may be similarly affected, although demographics and risk levels vary. Other than modification of iatrogenic immunosuppression, most skin cancer treatments are the same as those used in the general population. Virtually all immunosuppressed patients may benefit from regular dermatologic examination. Enhanced vigilance in this population can potentially reduce morbidity and death due to skin cancer.

Suggested Reading

Berg D, Otley CC. Skin cancer in organ transplant recipients: epidemiology, pathogenesis, and management. J Am Acad Dermatol. 2002;47(1):1–17; quiz 8–20; Epub 2002/06/22.

Butler GJ, Neale R, Green AC, Pandeya N, Whiteman DC. Nonsteroidal anti-inflammatory drugs and the risk of actinic keratoses and squamous cell cancers of the skin. J Am Acad Dermatol. 2005;53(6):966–72. Epub 2005/11/29.

Euvrard S, Kanitakis J, Claudy A. Skin cancers after organ transplantation. N Engl J Med. 2003;348(17): 1681–91. Epub 2003/04/25.

Euvrard S, Kanitakis J, Decullier E, Butnaru AC, Lefrancois N, Boissonnat P, et al. Subsequent skin cancers in kidney and heart transplant recipients after the first squamous cell carcinoma. Transplantation. 2006;81(8):1093–100. Epub 2006/04/28.

Gu YH, Du JX, Ma ML. Sirolimus and non-melanoma skin cancer prevention after kidney transplantation: a meta-analysis. Asian Pac J Cancer Prev. 2012;13(9): 4335–9. Epub 2012/11/22.

Hollenbeak CS, Todd MM, Billingsley EM, Harper G, Dyer AM, Lengerich EJ. Increased incidence of melanoma in renal transplantation recipients. Cancer. 2005;104(9):1962–7. Epub 2005/09/28.

Kalinova L, Majek O, Stehlik D, Krejci K, Bachleda P. Skin cancer incidence in renal transplant recipients -a single center study. Biomed Pap Med Fac Univ Palacky Olomouc Czech Repub. 2010;154(3):257–60. Epub 2010/11/05.

Kanitakis J, Alhaj-Ibrahim L, Euvrard S, Claudy A. Basal cell carcinomas developing in solid organ transplant recipients: clinicopathologic study of 176 cases. Arch Dermatol. 2003;139(9):1133–7. Epub 2003/09/17.

Kasiske BL, Snyder JJ, Gilbertson DT, Wang C. Cancer after kidney transplantation in the United States. Am J Transplant. 2004;4(6):905–13. Epub 2004/05/19.

Koljonen V, Kukko H, Tukiainen E, Bohling T, Sankila R, Pukkala E, et al. Incidence of Merkel cell carcinoma in renal transplant recipients. Nephrol Dial Transplant. 2009;24(10):3231–5. Epub 2009/07/10.

Leveque L, Dalac S, Dompmartin A, Louvet S, Euvrard S, Catteau B, et al. Melanome chez le transplante. [Melanoma in organ transplant patients]. Ann Dermatol Venereol. 2000;127(2):160–5.

Molina BD, Leiro MG, Pulpon LA, Mirabet S, Yanez JF, Bonet LA, et al. Incidence and risk factors for nonmelanoma skin cancer after heart transplantation. Transplant Proc. 2010;42(8):3001–5. Epub 2010/10/26.

Moloney FJ, Kelly PO, Kay EW, Conlon P, Murphy GM. Maintenance versus reduction of immunosuppression in renal transplant recipients with aggressive squamous cell carcinoma. Dermatol Surg. 2004;30(4 Pt 2):674–8. Epub 2004/04/06.

Moloney FJ, Comber H, O'Lorcain P, O'Kelly P, Conlon PJ, Murphy GM. A population-based study of skin cancer incidence and prevalence in renal transplant recipients. Br J Dermatol. 2006;154(3):498–504. Epub 2006/02/01.

Mudigonda T, Levender MM, O'Neill JL, West CE, Pearce DJ, Feldman SR. Incidence, risk factors, and preventative management of skin cancers in organ transplant recipients: a review of single- and multicenter retrospective studies from 2006 to 2010. Dermatol Surg. 2013;39(3 Pt 1):345–64. Epub 2012/11/30.

Webb MC, Compton F, Andrews PA, Koffman CG. Skin tumours posttransplantation: a retrospective analysis of 28 years' experience at a single centre. Transplant Proc. 1997;29(1–2):828–30. Epub 1997/02/01.

Weinstock MA, Bingham SF, Digiovanna JJ, Rizzo AE, Marcolivio K, Hall R, et al. Tretinoin and the prevention of keratinocyte carcinoma (Basal and squamous cell carcinoma of the skin): a veterans affairs randomized chemoprevention trial. J Invest Dermatol. 2012;132(6):1583–90. Epub 2012/02/10.

Zwald FO, Christenson LJ, Billingsley EM, Zeitouni NC, Ratner D, Bordeaux J, et al. Melanoma in solid organ transplant recipients. Am J Transplant. 2010;10(5): 1297–304. Epub 2010/04/01.

Radiation Therapy for Non-melanoma Skin Cancer in Immunosuppressed Patients and Cutaneous Toxicity from This Therapy

14

Adam D. Currey, Edit B. Olasz, J. Frank Wilson, and Zelmira Lazarova

Abstract

Cutaneous squamous cell carcinoma (SCC) is a common skin cancer affecting more than 3,000,000 individuals worldwide each year. The risk of SCC is strongly linked with immunosuppressive treatment in organ transplant recipients (OTR). Population-based standard incidence ratios for SCC are increased 65–250-fold and for basal cell carcinomas 10–16-fold in OTR compared with non-transplanted population. Skin cancers in immunocompromised patients tend to be more aggressive and metastasize more frequently. Therefore adjuvant radiotherapy and definitive radiotherapy for surgically incurable cancers plays an important role in the therapeutic options. In this chapter we discuss indications, approaches, planning, efficacy, and side effects of radiation treatment of non-melanoma skin cancer in OTR.

Keywords

Radiation therapy • Immunosuppression • Organ transplant recipients • Non-melanoma skin cancer • Cutaneous squamous cell carcinoma • Basal cell carcinoma • Keratoacanthoma • Radiation dermatitis

Skin Cancer in Immunosuppressed Patients

Over the last 40 years, the increasing success of organ transplantation and the AIDS epidemic have led to the realization that many human cancers occur more frequently in immunosuppressed individuals. Most recently it became evident that in addition to the aforementioned conditions, cancer risk is increased in lymphoproliferative disorders, iatrogenic immunosuppression, and

A.D. Currey, MD • J.F. Wilson, MD
Department of Radiation Oncology, Medical College of Wisconsin, Milwaukee, WI, USA

E.B. Olasz, MD, PhD • Z. Lazarova, MD (✉)
Department of Dermatology, Medical College of Wisconsin, 8701 Watertown Plank Road, Milwaukee, WI 53226-4801, USA
e-mail: zlazarov@mcw.edu

J.C. Hall (ed.), *Skin Diseases in the Immunocompromised*,
DOI 10.1007/978-1-4471-6479-1_14, © Springer-Verlag London 2014

with the use of certain new biologic agents. Skin cancer encompasses 42 % of all post-transplant malignancies. Population-based standard incidence ratios for squamous cell carcinomas of the skin are increased 65–250-fold and for basal cell carcinomas 10–16-fold in organ transplant recipients (OTR) compared with non-transplanted population. Increased incidence of melanoma in transplant patients has been reported, but recent studies have resulted in contradictory findings. Kaposi sarcoma has been reported in excess among OTR, especially from patient populations in which the disease is endemic, such as patients of Mediterranean, black African, or Caribbean origin. Lymphomas affect up to 5 % of all OTR, but purely cutaneous lymphomas are rare.

Merkel cell carcinoma (MCC) is a rare neuroendocrine tumor with very high mortality rate. The relative risk for the development of MCC in OTRs is estimated at five to ten times greater, compared to the general population. Five- year disease-specific survival in transplant patients is reported to be 46 %. Management is similar to that for the general population and includes excision, primary radiation therapy, and sentinel node mapping. Adjuvant radiation to the primary site and, if lymph nodes are involved, is generally recommended. Other types of skin cancer, such as atypical fibrous histiocytoma and dermatofibroma protuberans, have been also reported, but due to the rarity of these tumors, increased incidence in OTR has been difficult to quantify.

Exposure to chronic immunosuppression severely depresses specific components of host immunity, including both antitumor immune surveillance and antimicrobial host defense. The link between immunosuppression and cancer formation is further evidenced by observed reduction in skin cancer formation with reduction or cessation of immunosuppressive therapy. Additionally, there has been recent evidence that some immunosuppressive agents, most notably azathioprine, have direct pro-carcinogenic effects, whereas others may have anti-carcinogenic properties, as shown in the case of the mammalian target of rapamycin (mTOR) inhibitors, such as sirolimus. Conversion to sirolimus from calcineurin inhibitor-based regimen reduces the risk of development of squamous cell carcinoma (SCC) in kidney transplant recipients.

Skin cancers in immunocompromised patients tend to be more aggressive and metastasize more frequently, therefore adjuvant radiotherapy and definitive radiotherapy for surgically incurable cancers play an important role in the therapeutic armamentarium. In many instances these lesions represent significant oncological challenges and often carry the potential for disfigurement or even death of the patient if timely definitive measures are not implemented. Skillful application of definitive or adjunctive radiation therapy for selected lesions in OTR patients offers the advantages of high tumor control probability with anatomical and functional preservation. It is generally well tolerated by the patient. In this chapter we will focus on radiation treatment of cutaneous squamous and basal cell carcinoma, which are the most common skin cancers diagnosed in immunosuppressed patients.

Indications for Radiation Therapy in Immunosuppressed Patients

Obtaining optimal clinical outcomes from locally applied radiation therapy for skin cancer depends upon the histological type, clinical stage, location, specific anatomical configuration of the lesion, the adequacy of treatment, and whether it is primary or recurrent. Various patient-based factors (age, performance status, life expectancy, preferences) must also be taken into account in all management decisions that are made. Real-time decision making in a multidisciplinary context is key to optimal patient care delivery, particularly for OTR patients. General indications for radiation therapy in the OTR setting are essentially the same as those for other patients diagnosed with skin cancer.

Special awareness is due when considering radiation treatment for eruptive keratoacanthomas (KA). Although this treatment modality has been widely reported to be efficacious for KAs, specifically for giant type KAs, in our experience and in one previously published case, radiation therapy

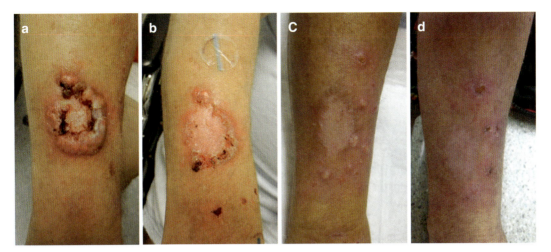

Fig. 14.1 Immunosuppressed patient with large SCC, keratoacanthoma-type on the right forearm treated with definitive radiation therapy. (**a**) Lesion at initial presentation. (**b**) Lesion during radiotherapy. (**c**) Original SCC was successfully treated, however patient developed multiple eruptive KAs in the radiation field. (**d**) Late findings of radiotherapy are demonstrated, with palor in the central region, hair loss, and fibrotic skin. Eruptive KAs effectively treated with intralesional 5-fluorouracil

may induce multiple eruptive KAs in the radiation field (Fig. 14.1).

There is no concern that standard radiation therapy regimens will additionally compromise the immune system of skin cancer patients or that their treatment tolerance will be reduced or atypical. Irradiation may be indicated either as definitive treatment or as an adjunct to primary surgery in selected high-risk cases. It is often the option of choice for medically frail patients or those with significant co-morbidities that render them poor surgical candidates or for patients who refuse surgery.

While OTR patients are much more at risk for the development of skin cancers on the torso or extremities than non-OTR patients, the majority of lesions that are suitable for radiation therapy will occur on the head and neck areas. These include, in particular, lesions overlying cartilaginous structures, large lesions involving cartilage or bone, and lesions extending beyond the confines of surgery that would not result in significant cosmetic or functional compromise of the patient.

Indications for adjunctive postoperative irradiation may include positive surgical margins, perineural invasion (PNI), and large tumor size,

particularly in the setting of poorly differentiated histology. When considering the relative risks and benefits of adjuvant radiation therapy, one must consider that it is much more difficult to control a recurrent lesion when compared to tumors with similar characteristics at first presentation. This is particularly true of SCC, as recurrent lesions can have a much higher propensity for nodal involvement. In any case, optimizing control of the index lesion is essential. In patients with positive surgical margins after resection of SCC, the risk of recurrence may be as high as 50 % depending on tumor size and location. The role of adjuvant radiation in cases of PNI has been controversial. In one review of the literature, the risk of local recurrence after surgery alone for patients with PNI was no different than that of patients treated with surgery followed by adjuvant radiation, provided negative margins were obtained. Other data has made the distinction between microscopic or incidental PNI versus more extensive PNI. While exact definitions across the literature vary, one review on this topic described microscopic PNI as disease involving smaller nerves (<1 mm) that exist in the reticular dermis in the absence of clinical symptoms. Extensive or clinical PNI is defined as disease involving "named" nerves, evidence of neural involvement on imaging, or patients with clinical symptoms of PNI. When such distinctions are made, the rates of recurrence tend to be markedly different. For patients with microscopic PNI, recurrence rates after radiotherapy with or without surgery vary from 75 to 90 %, while rates for patients with extensive PNI fall to 50–60 %. A recent study showed that SCC involving unnamed small nerves (<0.1 mm in caliber) may have a low risk of poor outcomes in the absence of other risk factors. Large-caliber nerve invasion is associated with an elevated risk of nodal metastasis and death, but this may be due in part to multiple other risk factors associated with large-caliber nerve invasion. These types of reported results have led the authors of the National Comprehensive Cancer Network Clinical Practice Guidelines to recommend adjuvant radiation therapy in the setting of extensive PNI or involvement of a large nerve. (http://www.nccn.org/professionals/physician_gls/pdf/nmsc.pdf).

In some cases, elective or definitive irradiation of draining lymphatic regions in conjunction with treatment to the primary site is also warranted. Indications for elective irradiation of clinically uninvolved draining lymph node regions will depend upon the same tumor-related factors. Following nodal surgery, postoperative irradiation may be indicated by dense lymph node involvement, incomplete dissection, or extracapsular disease extension. In cases with tumor extension beyond the lymph node capsule or unresectable nodal disease, concurrent radiosensitizing chemotherapy should be considered. Radiation therapy can also play an important role in palliation for patients with troublesome uncontrolled lesions.

Radiation Therapy Approaches

A modern radiation oncology technological armamentarium includes conventional X-rays, electron beam, and photon beam therapy. In rare instances, interstitial brachytherapy may be considered. All of these approaches should be available in centers that provide comprehensive care to OTR patients.

Using these types of irradiation as the sole radiation modality, or in appropriate combinations, the radiation oncologist creates a radiation therapy plan that tailors the radiation dose profile to the anatomical target area that is identified. Clinical inspection, relevant surgical and pathological findings and the results of any imaging studies provide information that is essential to the planning process. In this regard, precise definition of the extent of subclinical disease may be difficult. The situation requires the use of empirically derived, expanded target margins. Care is taken to adapt the radiation dosimetric plan to the size, shape, location, and extent of the target area while limiting dose to surrounding uninvolved normal tissues not at risk and maximally restricting dose to any proximate critical organs. Meticulous radiation therapy treatment planning is critical to obtaining desired clinical outcomes. Any treatment plan that is implemented must be closely monitored to confirm accurate and precise delivery over the entire course of treatment. This is especially true when, as is often the case, only a limited number of daily fractions is planned. Even a few "geographic misses" will risk compromising expected tumor control rates.

Superficial X-ray Therapy and Orthovoltage Treatment

Superficial X-ray therapy and orthovoltage treatment utilizes photons in the range of 50–150 and 150–250 kVp, respectively. This type of treatment is useful because of its characteristic dose distribution in tissue. For photons in this energy range, the maximal absorbed dose is at the skin surface, but then falls off rapidly at depth, thereby sparing tissues farther below the skin. The amount of normal surrounding tissue that is treated can be smaller with superficial X-ray therapy compared with other radiation modalities. Furthermore, the physical properties of these photons allow shielding of adjacent structures such as the cornea or nasal mucosa from dose is readily achievable with custom cut lead sheets. However, the absorbed dose of low-energy photons increases differentially in bone when compared to soft tissue. This may give one pause when using this particular modality to treat skin cancers directly overlying bone (i.e. the zygoma, skull, or shin) even though clinical problems related to this differential dose absorption are minimal. Another relative disadvantage of superficial X-ray therapy is that it is usually only available at high-volume radiation facilities.

Electron Beam Therapy

Treatment with electron beam therapy can be performed at most radiotherapy centers. Similar to superficial X-ray therapy, with electron beam therapy, dose falls off rapidly with increasing depth of tissue. But the dose distribution characteristics of electron beam irradiation are less favorable. This requires treatment of larger areas in order to adequately treat a given skin tumor, and can create difficulty in shielding sensitive adjacent structures such as those of the eye. Furthermore, treatment of skin cancers situated on highly irregular skin surfaces in the area being treated (i.e., nose, ear) can result in dose inhomogeneity. This inhomogeneity of dose can result in areas of inadequate or excess dose across portions of the targeted area that could lead to a higher risk of recurrence or treatment related toxicity, respectively.

Mega-Voltage Photon Therapy

For patients with large tumors, or lesions arising from the scalp and other difficult-to-treat locations, photons in the mega-voltage energy range can be used. With sophisticated technological improvements in radiation delivery (intensity-modulated radiation therapy or IMRT, and image-guided radiation therapy or IGRT), it is now possible to modulate photon beam delivery such that radiation dose to tumor can be given while keeping doses to the underlying critical organs acceptably low. A prime example of where this is useful is in treatment of larger areas of the scalp. With more conventional techniques, wrapping dose along the curvature of the scalp while sparing the underlying brain or nearby optic structures presents challenges. Newer technologies such as IMRT and helical delivery of radiotherapy (e.g. TomoTherapy) can generate dose distributions unattainable in years past that allow a radiation oncologist to treat these lesions that arise in difficult locations.

Treatment Planning

Dose–time–volume relationships require special attention in the radiation therapy of skin cancer in order to obtain desired clinical outcomes. Standard dose and fractionation schedules for the treatment of skin cancer are well established and are determined by the stage, location, and extent of the lesion. Overall treatment duration is dictated by the size of the target area and by the tumor and normal tissue responses observed during treatment. In most instances, the treatment course is protracted over a total of 3–6 weeks to achieve optimal cosmetic outcome with low risk of complications. However, treatment duration may be shortened when treating frail or invalid patients with transportation difficulties. Daily fractions of 200–250 cGy are usually administered five times per week. Doses are prescribed either at the surface of superficial lesions or at an appropriate depth when treating larger lesions. Total doses equivalent to 5,000 cGy are appropriate in most cases when treating subclinical disease. Higher doses equivalent to 6,000–6,500 cGy are necessary for larger lesions.

Efficacy of Radiation Therapy in OTR

When expertly executed, radiation therapy in the non-OTR setting has been shown to provide excellent rates of tumor control with very acceptable complication rates. In a series of 468 patients with 531 skin cancers treated at the Mallinckrodt Institute, overall local control rate was 89 % for all cases, and 93 % for previously untreated tumors. Slightly better local control rates were seen for basal cell carcinomas. Similarly, Mendenhall et al. have published a series from the University of Florida using radiation therapy for carcinomas of the skin. For lesions 2–5 cm in size, 5-years local control rate was 93 %. For tumors larger than 5 cm, recurrent lesions, or those invading cartilage or bone, control rates decreased. At Princess Margaret Hospital, several series have been reported for radiation therapy for carcinomas of the eyelid, ear, and nose with control rates over 90 %.

While these excellent control rates have been reported for all patients with basal cell and squamous cell carcinoma, there is relatively little literature on efficacy of radiation therapy in OTR. Bradley et al. have reported our experience in treating these patients at the Medical College of Wisconsin. From 1996 to 2008, 22 OTR were treated for 262 squamous cell carcinomas of the skin, at least one of which was treated with radiation therapy in either the definitive or adjuvant setting. The 3-years overall survival after first skin cancer diagnosis was 73 % and 12 patients developed a loco-regional recurrence at the initial site of failure. Of those, eight recurred locally, two regionally, and two with a combination of the two. Overall survival and cause-specific survival from first skin cancer diagnosis were both improved with radiation doses greater than or equal to 60 Gy. Location of the primary lesion on the ear/preauricular area, size of the treated lesion, and perineural invasion were all predictive of recurrence. The higher rate of local recurrence in our series is reflective of the more aggressive nature of these lesions in the OTR population.

Side Effects of Radiation Therapy

Clinically observed radiation reactions of the skin may be divided into early or acute and delayed or late changes. The severity of these reactions depends upon the dose–time–volume factors mentioned above. Early phase reactions include initial include erythema, followed by gradually increasing hyperpigmentation and dry desquamation that may progress to moist desquamation as treatment continues. Clinically, erythema typically appears in the second or 3rd week of treatment during treatment using standard radiation fractionations (1.8–2 Gy per day). Histologically, the onset of dermatitis coincides with a loss of epidermal cell density and loss of mitotic activity within the basal layer of the epidermis. However, with standard fraction sizes, these changes do not occur until total doses of 20–25 Gy have been achieved.

For carcinomas of the skin to be adequately controlled it is usually necessary to treat to doses that result in a moderate moist reaction. However, when appropriately fractionated, these reactions are all transient and resolve within a short time frame with conservative management once treatment is completed. After treatment is completed, areas of desquamation will be repopulated with survival stem cells. This will often manifest clinically as "skin islands" growing in the areas of desquamated tissue.

In patients treated for cancers of organs other than the skin, advances in radiation delivery using megavoltage and intensity-modulated radiation therapy have permitted delivery of high doses of radiation to tumor tissues with relative skin sparing compared to treatment with modalities of the past. However, even with the most modern radiotherapy techniques, up to 95 % of patients will experience a dose-dependent skin reaction at the treated area. Thus an injury to skin can pose a morbidity risk, especially when radiation is administered in combination with chemotherapy and immunosuppressive treatment. As mentioned above, the radiation-induced changes are graded as acute or chronic and may manifest at the entrance and exit portals. Acute injury occurs within hours to weeks after radiation insult, while late injury persists month to years after radiation exposure. Different areas of the body have different sensitivities to radiation; nevertheless, the dose of radiation on the skin is directly related to the severity of injury. Fractionation of the total dose can increase the skin tolerance, but tolerance for the subsequent exposure may decrease.

Since radiation skin injury has distinct pathophysiological presentation with a dose dependent pattern, a new scoring system has become available to evaluate and classify acute and late effects of radiation-induced skin injury: common terminology criteria for adverse events v4.0 (CTCAE, http://ctep.cancer.gov/reporting/ctc.html). Grade 1 skin changes are characterized by faint erythema, mild dry desquamation, and localized pigment changes. Dryness, pruritus, and hair loss result from destruction of sebaceous glands and hair follicles of the dermal layer. The onset of these changes is 7–10 days after irradiation with a skin dose of 6–10 Gy. Grade 2 changes include edematous erythema progressing into patchy

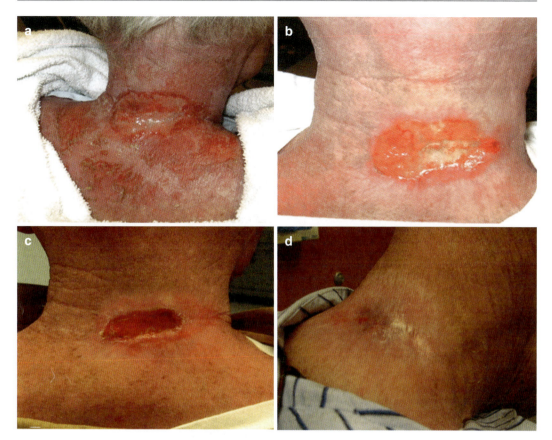

Fig. 14.2 Patient presented with a 10 cm basal cell carcinoma on posterior neck. Patient was treated with definitive radiation therapy using tomotherapy and received 60Gy at 2Gy per fraction. (**a**) Appearance of the patient's skin at the end of radiation therapy. The tumor has completely regressed; skin changes illustrate Grade 2 moist desquamation in the treatment field. The central ulceration was present at the beginning of treatment and was not a result of radiotherapy. (**b**) Clinical presentation 2 weeks post-treatment. (**c**) Three weeks post-treatment the ulceration is substantially smaller. (**d**) Six months later, the ulcer has completely healed

moist desquamation with persistent fibrinous exudates localized mostly in skin folds, after irradiation with a skin dose of 20–30 Gy (Fig. 14.2). This process peaks at 10–14 days after last radiation exposure and heals within 1–3 months. It is important to recognize that moist desquamation indicates impairment of skin integrity and thus increased risk for skin infection. Grade 3 changes are characterized by confluent moist desquamation with shallow erosions outside of skin folds with a skin exposure of 30–40 Gy in a single treatment. Grade 4 changes appear after radiation dose to the skin of more than 40 Gy in a single treatment and they are distinguished by tissue necrosis, ulcers, and hemorrhage. The ulcerations are very painful and do not heal well. Chronic changes are those that are present more than 90 days after completion of radiotherapy and characterized by epidermal atrophy, dyspigmentation, telangiectasias, and dermal fibrosis (Fig. 14.3). The Radiation Therapy Oncology Group (RTOG) has established grading criteria specific for chronic radiodermatitis. Grade 1 is characterized by slight atrophy. In grade 2 (Fig. 14.4) there are patchy areas of atrophy, epilation, and telangiectasias. Distinct atrophy and gross telangiectasias are specific for Grade 3 (Fig. 14.5). Grade 4 (Fig. 14.6) involves persistent ulceration.

Acute and late effects of radiation therapy are highly dependent upon total radiation dose

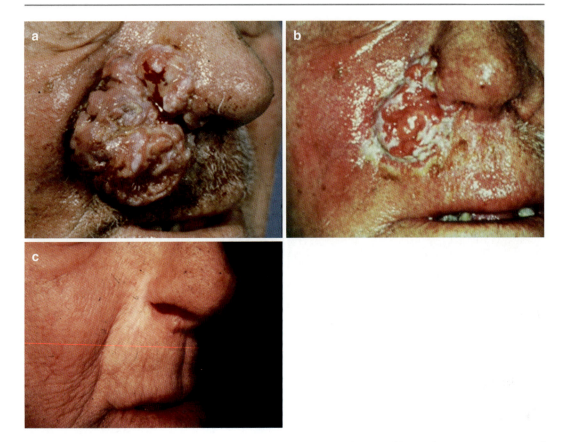

Fig. 14.3 Patient with large exophytic basal cell carcinoma treated with definitive radiation therapy. (**a**) Lesion at initial presentation. (**b**) Mid-treatment demonstrated tumor regression and Grade 1 erythema in lateral aspect of treatment field. (**c**) Six months post-treatment treated area shows depigmentation, alopecia, and dermal fibrosis representing late effects of radiation therapy

delivered, the total duration of the treatment course, as well as upon the daily dose per radiation treatment. This was well demonstrated in a randomized phase III RTOG study treating squamous cell carcinoma of the upper aerodigestive tract. Patients received one of four treatment regimens: (1) conventional fractionation [2 Gy per day over 7 weeks to 70 Gy]; (2) hyperfractionation [1.2 Gy per fraction given twice daily over 7 weeks to 81.6 Gy]; (3) split course accelerated fractionation [1.6 Gy per fraction twice daily over 6 weeks to 67.2 Gy with a 2-week break]; or (4) accelerated fractionation with concomitant boost [1.8 Gy per day with 1.5 Gy as a second daily treatment at the end of therapy, to 72 Gy over 6 weeks]. The incidence of any Grade 3 or worse of acute side effects was 35 % for conventional fractionation and 54.5, 50.4, and 58.8 % for hyperfractionation, split course accelerated fractionation, and accelerated fractionation with concomitant boost, respectively. Most of this acute toxicity was related to oropharyngeal mucositis. Acute Grade 3 or worse skin toxicity was 7 % for standard fractionation, 12 % for hyperfractionation, 3 % for split course, and 11 % for accelerated fractionation with concomitant boost. Interestingly, the incidence of Grade 3 or worse late toxicity (defined as >90 days from completion of treatment) did not follow this same trend, and were only slightly higher in the concomitant boost arm of treatment. Grade 3 or worse late effects in the skin even with these high doses were only 2–4 % in all arms. These different rates of acute

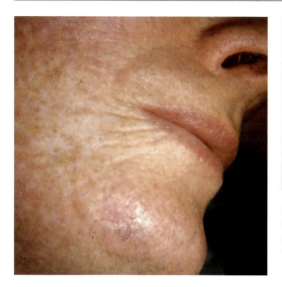

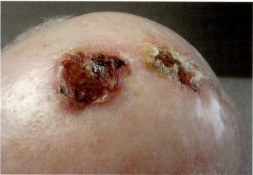

Fig. 14.6 Type 4 chronic radiation damage in a patient treated with radiation for Merkel cell cancer. The scalp showed non-healing ulcers for over 2 years with failure of wound care to cause significant healing

Fig. 14.4 Type 2 chronic radiation dermatitis with an ill-defined plaque on right chin indicating a basal cell cancer. This is a patient treated as a teenager with radiation for acne. This practice of treating acne with radiation was not completely stopped until the late 1970s, so we will continue to see these patients. There is some atrophy and telangiectasia

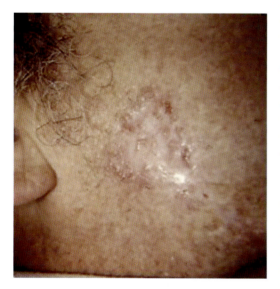

Fig. 14.5 Type 3 chronic radiation dermatitis with gross telangiectasias, atropy, and a bleeding basal cell cancer in the right preauricular area in a patient treated as a teenager with radiation for acne

versus late effects demonstrate the radiobiologic principle that radiation dose and fraction size have differing effects on acute versus late toxicity.

Biology of Radiation-Induced Skin Injury

The cutaneous symptoms after radiation exposure are based on combination of five main effects. Type I radiation effects involve cellular death and cellular depletion, followed by a proliferative response of stem cells. The damage depends on the total physical dose and less on the dose per fraction. Repetitive exposure delivers a series of insults to the skin that has no time to repair previous damage, leading to an increased radiosensitivity of surviving skin stem cells. Since adult stem cells self-renew in tissue over long periods of time, they are at high risk of accumulating harmful mutations. In the skin, stem cells are localized in two compartments; in epidermal basal layer and in bulge area of hair follicle. In a recent study, Sotiropoulou et al. demonstrated that irradiation of murine skin caused cell cycle arrest and apoptosis in both epidermal cells and bulge stem cells, but bulge stem cells showed reduced apoptosis after irradiation when compared to epidermal cells. Authors point out that bulge stem cells' resistance to DNA damage-induced cell death is a consequence of higher expression of anti-apoptotic gene Bcl-2 and rapidly attenuated activation of p53, which is correlated with an enhanced DNA repair activity by non-homologous end joining. These data implicate that efficient DNA repair in the buldge stem cells could be a double-edged sword promoting short-term survival after radiation-induced DNA damage at the expense of long-term preservation of genomic integrity.

Type II radiation effects are based on reactive activation of genes involved in multiple pathways including inflammation, angiogenesis, apoptosis, and oxidative stress. These effects strongly depend on the dose per fraction. In the skin, damage to the keratinocytes and burst of free radicals results in production of multiple cytokines and chemokines such as interleukin (IL) IL-8, IL-6, IL-1α, IL-1β, TNFα, CCL4, CXCL10, and CCL2. These cytokines affect the endothelial cells of dermal vessels, causing upregulation of multiple adhesion molecules. It has been shown that up-regulation of epidermal growth factor receptor may influence epidermal tissue repair while up-regulation of intercellular adhesion molecule 1 can contribute to cutaneous barrier dysfunction. Importantly, the trans-endothelial migration of immune cells from circulation to irradiated skin is considered a "hallmark" of radiation-induced skin injury.

It is well known that irradiation causes the immediate generation of short-lived reactive oxygen species (ROS), but the role of chronically generated ROS in longer-term damage, though hypothesized and increasingly implicated, was not well documented. A recent study published by Lazarova demonstrated that chronic oxidative stress occurs in irradiated skin, even a month after exposure. Furthermore, the dramatic reduction of skin injury by a synthetic superoxide dismutase/catalase mimetic, EUK-207, concomitant with its abrogation of oxidative stress indicators, demonstrated that oxidative stress is causative in both chronic radiation dermatitis and impaired wound healing in irradiated skin. These data support the concept that selected ROS-scavenging agents such as EUK-207, having the appropriate specificity and given under the right circumstances, can mitigate radiation-induced skin injury, including facilitating wound healing. The role of oxidative stress damage in radiation-induced mucosal injury was elucidated by Iglesias-Bartolome et al. Inhibition of the mTOR with

rapamycin protected proliferative basal epithelial stem cells upon ionizing radiation in vivo, thereby preserving the integrity of the oral mucosa. This protective effect of rapamycin was mediated by the increase in expression of mitochondrial superoxide dismutase, and the consequent inhibition of ROS formation and oxidative stress damage. Special considerations should be given with certain immunosuppressive and chemopreventative agents when planning radiotherapy in organ transplant patients. There is a need to study the potential radiosensitizing or radioprotective properties of these medications. For example azathioprine acts as a type II UVA photosensitizer due to the ability of its metabolites incorporating into the patients' DNA and thereby increasing skin sensitivity to UVA. There are no studies showing a potential influence of ionizing radiation. Interestingly it has been shown that mTOR inhibition augments radiation-induced autophagy. Further studies are needed to compare radiation therapy for skin cancer on patients with mTOR inhibitors. In addition, capecitabine, an oral prodrug of 5-fluorouracil and acitretin, is recommended to use in patients with high SCC burden for chemopreventative purposes. In the management of rectal cancer, capecitabine appears feasible when given with radiosensitizing chemotherapy. Capecitabine has been studied as adjuvant chemoradiation in several cancer therapies including pancreatic adenocarcinoma and rectal cancer.

Type III radiation effects are based on permanent tissue disorganization and they are built on the malfunction of fibroblasts, mesenchymal, epithelial, and endothelial cells. Transforming growth factor (TGF)-β1/Smad cascade is involved in the initiation and maintenance of radiation-induced fibrosis. Up-regulation of TGF-β has been found in multiple models of radiation-induced skin injury as well as in the fibrotic tissues following radiotherapy. In the presence of TGF-β1, cutaneous fibroblasts stimulated connective tissue growth factor synthesis and extracellular matrix production and deposition. Importantly, mice lacking a downstream mediator of TGF-β demonstrated decreased radiation-induced skin fibrosis and accelerated wound healing.

Type IV effects are characterized by accumulation of somatic cell mutations leading to development of solid tumors. It has been shown that frequency of DNA mutations is dose dependent and appears to increase linearly for doses between 0.1 and 5 Gy. The risk of second carcinomas following radiotherapy in immunosuppressed patients is not negligible. The lung cancer incidence following breast radiotherapy has been reported as high as 2 %, while up 18 % of deaths after successful treatment of Hodgkin's lymphoma are due to secondary carcinomas.

Type V radiation effects are in the category of bystander effects, referring to the radiation damage induced in cells or organs that have not been directly exposed to radiation.

Management of Radiation Dermatitis

Radiation dermatitis occurs in most immunocompromised patients receiving radiation therapy for skin cancer. In our experience there is no difference in the severity of radiation dermatitis in the immunocompetent vs. immunosuppressed patients, but no definitive studies have been published to support this.

Therapeutic strategies have been developed to ameliorate the symptoms of radiation dermatitis and they include topical regimens such as powders, emollients, cooling gels, creams, and topical steroids. In a prospective randomized, double-blind study Schmuth et al. provided evidence that prophylactic and ongoing use of topical steroids with either topical corticosteroid or a dexpanthenol-containing emollient ameliorates, but does not prevent, radiation dermatitis. The general consensus is that the majority of patients benefit from bland moisturizers. In breast cancer patients, several phase III randomized studies have demonstrated that using a moisturizing product can reduce the severity and duration of radiation dermatitis. The oil-in-water creams and ointments are better tolerated than lotions, however approximately 10 % of patients can develop allergic-type reactions to topical agents, further exacerbating radiation dermatitis.

Conclusion

Immunosuppression in organ transplant recipients is associated with an increased risk of developing skin cancer. Obtaining optimal clinical outcomes for these patients depends on the multidisciplinary team, including radiation oncologists, dermatologists, and surgeons. Skillful application of radiation therapy for selected cancer lesions in OTR patients is generally well tolerated and it remains an effective treatment modality.

Historically, radiation damage was seen in physicians, caused by lack of protection when treating patients with ionizing radiation. Now the majority of radiation damage to the skin is due to ionizing radiation therapy on the patient's skin. There is now a new, growing group of physicians exposed to ionizing radiation through fluoroscopic examinations. Caution is needed in all three groups, and signs of acute and chronic radiation dermatitis need to be recognized and treated. Follow-up is essential due to late-onset skin malignancies, most commonly squamous cell carcinomas.

Suggested Reading

Brown KR, Rzucidlo E. Acute and chronic radiation injury. J Vasc Surg. 2011;53(1 Suppl):15S–21.
Brown LM, Howard RA, Travis LB. The risk of secondary malignancies over 30 years after the treatment of non-Hodgkin lymphoma. Cancer. 2006;107(11):2741–2.
Euvrard S, Morelon E, Rostaing L, Goffin E, Brocard A, Tromme I, et al. Sirolimus and secondary skin-cancer prevention in kidney transplantation. N Engl J Med. 2012;367(4):329–39.
Greenberg JN, Zwald FO. Management of skin cancer in solid-organ transplant recipients: a multidisciplinary approach. Dermatol Clin. 2011;29(2):231–41, ix.
Halperin EC, Perez CA, Brady LW. Perez and Brady's principles and practice of radiation oncology. 5th ed. Philadelphia: Lippincott Williams & Wilkins; 2008.
Herman S, Rogers HD, Ratner D. Immunosuppression and squamous cell carcinoma: a focus on solid organ transplant recipients. Skinmed. 2007;6(5):234–8.

Hymes SR, Strom EA, Fife C. Radiation dermatitis: clinical presentation, pathophysiology, and treatment 2006. J Am Acad Dermatol. 2006;54(1):28–46.

Koenig TR, Mettler FA, Wagner LK. Skin injuries from fluoroscopically guided procedures: part 2, review of 73 cases and recommendations for minimizing dose delivered to patient. AJR Am J Roentgenol. 2001a; 177(1):13–20.

Koenig TR, Wolff D, Mettler FA, Wagner LK. Skin injuries from fluoroscopically guided procedures: part 1, characteristics of radiation injury. AJR Am J Roentgenol. 2001b;177(1):3–11.

Kwan W, Wilson D, Moravan V. Radiotherapy for locally advanced basal cell and squamous cell carcinomas of the skin. Int J Radiat Oncol Biol Phys. 2004;60(2):406–11.

Mendelsohn FA, Divino CM, Reis ED, Kerstein MD. Wound care after radiation therapy. Adv Skin Wound Care. 2002;15(5):216–24.

Olasz EB, Neuuburg M. Skin disease in transplant patients. Sauer's manual of skin diseases. 10th ed. Philadelphia: Lippincott Williams & Wilkins; 2010. p. 195–210.

Roychoudhuri R, Evans H, Robinson D, Moller H. Radiation-induced malignancies following radio-therapy for breast cancer. Br J Cancer. 2004;91(5): 868–72.

Ryan JL. Ionizing radiation: the good, the bad, and the ugly. J Invest Dermatol. 2012;132(3 Pt 2):985–93.

Salvo N, Barnes E, van Draanen J, Stacey E, Mitera G, Breen D, et al. Prophylaxis and management of acute radiation-induced skin reactions: a systematic review of the literature. Curr Oncol. 2010;17(4): 94–112.

Wickline MM. Prevention and treatment of acute radiation dermatitis: a literature review. Oncol Nurs Forum. 2004;31(2):237–47.

Zwald FO, Brown M. Skin cancer in solid organ transplant recipients: advances in therapy and management: part II. Management of skin cancer in solid organ transplant recipients. J Am Acad Dermatol. 2011a;65(2):263–79; quiz 80.

Zwald FO, Brown M. Skin cancer in solid organ transplant recipients: advances in therapy and management: part I. Epidemiology of skin cancer in solid organ transplant recipients. J Am Acad Dermatol. 2011b;65(2):253–61; quiz 62.

Index

A

Abacavir, 28
Acne, 83
Acral erythema. *See* Hand-foot syndrome
Actinic keratosis (AK), 56, 136, 137, 158
Actinomyces isrealii, 102
Acyclovir, 16, 17, 35
Adalimumab, 80
Afatinib treatment, 111, 112, 114
Aggressive squamous cell carcinoma
    with in-transit cutaneous metastasis, 159
    with palpable lymphadenopathy, 160
    without metastasis, 159
Aging
    angular cheilitis, 131–132
    candida albicans, 132–133
    damage theory of, 125, 126
    definition of, 124–125
    herpes zoster, 128–130
    HIV, 133–135
    and immunity, 125
    and inflammation, 126–128
    life expectancy, 124
    life span, 124
    seborrheic dermatitis, 130–131
    seborrheic keratoses, 135–137
    and skin cancers, 133
AIDS. *See* Human immunodeficiency virus/acquired
        immunodeficiency syndrome (HIV/AIDS)
AIDS-defining illnesses
    bacterial infections
        bacillary angiomatosis, 23
        mycobacterial infection, 24
        staphylococcal skin disease, 23–24
        syphilis, 22–23
    CD4 count, 14
    fungal infections
        coccidoidomycosis, 22
        cryptococcosis, 22
        histoplasmosis, 22
        onychomycosis, 21
        oral candidiasis, 21
    infectious etiologies, 15
    inflammatory disorders, 27
    neoplastic lesions, 25–27
    parasites/infestations, 24–25

    systemic infections, 21
    viral infections
        anal cancer, 19–21
        CMV, 17–18
        EBV, 18
        HPV, 19–21
        HSV, 15–16
        HZ, 16–17
        molluscum contagiosum, 18–19
        VZV, 16–17
AIN. *See* Anal intraepithelial neoplasia (AIN)
Alefacept, 80
Algae, and skin disorder, 10–11
Allogenic transplants, 55, 61
Alopecia, 88
    CMC, 41
    hair disorders, 66
    NRTI, 28
Alopecia areata (AA), 84
Aminolevulinic acid (ALA), 153
Amyotrophic dermatomyositis, 51
Anagen effluvium, 88
Anal cancer, 19–21
Anal intraepithelial neoplasia (AIN), 19
Angular cheilitis, aging in, 131–132
Antifungal therapy, 42
Antihistamines, 37
Antiretroviral therapy, 27
Anti-thymocyte globulin (ATG), 156
Anti-TNF therapy
    cutaneous adverse events, 82
    HBV, 76
    HCV, 75–76
    leprosy, 73
    psoriasis/psoriasiform eruptions, 80–82
    TB, 72–73
Aspirin, 4
Aspregillus, 103–104
Astemizole, 27
Ataxia-telangiectasia (AT), 35–36
Atopic dermatitis
    HIES, 36
    phototherapy treatment for, 149
Autoimmunity
    disorders, 80–85
    in IgA deficiency, 38

Autosomal recessive, 32, 34, 36–37
Azathioprine, 156, 157
Azoles, 42

B
Bacillary angiomatosis, 23
Bacterial infection
    AIDS-defining illnesses
        bacillary angiomatosis, 23
        mycobacterial infection, 24
        staphylococcal skin disease, 23–24
        syphilis, 22–23
    corticosteroids, 101–102
    and HIES, 36
    less-common, 75
    mycobacterial infection
        leprosy, 73
        TB, 72–73
    and skin disorder, 6–7
    staphylococcal infection, 74
    streptococcal infection, 74–75
Basal cell carcinoma (BCC). *See also* Radiation therapy
    flendrie, 79
    in OTRs, 164–165
    SCC and, 27
Bazex's syndrome, 51
Bell's palsy, 129
Biological therapies, 72, 73, 80
Biologics
    anti-TNF therapy, 72
    bacterial infection (*see* Bacterial infection)
    fungal infection, 77–78
    infection, 72
    inflammatory/autoimmune disorders, 80–85
    malignant disease, 79–80
    parasitic infection, 79
    viral infection (*see* Viral infection)
Birt-Hogg-Dubbe syndrome, 51
Bleomycin, 93
B lymphocytes
    aging/skin cancers, 133
    organ transplantation, 157
    SCID and, 32
Bone marrow transplants, 61
Bordetella holmesii, 75
BRAF TKI inhibition
    follicular hyperkeratotic rash, 118
    photosensitivity, 119
    side effects of, 118–119
    skin rash management, 119
Bruton's agammaglobulinemia (XLA), 37–38

C
Calciphylaxis, 57, 58
Cancer
    candidiasis, 46
    cellulitis, 46–47
    chemotherapy (*see* Chemotherapy)

corticosteroids, 104
herpes zoster/simplex, 47
hypercoagulability syndromes, 51–52
infections, 45–46
paraneoplastic skin disease, 47
    inflammatory (*see* Inflammatory paraneoplastic skin disease)
    metabolic, 52
    nonspecific inflammatory, 52
paraneoplastic tumors, 51
pigmentary changes, 51
Candida albicans
    aging in, 132–133
    CMC, 41–42
Candida sepsis, 8
Candidiasis, 7–8, 15, 46, 103
Capecitabine, 160
Capnocytophaga cynodegmi, 75
Carbon dioxide laser surgery, 20
C2 deficiencies, 43
Celecoxib, 164
Cellular proteins, phosphorylation, 108
Cellulitis, 10, 11, 46–47
Chediak-Higashi syndrome (CHS), 39–40
Chemoprevention, SCC
    goal of, 160
    indications, 160
    retinoids, 161
Chemotherapy, 87–88
    mucocutaneous side effects
        acral erythema, 91–92
        chemotherapy-induced alopecia (CIA), 88–89
        drug reactions, 93–94
        dyschromia, 90–91
        extravasation reactions, 90
        mucositis/stomatitis, 89–90
        neutrophilic eccrine hidradenitis (NEH), 92–93
        onychodystrophy, 93
    timeline for cutaneous reactions, 97
Chemotherapy-induced alopecia (CIA), 88–89
Chronic actinic dermatitis, 152
Chronic granulomatous disease (CGD), 40–41
Chronic mucocutaneous candidiasis (CMC), 32, 41–42
Clostridium perfringens, 6–7
CMV. *See* Cytomegalovirus (CMV)
Coccidioides, 22
Coccidioidomycosis, 10, 15, 22, 78
Common terminology criteria for adverse events v4.0 (CTCAE), 176
Common variable immunodeficiency (CVID), 38–39
Condyloma acuminata, 19
Connective tissue disease
    C2 deficiencies, 43
    phototherapy treatment for, 148
Corticosteroids
    bacterial infections, 101–102
    cancer, 104
    direct drug effects, 100
    fungal infections, 103–104
    HIES, 37

hypersensitivity, 99–100
immunosuppression, 100–101
organ transplantation, 156, 157
systemic, 27
viral infections, 102–103
Cowden's syndrome, 51
C-reactive protein (CRP), 4, 127
Cryotherapy, 19
Cryptococcosis, 9–10, 15, 22
Cryptococcus, 22, 103
Cryptosporidium, 34
CTCL. *See* Cutaneous T-cell lymphoma (CTCL)
Curettage, 19
Cutaneous graft versus host disease (GVHD), 148
Cutaneous lymphoma, 26–27, 79
Cutaneous mucormycosis, 9
Cutaneous nocardiosis, 75
Cutaneous T-cell lymphoma (CTCL), 79, 149
Cutaneous tuberculosis, 7
Cyclosporine, 156, 157
Cytarabine, 91, 92
Cytomegalovirus (CMV), 17–18, 77, 102

D
Dabrafenib, 85
Damage theory, of aging, 125, 126
Dedicator of cytokinesis 8 (DOCK8) gene, 36
Dermatological toxicity, TKI
hair/skin, discoloration of, 117, 118
hand-foot syndrome, 115–117
skin rashes, 117
Dermatomyositis, 50–51
Diabetes mellitus
dermatologic conditions, 3
etiological factors, 5
metabolic dysregulation, 4
prevalence of, 3
type I, 3–5
type II, 3–5
xerosis, 5
Diabetic foot, 5
Diabetic patients, skin disorder in, 5, 6
algae
parasites, 11
protothecosis, 11
bacteria
clostridium perfringens, 6–7
Escherichia coli, 7
group B streptococcus, 6
klebsiella, 7
morganella, 7
mycobacterium tuberculosis, 7
staphylococcus, 6
mycosis
candidiasis, 7–8
coccidioidomycosis, 10
cryptococcosis, 9–10
sporotrichosis, 10
zygomycosis, 8–9

viral
herpes simplex, 10
herpes zoster, 11
Didanosine, 27
Disseminated infections, 102
Doxyrubricin, 64
Drug eruptions, 63
Drug reactions, 27–28
Dyschromia, 90–91

E
Ecthyma gangrenosum, 38
Eczema, 82–83, 149
Efalizumab, 80
Electrodessication, 19
Electron beam therapy, 175
Emollient, 37
Engraftment syndrome, 63
Entropy, 125
Eosinophilia, 33
Eosinophilic pustular folliculitis (EPF), 27, 152
Eosinophilic pustulosis, 27
Epidermal growth factor receptor (EGFR) inhibitor, 94–95
BCCA guidelines for, 112, 113
management recommendations for
dry skin, 113
eyelash growth, 113–114
nail changes, 113
scaling and hyperkeratosis, 113
scalp rash, 113
skin rash, 111–113
pathophysiological effects of, 110
patient outcome, rash *vs.* efficacy, 114
randomized clinical trials, 109
rashes on face and chest, 111
stage IV non-small cell lung cancer, 111, 112
Epstein-Barr virus (EBV), 18
Erlotinib treatment
grade II papulopustular eruption on face, 111
papulopustular eruption on chest, 111
TKI-induced eyelash growth, 114
Erythema, 6
gyratum repens, 49
multiforme, 64
nodosum, 49–50
Erythroderma, 32
Escherichia coli, 7
Etanercept, 80, 82
Etretinate, 29
Exanthems, 32
Extracorporeal photophoresis, 66
Extramammary paget's disease, 51
Extravasation reactions, 90

F
Figurate erythemas, 48–49
Fluorescent activated cell sorter (FACS), 33

Folliculitis, 37
Foscarnet, 18
Fungal infection
    AIDS-defining illnesses
        onychomycosis, 21
        oral candidiasis, 21
    corticosteroids, 103–104
    mycoses, 77–78

G
Ganciclovir, 18
Genital condylomata, 77
Gingivitis, 34
Glucagonoma syndrome, 51
Graft-versus-host disease (GVHD), 61–62
    acral erythema, 91
    acute, 62–64
    chronic, 64–66
    classification, 62
    cutaneous, 148
    management, 66–67
    SCID, 32
Gram stain, 24
Granulomata, 35, 39, 41
Granulomatous disorders, 83
Group B streptococcus, 6
GVHD. *See* Graft-versus-host disease (GVHD)

H
HAART. *See* Highly Active Antiretroviral Therapy
    (HAART)
Hair loss
    by chemotherapy, 88
    chronic GVHD and, 65, 66
Hairy leukoplakia, 18
Hand-foot syndrome, 63, 64, 91–92
    axitinib therapy, 115, 116
    management recommendations for, 117
    sunitinib treatment, 115, 116
    VEGFR, 117
HBV. *See* Hepatitis B virus (HBV)
HCV. *See* Hepatitis C virus (HCV)
Hedgehog (Hh) signaling pathway, 165
Hematopoietic cell transplantation (HCT), 61, 62
Hematopoietic stem cells (HSC), 62
Hematopoietic stem cell transplantation (HSCT), 33
Henoch-Schoenlein purpura, 43
Hepatitis B virus (HBV), 76
Hepatitis C virus (HCV), 75–76
Hepatitis viruses, 75–76
Hepatosplenomegaly, 34, 35
Hereditary polyposis syndrome, 51
Herpes simplex virus (HSV)
    in AIDS patients, 15–16
    biologics, 76
    in cancer patients, 47
    corticosteroids, 102
    in diabetes patients, 10

Herpes zoster (HZ)
    aging in, 128–130
    in AIDS patients, 16–17
    in cancer patients, 47
    in diabetes patients, 11
Highly active antiretroviral therapy (HAART),
    14, 20, 26
Histoplasmosis, 15, 22
HPV. *See* Human papillomavirus (HPV)
HSV. *See* Herpes Simplex Virus (HSV)
Human epidermal growth factor receptor (HER)
    inhibitors, 110
Human herpesvirus 8 (HHV-8), 25, 26
Human herpes virus (HHV) infections
    CMV, 77
    HSV, 76
    Kaposi's sarcoma-associated herpes virus, 77
    VZV, 76
Human immunodeficiency virus/acquired
    immunodeficiency syndrome (HIV/AIDS)
    and aging, 133–135
    skin cancers in, 169–170
    skin disorders
        AIDS-defining illnesses (*see* AIDS-defining
        illnesses)
        drug reactions, 27–28
        etiology, 13–14
        inflammatory skin diseases, 28–29
        pruritic papular dermatitis of, 29
    UV therapy for, 152
Human leukocyte antigens (HLA), 62
Human papillomavirus (HPV)
    in AIDS patients, 19–21
    biologics, 77
    carcinogenic effect, 56
    corticosteroids, 102–103
Hypercoagulability syndromes, 51–52
Hyperglycemia, 3
Hyper immunoglobulin E syndrome
    (HIES), 36–37
Hyper immunoglobulin M syndrome, 34
Hyperpigmentation, 90
Hypersensitivity reactions, 99–100
Hypogammaglobulinemia, 33
Hypopigmentation, 39

I
Immune-mediated inflammatory diseases
    (IMIDs), 168–169
Immune reconstitution inflammatory syndrome
    (IRIS), 28
Immunity
    and aging, 125
    cellular/humoral, 51
    dermatologic conditions, 3
Immunodeficiency
    aging and (*see* Aging)
    HIV and, 15, 20
    well-defined syndromes with, 34–37

Immunoglobulin (IgA) deficiencies, 38
Immunosuppression
    corticosteroids, 100–101
    diabetes mellitus associated with, 5, 6
    drugs, 152
    patients
        radiation therapy (*see* Radiation therapy)
        skin cancer in, 171–172
    phases, in organ transplantation, 156
    pyoderma gangrenosum, 48
    SCC
        reduction of, 162, 163
        regimen adjustment, 161–162
    and skin cancer, 79
    syphilis, 22–23
Indinavir, 28
Infestations, 24–25
Inflammatory disorders
    acne, 83
    and aging, 126–128
    in AIDS patients, 27–29
    alopecia areata, 84
    eczema, 82–83
    granulomatous disorders, 83
    lichenoid disorders, 82
    lupus erythematosus, 84
    psoriasis/psoriasiform eruptions, 80–82
    in transplant patients, 57–59
    vasculitis, 83–84
Inflammatory paraneoplastic skin disease, 47–48
    dermatomyositis, 50–51
    erythema nodosum, 49–50
    figurate erythemas, 48–49
    glucagonoma syndrome, 51
    paraneoplastic pemphigus, 49
    pyoderma gangrenosum, 48
    sweet's syndrome, 48
    vasculitis, 49
Infliximab, 73, 78, 83
Injection site reaction, 84–85
Innate immune system, 4
Interferon (IFN) gamma therapy, 37
Interleukin (IL)-6, 4
In-transit cutaneous metastasis, 159
Invasive BCC treatment, 165

J
Job's syndrome, 36, 37

K
Kaposi's sarcoma (KS), 15, 25–26, 104
    associated herpes virus, 77
    in OTRs
        clinical features of, 168
        management of, 168
        pathogenesis of, 167–168
        risk factors, 167

Keratoacanthomas, 79, 172, 173
Kinases, 108
Klebsiella, 7

L
Lamivudine, 27–28
Leiomyomas, 51
Leishmaniasis, 79
Lentigo, 51
Leprosy, 73
Lesar Trelat sign, 51
Leukocyte adhesion deficiency (LAD), 40
Leukocytoclastic vasculitis (LCV), 83–84
Lichenoid disorders, 82
Lichen planus, 65, 149
Lupus erythematosus, 84
Lymphadenopathy, 34, 35
Lymphocyte recovery, 63
Lymphomas, 26–27

M
Malignant disease
    cutaneous lymphoma, 79
    melanoma, 80
    non-melanoma skin cancer, 79–80
Mammary paget's diseases, 51
Mega-voltage photon therapy, 175
Melanoma
    in OTRs, 165–166
    transplant patients, 80
    UVA and UVB, 150
Merkel cell carcinoma (MCC), 167, 172
Metabolic paraneoplastic skin disease, 52
Methicillin-resistant *Staphylococcus aureus* (MRSA), 74
Methicillin-sensitive *Staphylococcus aureus* (MSSA), 6, 74
Methotrexate, 29, 78
5-methoxypsoralen, 146
8-methoxypsoralen (8-MOP), 146
Methyl ester methyl aminolevulinate (MAL), 153
Molluscum contagiosum virus (MCV), 18–19, 56, 77, 102
Monoclonal antibodies, 94–95
Morganella, 7
Muckle-Wells syndrome (MWS), 42–43
Mucocutaneous side effects
    of chemotherapy, 88–94
    of monoclonal antibodies, 94–95
    of tyrosine kinase inhibitors, 94–95
Mucormycosis. *See* Zygomycosis
Mucosal candidiasis, 21
Mucositis, 89–90
Muir Torre Syndrome, 51
Multicentric reticulohistiocytosis, 51
Muromonab-CD3 (OKT3), 156
Mycobacterial infection, 24
    leprosy, 73
    TB, 72–73

Mycobacterium kansasii, 73
Mycobacterium marinum, 73
Mycobacterium tuberculosis, 7
Mycophenolate mofetil, 156, 157
Mycosis
    fungoidesm, phototherapy treatment, 149
    and skin disorder, 7–10
    subcutaneous, 78
    superficial, 77–78

N
Nail disorders, 66
Narrowband UVB (nbUVB), 142–153
Necrosis, 90
Necrotizing fasciitis, 7, 9, 10
Nelfinavir, 28
Neoplastic lesions, 25–27
Neuropathy, 5
Neutrophilic eccrine hidradenitis (NEH), 92–93
Nevirapine, 28
Nikolsky's sign, 64
NNRTI, 28
Nocardia
    N. asteroides, 102
    N. farcinica, 75
    N. otitidiscaviarum, 75
Nocardiosis, 75
Non-Hodgkin's lymphoma, 79
Non-melanoma skin cancer (NMSC), 79–80
Nonspecific inflammatory paraneoplastic
        skin disease, 52
Nontuberculous mycobacteria (NTM), 73
NRTI, 27–28
Nuclear factor kappa beta, 127, 128

O
Ofuji's disease. *See* Eosinophilic pustular
        folliculitis (EPF)
Onychodystrophy, 93
Onychomycosis, 21
Opportunistic infections, 100, 102, 103
Oral candidiasis, 21
Oral difluoromethylornithine (DFMO), 164
Oral lesions, 66
Orbital cellulitis, 74
Organ transplant patients, skin disease in, 55–56
    allogenic transplants, 55
    calciphylaxis, 57, 58
    infections, 56–57
    inflammatory skin diseases, 57–59
    pruritis, 58
    tumors, 56
Organ transplant recipients (OTR)
    HIV and AIDS, 169–170
    iatrogenic immunosuppression, 156
    immune-mediated inflammatory disease, 168–169
    skin cancer

basal cell carcinoma (*see* Basal cell carcinoma
        (BCC))
    Kaposi's Sarcoma, 167–168
    melanoma, 165–166
    Merkel cell carcinoma, 167
    risk factors for, 156
    squamous cell carcinoma (*see* Squamous cell
        carcinoma (SCC))
Oropharyngeal candidiasis, 21
Orthovoltage treatment, 174–175
OTR. *See* Organ transplant recipients (OTR)

P
Palpable lymphadenopathy, 160
Palpable purpura, 49
Paraneoplastic pemphigus, 49
Paraneoplastic skin disease
    inflammatory, 47–48
    metabolic, 52
    nonspecific inflammatory, 52
Paraneoplastic tumors, 51
Parasites, 11, 24–25
Parasitic infection, 79
PASI score. *See* Psoriasis Area and Severity Index
        (PASI) score
Pathogen-associated molecular patterns (PAMPs), 4
Pattern recognition receptors (PRRs), 4
Perineural invasion (PNI), 173–174
Peripheral T lymphocytes, 33
Permethrin, 25
Peutz Jeghers syndrome, 51
Phagocytes, 40
Photodermatoses, 149–150
Photodynamic therapy (PDT), 153, 162
Photosensitivity dermatitis. *See* Chronic actinic
        dermatitis
Phototherapy, 66
    challenges of, 142–143
    history of, 143
    narrowband UVB, 142
    and photochemotherapy, 144
    treatment for
        atopic dermatitis, 149
        connective tissue disease, 148
        cutaneous graft versus host disease, 148
        cutaneous T-cell lymphoma, 149
        lichen planus, 149
        mycosis fungoides, 149
        photodermatoses, 149–150
        Sezary syndrome, 149
        vitiligo, 150
    types of, 142
    UVB, 148
Pigmentary changes, 51
Piloleiomyomas, 51
Plasmablastic lymphoma, 26–27
Platelet-derived growth factor receptor (PDGFR)
        inhibitors, 114, 117

Platelet transfusions, 35
Podophyllin, 18
Poikiloderma, 65
Polymerase chain reaction (PCR), 47
Porokeratosis, 56
Positive Hutchinson sign, 129
Post-herpetic neuralgia, 17, 129, 130
Primary immunodeficiencies (PIDs)
    autoinflammatory disorders, 42–43
    combined immunodeficiencies, 31–32
        Hyper IgM, 34
        SCID, 32–34
    complement deficiencies, 43
    congenital defects of phagocyte number/function
        CGD, 40–41
        LAD, 40
    defects in innate immunity, 41–42
    immune dysregulation diseases, 39–40
    predominantly antibody deficiencies
        CVID, 38–39
        selective IgA deficiencies, 38
        XLA, 37–38
    well-defined syndromes with immunodeficiency
        AT, 35–36
        HIES, 36–37
        WAS, 34–35
Protease inhibitors, 28
Protothecosis, 11
Pruritic papular dermatitis, 29
Pruritus, 58, 83, 85
Pseudomonas aeruginosa, 75
Psoralen plus UVA (PUVA), 153
    atopic dermatitis/eczema, 149
    contraindications, 151
    cost of, 148
    human papilloma virus, 150
    keratoacanthoma incidence, 150, 151
    and nbUVB (*see* Narrowband UVB (nbUVB))
    negative cosmetic effects, 143, 150
    oral, 144
    SCC, 143, 150
    uses of, 146
    vitiligo, 150
Psoralens
    advantage of, 146
    cost of, 148
    light absorption, 146
    light exposure, 147
    5-methoxypsoralen, 146
    8-methoxypsoralen, 146
    minimal phototoxic dose, 147
Psoriasis, 29
    classification of, 144
    clinical presentation of, 144
    excimer laser treatment, 145
    Goeckermann therapy, 146
    medical management of, 145
    narrowband UVB, 145
    PASI score, 144, 145

patient convenience, 146
    psoralens for, 142
    PUVA, 145
Psoriasis Area and Severity Index (PASI)
    score, 144, 145
Psoriasis/psoriasiform eruptions, 80–82
Pyoderma gangrenosum, 48
Pyridoxine, 92

R
Radiation dermatitis, 64
    chronic, 177, 179
    management of, 181
Radiation enhancement, 96
Radiation-induced skin injury, biology of
    type I radiation effects, 179–180
    type II radiation effects, 180
    type III radiation effects, 180–181
    type IV radiation effects, 181
    type V radiation effects, 181
Radiation recall dermatitis, 95–96
Radiation therapy
    approaches, 174
    efficacy of, 175–176
    electron beam therapy, 175
    indications
        keratoacanthomas, 172, 173
        large tumor size, 173
        perineural invasion, 173–174
        positive surgical margins, 173
    mega-voltage photon therapy, 175
    orthovoltage treatment, 174–175
    side effects
        chronic radiation dermatitis, 177, 179
        dry to moist desquamation, 176
        erythema, 176
        grade 1 skin changes, 176
        grade 2 skin changes, 176–177
        grade 3 and 4 skin changes, 177
        hyperpigmentation, 176
        radiation enhancement, 96
        radiation recall, 95–96
        upper aerodigestive tract, SCC of, 178
    superficial X-ray therapy, 174–175
    treatment planning, 175
Ramsay Hunt syndrome, 129
Rapamycin inhibitors, 156
Rearranged during transfection (RET)
    inhibitors, 119
Retinoids, 161
Rhinocerebral mucormycosis, 9
Rituximab, 74, 169

S
Saquinavir, 28
Scabies, 24–25
Scleroderma, 65

Sclerosing skin diseases. *See* Connective tissue disease
Sclerotic manifestations, 65–66
Seborrheic dermatitis (SD), 28–29
    and aging, 130–131
    characteristics of, 131
    immobility, 131
    pathogenesis of, 130
    secretion rate, 130, 131
Seborrheic keratoses, 135–137
Selective immunoglobulin (IgA) deficiencies, 38
Severe combined immunodeficiency (SCID), 32–34
Sezary syndrome, 149
Shingles. *See* Herpes zoster
Sicca syndrome, 66
Signal transducer and activator of transcription 3
        (STAT3) gene, 36
Skin atrophy, 100
Skin cancer
    and aging, 133
    in immunosuppressed patients, 171–172
Sorafenib, 95
Splenectomy, 40
Sporothix schenkii, 10
Sporotrichosis, 10
Squamous cell carcinoma (SCC). *See also* Radiation
        therapy
    actinic keratosis, 158
    aggressive SCC
        with in-transit cutaneous metastasis, 159
        with palpable lymphadenopathy, 160
        without metastasis, 159
    celecoxib role, 164
    chemoprevention
        goal of, 160
        retinoids, 161
    clinical features, 158
    cutaneous, 67
    immunosuppression
        reduction of, 162, 163
        regimen adjustment, 161–162
    management of, 158
    metastatic risk, 157
    neoplastic lesions, 27
    non-melanoma skin cancer, 79
    oral difluoromethylornithine, 164
    pathogenesis of, 157–158
    photodynamic therapy, 162
    risk factors, 159
    topical diclofenac sodium, 164
    topical 5-fluorouracil, 162
    topical imiquimod, 162, 164
    warts, 158, 162
Staphylococcal skin disease, 23–24, 74
Staphylococcus, 6
    S. aureus, 23, 46, 74
Steroid acne, 100
Steroid rosacea, 100
Stomatitis, 34, 89–90
Streptococcal infection, 74–75

Sunitinib, 95
    blister formation on foot, 115
    hair
        depigmentation, 117, 118
        discoloration of, 117
    hand-foot syndrome, 115, 116
    skin, discoloration of, 117
Superficial BCC treatment, 165
Superficial X-ray therapy, 174–175
Sweet's syndrome, 48
Syphilis, 22–23
Systemic corticosteroids, 66–67
Systemic lupus erythematosus (SLE), 43
Systemic retinoids, 161

T
Tacrolimus, 156, 157
TB. *See* Tuberculosis (TB)
T cells, and GVHD, 62, 63
Tegretol, 63
Telogen effluvium, 88
Tinea incognito, 103
TKIs. *See* Tyrosine kinase inhibitors (TKIs)
T lymphocytes
    aging/skin cancers, 133
    organ transplantation, 157
    SCID and, 32
    and type I diabetes, 4
Tocilizumab, 169
Toll-like receptors (TLRs), 4
Topical diclofenac sodium, 164
Topical 5-fluorouracil, 162
Topical imiquimod, 162, 164
Topical retinoids, 161
Toxic epidermal necrolysis, 63
Toxic shock syndrome (TSS), 6
Transplantation, 40, 55–59
Trichophyton rubrum, 78
Tripe palms, 51
Tuberculosis (TB), 72–73
Tumor necrosis factor (TNF)-α, 4, 72
Tyrosine kinase inhibitors (TKIs), 94–95
    BRAF inhibitors, 118–119
    cellular molecular pathways, 110
    description of, 108, 109
    EGFR and HER family inhibitors, 110–114
    RET Inhibitors, 119
    side effects, 109
    VEGF/PDGF/mixed inhibitors, 114–118

U
Ultraviolet A/ultraviolet B (UVA/UVB) therapy
    photodynamic therapy, 153
    phototherapy (*see* Phototherapy)
    side effects of, 150–151
Urticaria-deafness-amyloidosis (UDA) syndrome.
        See Muckle-Wells syndrome (MWS)
Ustekinumab, 169

V
Valley fever. *See* Coccidioidomycosis
Varicella zoster virus (VZV), 16–17, 76
Vascular endothelial growth factor receptor (VEGFR)
       inhibitors, 114, 115, 117
Vasculitis, 49, 83–84
Vemurafenib, 85
Viral exanthems, 63
Viral infection
   AIDS-defining illnesses
     anal cancer, 19–21
     CMV, 17–18
     EBV, 18
     HPV, 19–21
     HSV, 15–16
     HZ, 16–17
     molluscum contagiosum, 18–19
     VZV, 16–17
   corticosteroids, 102–103
   hepatitis viruses
     HBV, 76
     HCV, 75–76
   human herpes virus infections
     CMV, 77
     HSV, 76

     Kaposi's sarcoma-associated herpes
       virus, 77
     VZV, 76
  and skin disorder, 10–11
Vismodegib, 165
Vitiligo, 150

W
Warts, 56
Wickham's striae, 66
Wiskott–Aldrich syndrome (WAS), 34–35

X
X-linked neutropenia (XLN), 34, 35
X-linked thrombocytopenia (XLT), 34, 35

Z
Zalcitabine, 28
Zidovudine, 27
Zygomycosis, 8–9